An Animal Life:
The Beginning

written by

Howard Krum

with

Roy Yanong and Scott Moore

illustrated by

Patty Hogan

An Animal Life: The Beginning

Howard Krum

Published 2012 by Fluid Design Foundation (FDF)
890 Hunt Road
Windsor, Vermont 05089

Book cover and interior design by Carrie Fradkin

Full-sized versions of all illustrations available at: AnAnimalLife.com

ISBN: 978-0-9884885-0-2

First Edition

DISCLAIMER

This book is a work of fiction. As such, this book is not a veterinary or human medical reference text and is not to be used as a guide for the diagnosis and/or treatment of any animal or human disease. This work of fiction was inspired by the authors' real-life experiences as veterinary students; however, names, characters, places, and incidents either are products of the authors' imaginations or are used fictitiously. Any resemblance to actual events or persons, living or dead, is entirely coincidental.

DEDICATION

To the University of Pennsylvania School of Veterinary Medicine Class of 1992 — we love you guys!

To Mary Margaret — you made it all possible.

Table of Contents

An Animal Life

People ask: "So what's this book about?"

We usually reply: "It's about 300 pages…"

Also, it's about life, death, and finding your place in this world. And veterinary medicine. But that's it, just those three things: a medical mystery, finding True Love, and becoming a veterinarian. Promise.

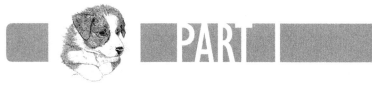

PART 1

Veterinary School Interviews

Two adjacent rooms in the old veterinary school building at the University of Philadelphia, School of Veterinary Medicine

Interviewer, Room 1: "As succinctly as you can, please tell me why you want to be a veterinarian."

Applicant: "Yes sir, good question." John "Jack" Fitzgerald Doyle took a moment to compose his thoughts — this was easily the biggest moment in his adult life. "For me, it's about helping those who can't help themselves." Then Jack nearly snickered because he didn't quite believe what he was about to say, "I've been told I have a need to rescue things."

The vet school professor returned a blank stare. He was considering a follow-up to the applicant's response, but Jack mistook the hesitation for evasion so he countered with, "Why did *you* become a veterinarian?" then rose from his seat and began casing the evidence. "I'm guessing by these X-rays of a shattered K-9 foreleg and, beside it, the same leg miraculously repaired, the 44, no, make it 45 thank-you cards on your desk, that cot and those work/life balance self-help books that you and I suffer a similar affliction. You fix broken animals and serve others no matter the cost. So…"

Jack paused with a light laugh, shook his head and sat down. "I'm sorry. I should have exercised my right to remain silent. This is your interrogation." He bowed his head in deference then concluded, "Next question?"

Interviewer, Room 1: "Well, clearly, service is important to you so why not stay on the police force?"

Applicant: Jack's sharp hazel eyes danced as he imagined the risk. Rolling up a sleeve, he revealed three purple scars disfiguring the meat of his right forearm. "Because I hear that veterinarians take fewer bullets than Philly beat cops."

Interviewer, Room 1: The professor smiled, nodded without comment and placed a check mark in Jack's file.

◄ • ►

Interviewer, Room 2: "I see that you've applied to our dual DVM/PhD program. Vet school can be stressful. There's a lot of studying, tests and late nights in the lab that can be demanding emotionally and otherwise. Confidentially, we'd like to know if you've faced any personal challenges that might prepare you for this professional experience." The professor paused then added, "Have you ever been forced to give up something that's important to you?"

Applicant: After nearly 10 full seconds of complete silence, Anna Heywood looked her interviewer square in the eye and replied, "I've lost everyone I have ever loved — I lost my parents not once but twice." She swallowed hard but continued, "A year ago I was diagnosed with Lou Gehrig's disease. It's slowly eroding my fine motor control so I had to give up training for the Olympic gymnastics team." Anna paused, cocked her head to one side and didn't break the stare, "Should I go on?"

Interviewer, Room 2: The professor coughed, fidgeted with her notes, placed a check mark next to Anna's name and then replied, "Uh, no, that's fine."

CHAPTER ONE

Dr. Green

In a helicopter over an "African Savannah," the keystone exhibit at the Peaceable Kingdom animal park in Chadds Ford, Pennsylvania

Z oo vets — ironically — are a mysterious, exotic and routinely endangered species of animal doctor.

Zoo vets toil inconspicuously, often nomadically through the fringe habitats where research, clinical medicine and environmental conservation overlap. They are, in a compound word, stereo-atypical — having no unifying personality, corporal configuration or political persuasion. This is not normal. For example, how common are: plumbers with suspenders, dancers with potbellies, or Republican Green Peace activists?

Zoo veterinarians can be elephantine, wolfish, or mousy. They can display a bovine warmth, a hawkish stare, or crocodilian resolve. They can plow through their never-ending caseload with bullish intensity or a slothful inevitability. Some — on rare occasion — can be pigheaded, waspish, or even downright crabby, while others remain unflappable saints in any emergency and are surely destined to be lionized. There are deer-hunting carnivores, wildly-grazing omnivores, and strict lacto-, ovo-, *everything's a "no-no,"* vegetarians. When the latest version of zoo vet was minted, there was no mold to be broken. Only one quality binds them all: a sacrificial fidelity to the Mission.

Dr. Violet Marie Green was identical to every other zoo vet in the world, she was unique. Her mom, Miss Florida 1961, and her dad, a question mark, Violet last wore lipstick and big hair on July 4th, 1963. She was six years old when, after breaking a 2x4 with her fist (karate being her 'talent') and winning the overall contest, a Mini Miss pageant judge defined the word 'independence' for her. After careful consideration, as was her way, she replied, "Thank you sir, I understand," and handed back her crown and scepter.

After college, she suited up and excelled as a Peace Corps elementary school teacher in Haiti. Later, clad in formfitting neoprene, she was a Sea World dolphin trainer in Orlando — but was again unfulfilled.

Today, she owns one unworn dress (little and black, a gift from her mom), one dark skirt, a lightweight V-neck sweater, seven pairs of Lycra running tights and a dozen holey (she would write it "Holy") tees. Other than that, her absolutely everyday wear could be sorted into three piles: pile 1 — loose-fitting jade scrub tops; pile 2 — size two khaki cargo shorts; and, pile 3 — jog bras, hiking socks and Victoria's Secret mini briefs.

Although a fashion-unconscious accessorizer, she at least made an attempt: a stethoscope, mini Maglite, pocket calculator, wristwatch and pager (all in matching flat black) rested for 3-4 hours most nights atop her bedroom dresser. The more frilly stuff, like an 18-inch string of natural pearls, a gift from one unrequited admirer or another, sat in a box labeled "For Charity."

Dr. Violet Marie Green exhibits a cool warmth and dogged determination that has a gravity well beyond her toned and tanned, compact mass. Every person she has ever met would sum up her demeanor with one word: focused. Her focus is her patient, and everything flows from that point source — the research, the teaching and ultimately the Mission.

—◄ ◉ ►—

The slender blades throbbed as they churned the humid, morning air. Dr. Violet Marie Green sat sideways, both feet resting on the M*A*S*H style chopper's right runner as they skimmed the sassafras tops at 60 miles an hour. It was the perfect vehicle for the project and Mr. Davaris hadn't even paused at her request. He simply barked over the walkie talkie, "You'll have one by the end of the week." The seamless cockpit bubble yielded panoramic views while the wide-open sides gave her easy outboard access and plenty of room to shoot.

Her back straightened when she caught sight of their target and her sky-blue irises constricted to narrow her pupils, excluding the extraneous. The animal with the fluorescent orange number "7" spray-painted on its neck was now in full view.

Poking the pilot in the shoulder with her left hand, she pointed with her right to the giraffe. Violet reached to her belt, flipped on her walkie talkie and pulled the headset over her golden blonde hair, "William, you guys in position?"

The speaker crackled in response, "Hey, Doc. We're about one click behind you at 5 o'clock."

She swiveled, looking back through the tail rotor and picked out the Range Rover's dust trail. "Gotcha, 10-4. Listen, keep your heads up, you have a small herd of elephant and two zebra out about 800 meters at 3 o'clock. Otherwise, it's just like we expected, Lucy and her family are in the dense brush near the main water hole in sector 12." She paused, then added, "I don't like it. There's too much water out here."

A hiss came to her left ear, "That's what we're here for — you know, to save the day! You gently push her towards that open space to the east, get the meds on board, and we'll keep her dry." He added, "Doc, you worry too much."

Violet pulled her strong smooth legs back into the cockpit, lifted the rifle from the rack, laid it across her lap and pulled open the bolt to expose the empty chamber. She heard the pilot whistle over the headset and say, "Damn, that's hot stuff." He wasn't referring to the rifle but she didn't catch the subtle pass.

"A six-thousand-dollar, laser-guided, long-range, drug delivery device." She focused on the trigger for a moment and then added, "We're lucky to have it — I hate it." The pilot, like the chopper, was new to the project so he did not yet know that, if possible, Dr. Green would practice veterinary medicine with just her bare hands, a pencil and a waterproof journal to take notes. She didn't trust modern technology: it seemed dangerous to her and had the potential to really leave you hanging.

A bandoleer of red-tufted, pressurized syringe darts was taped to the inside of the cockpit bubble. They were labeled and arranged sequentially with increasing amounts of M99. She slipped on safety goggles and latex gloves. If an errant drop of the stuff touched human skin, cardiac arrest would be only minutes away. Violet mumbled, "There's gotta be a better way," and then spoke into the mic, "William, I'm dosing her at 1800 pounds."

From the ground came the rumble of the vehicle and an Aussie twang, "Sounds about right to me, Guv', especially considering she's only two months along."

Violet carefully removed the needle's protective cap, laid the dart in the chamber and slid the bolt closed with a clack. Violet hated darting, not only because of the intrinsic risk for patient overdose and traumatic injury, but because it was too much like hunting for her. She checked her harness connections and yelled to the pilot, "Try to give me a range of 100 yards, but if she spooks pull back." She rotated to her right, planted both feet on the runner and without a second thought said, "I'm going out," and pushed off into the not-so-thin air. When her 110-pound mass reached the end of its tether, the jolt slammed the chopper's center of gravity to starboard. The pilot gunned the gas and jammed the stick to port to compensate for the tilt and mumbled, "Easy there, Rambo."

Violet strained at the end of her leash with the single-mindedness of a Pointer on a grouse and replied, "This is perfect." Cantilevered out over the landing gear she clicked on the laser sight, raised the rifle to her shoulder and lit up the patient's left rump with a bright red dot.

Then suddenly, in her left ear she heard, "Doc! Flamingoes at 11 o'clock!" Automatically raising her left eyebrow to widen her field of view, she was instantly engulfed by a pink blur and then a fine red mist plastered her goggles. The pilot banked intuitively to the right but the rapid acceleration and pivot spun his passenger, slamming her face-first into the plexi cockpit. She scrambled briefly for footing on the slick bar and then fell.

William shouted over the walkie talkie, "Vi!"

Dangling from her harness under the chopper's belly, with the dart gun still firmly in her left hand, Violet watched as her stethoscope tumbled, earpiece over bell, toward the ground 200 feet below. It landed with a sharp puff of dust and she winced, "That would have hurt…" The lost instrument exposed a pale tan line that ringed the back of her neck.

"Violet…! Are you okay?"

She reported to everyone, "I'm fine. Hold your location."

Without a pause she reached up, grabbed the landing gear, and with a one-handed pull up got her torso over the bar. She slid the gun into the cockpit and clambered like a chimp back into position. Readjusting her headset she said, "Thanks for the heads up, William. You saved our butts and most of that flock," then added, "Chilean flamingoes… cotton candy pink and they eat with their heads upside down. After all I do for them they still try to kill me."

William questioned, "We should probably call this off."

"Nope, I'm good," she scanned the horizon, "and Lucy's still in place. Let's go."

The pilot hovered briefly over the milling, confused family of giraffe and Dr. Green squeezed off the shot. This time nothing pink or red or any other color intervened. Like any good marksman, she could visualize the dart through its slight arc connecting with the target. She imagined the pressure surging away as the projectile dispensed the drug into the gluteus muscle group. Depressing a button on her black-lugged Timex to start the countdown, she reported into the microphone, "Okay folks, 8 minutes and 30 seconds until full effect. She's all yours, William."

Violet stepped back inside the chopper and signaled to the pilot with the swirling motion of her index finger, "Let's land."

The black and white, vertically-striped Range Rover surged toward the now accelerating giraffe herd. "African guides" with 25-foot-long, lasso-tipped capture poles balanced on each front corner of the swaying vehicle. The truck was packed with overstuffed tackle boxes containing emergency meds such as: atropine, epinephrine, and naloxone; treatments including: antibiotics, anti-inflammatories and even dewormers; and other supplies like syringes, needles, gauze, scalpels, retractors, hemostats, hand pump ventilators and endotracheal tubes. It was a hospital on wheels, a full-service mobile veterinary clinic.

Despite the rough terrain, William easily slalomed the Rover through a staggered series of faux termite towers, positioning the vehicle between the long-striding giraffe and the water hazard. Guiding the animal toward the open plain, he turned to the fourth year riding shotgun, "Mate, you ready on the hay bales?" The ashen, profusely sweating vet student stammered weakly, "Um, yes, uh, I place the bale under Lucy's head as she goes down." Then remembering the procedure briefing from 4 AM, "But I don't do anything," he repeated while punching his fist on his knee, "I don't do anything, until you say so."

The Aussie gave him a wink and a nod then turned to the young woman in the back, "…and Trisha, luv, you assist Doctor Green with the transmitter placement. I'll be gofer and transcriber."

Trisha Maxwell replied efficiently, "Got it."

The Rover's speedometer read 35 mph as they sidled up to the giraffe. Although Lucy's mammoth pistons continued to propel her solidly forward, William now noticed a slight hyperextension of the animal's front fetlocks with each stride. When the speed dropped to 30, he knew it was time. The right fender "guide" leaned outboard, expertly looping the lead rope over the horns and then behind the ears. William eased off the gas and slowed Lucy to a gentle stop. The animal swung around to face the

Rover, her head towering 17 feet above them. She stood calmly for about five seconds, blinked her gorgeous thick lashes once, twice, and then gingerly kneeled down in the front. William said softly, "That's a good girl, you're gonna take a little nap and get a pretty necklace."

The hay bales were positioned so that Lucy's head rested two feet above her prone thorax. When Violet came trotting up she pressed a second button on her watch. "Perfect positioning with her right side up. Okay, we've only got about 12 minutes — I don't want to re-dose her. As we practiced, William and you," she pointed to the male student, "are on vitals: heart rate, resps and then blood pressure." Violet unlatched and flipped open a massive green tackle box with multiple tiers of gear; she could teach and work simultaneously. "Normal resting BP?"

The pasty white student wiped his brow with the back of his wrist and squeaked, "Uh, about 240 systolic over 160 diastolic millimeters of mercury."

"Fabulous! Now, what could happen if her head drops below the horizontal plane of her stomach while anesthetized?"

The fourth year took a deep breath and then replied dramatically, "Our primary concern is regurgitation leading to aspiration pneumonia, but hypertensive decompensation while under anesthesia could possibly lead to retinal detachment and intracranial hemorrhage — I suppose with that kind of pressure her brain could be pulverized."

"Fantastic! Regurgitation was the answer I was looking for but 10 extra points for vivid word choice. You just don't get to use *pulverized* all that often." Some color flowed into the student's face and he flashed a quick smile. There were no actual grade points at stake but the gesture had its desired effect. "You let me know immediately if her vitals deviate from the normal limits."

The kid replied with something resembling a confident tone, "Got it."

As Violet reached into the box for a battery-operated clipper, she noticed a squadron of mosquitoes drilling into her forearm. In one fluid motion and with zero wasted effort, she shooed nearly a dozen of the tiny blood suckers by dragging her free arm over the other and turned to face Trisha Maxwell, "Now, with your mind's eye, visualize where the right jugular should lie and then point it out."

The girl blinked as she transitioned into the mental zone of overlapping anatomical drawings and extended her right index finger to a trough between the sternocephalicus and trachea. "It should be here."

"Perfect, now press down with the palm of your hand and watch for the fill."

Trisha did as directed, saw the two-inch fire hose distending cranially and reacted, "Wow, even I could hit that."

"Great, then I'll clip and prep the site so you can place the catheter."

"Me?"

"See one. Do one. Teach one."

"But this is my first giraffe and Lucy's your…"

Violet cut her off, "You did great on those zebra yesterday and you can do this, too." Wasting no time, she clipped a linear swath leaving a tuft of hair to glue the catheter hub in place and drenched the site in Betadine. Then, with a sterilely-gloved hand, Violet suggested, "I'd probably go right about there. Bevel up, at about a 50-degree angle." Trisha held off the enormous vein with her left palm and angled the needle through the rawhide epidermis, dermis and subcutis, and then the vascular tunic until a red flash appeared in the hub. "Again, perfect. Now advance it about two millimeters, slide in the catheter and then remove the stylet."

They connected and flushed a short IV extension set, glued the catheter hub and transmitter collar in place and turned on a radio receiver — it beeped a steady and rapid heart rate of 150. "The UV light will degrade the glue in 24-26 hours and the whole unit will drop off for retrieval. Until then it will record heart rate, pressure and take serial blood aliquots every 30 minutes. And, just to be safe, I programmed it to upload location, core body temp and the other data to the Argos satellite." She paused, "Oh yeah, I almost forgot the temperature transducer."

The male vet student was stationed at the head when suddenly the radio receiver reported a monotone beeeeeeeeep for several seconds and then fell silent. The fourth year's ephemeral composure disintegrated, "Doctor Green, EMERGENCY!" Violet glanced over her left shoulder noting the rise and fall of the golden-brown patchwork of fur. He continued, "She's in cardiac arrest! We need the paddles from the Rover…" Then, as he started to dash, he caught his foot on the hay bale and Lucy's elegant, six-foot-long neck began to slump and slide off the yellow straw. Even in the fog of a frenetic, presumed crisis, the student instantly realized his mistake and dove for the catch. He looked up, more than wide-eyed, at Violet and Trisha. "I'm sorry, I…"

"You did fine. Now, let's focus." Violet paused to let the words sink in. "What's her CRT?"

The student numbly elevated the squishy soft, warm muzzle and momentarily depressed a small section of the exposed gums with his thumb. It must have blanched white and turned quickly pink again because he reported, "The capillary refill time is less than two seconds."

"Good, and how about her resps?"

The fourth year eyed the thoracic wall excursions. Counting and calming down he said, "10 breaths per minute…" and then concluded sheepishly, "She's not in cardiac arrest."

"Wonderful. Excellent deduction." Dr. Green reversed the polarity of the situation. She had a knack for coaxing the best out of her students. "Remember, never rely solely on technology — for anything. Your eyes, ears, and hands are by far the best diagnostic tools your brain could ever have." Then, using a heparin flush, she quickly unclogged the catheter and began to pack up.

"What about your nose?" William chimed in.

"No nose knows more than yours." Cracking a smile, Violet checked her watch and administered the reversal agent, "It's time. We gotta get out of here." A moment later, Lucy snorted and began raising her head.

They loaded the vehicle in seconds and, with Violet now riding shotgun, the Rover backed to a safe distance to observe. Lucy's recovery, although ungainly, was uneventful. She returned safely to her family for a sniffing inspection. William said, "Speaking of noses, I think something smells funny with one of the "Arabian" Przewalski's in quarantine; she's almost ataxic."

Violet waved away another flight of mosquitoes and now noticed that both of her forearms were riddled with welts. She shook her head in annoyance at both the bugs and her boss and pursed her lips, "Davaris… He buys 39 *extinct* Mongolian horses from a sheik in Dubai and doesn't even tell me."

"Yeah, well, when you're the President and Chief Exec of the E.G.O. corporation you've simply got to have the World's Biggest, Fastest, Smallest, and Tallest of just about everything."

"In this case, the world's largest private collection of Przewalski's horses, in the largest and most successful animal park in the world." Again shaking her head she added, "But why?"

"Doc, at least it gives you the chance to do real science and run solid trials of field hardware. I reckon, for this kind of easy grant money, you gotta be willing to believe that the ends justify the BS. You do keep saying that it's all about the bloody *'Mission.'*"

With her lips still pursed, Violet Marie Green looked down at the complicated logo on her scrub top. It half overlapped her heart and, from her point of view, was upside down and backwards. The blue and green globe composed of antelope, elephant, gazelle and other animal silhouettes was stitched together like a puzzle and underscored with the park's name, "The Peaceable Kingdom." Embroidered words ringed the image like a halo: "Saving the Wild, One Animal at a Time."

Dr. Violet Marie Green sighed and then said, "Okay, let's go check out that Przewalski's, but after that I've gotta get back to the school for first-year orientation."

William, instantly bolt upright and feigning shock, nodded his head back towards the rear seat, "Crikey, you mean newbie versions of *them?*"

CHAPTER TWO

Orientation

*Room A1 of the old veterinary school building at the
University of Philadelphia, School of Veterinary Medicine*

N eurons (when functioning properly) are living, breathing conduits — the stuff of animal wiring. Like leaden batteries and lifeless capacitors, they exploit the positive and negative. Pluses and minuses and a sub-cellular ionic gap can be used to telegraph discomfort, trigger muscles and even dream dreams. On rare occasions and in special situations humans report, "You could feel the excitement in the air." We use words such as *palpable* and *electric* to describe the invisible hum of shared expectation. Today, the air in Room A1 absolutely pulsed.

Room A1 was aptly named. It was the first veterinary teaching hall chartered for the New World. Every first-year veterinary student knew the story about Benjamin Franklin. The gifted statesman, kite-flying scientist, envied philanderer, and national founding father passionately championed the construction of this hall, stating, "If this edifice is not so built, then God save these 13 United States." Unfortunately, it was just fiction. He never said any such thing, but the pervasive legend seemed to fit the time frame, as well as the real-life tenor and esteemed goals of the institution, so it stuck.

At the time of construction, A1 and the professors lecturing in it were expected to produce animal doctors for a newly emerging agricultural powerhouse. The infant American Union was in dire need of animal medical care. In the cleared fields of nearby Penn's Woods, herds of cattle just dropped over dead and no one knew why. Of course, when animals died in great numbers so did people, their livelihoods decimated. So the impetus for a veterinary teaching hospital in this country was human survival, not altruism toward nature or animals. Nature was the enemy. Veterinarians were the foot soldiers expected to wage and win the war. The best of the finest students — the cream of the crop — were installed in this space and nurtured by scholars from the Old World and New.

The interior of Room A1 has been modified only slightly over the years — electric lights have been bolted alongside gas fixtures which flank the original candlestick holders (still holding candles); a motorized projection screen and sliding blackboard conceal a bricked-up, center-stage archway. This archway allowed for the entry of animal patients used in disease demonstrations. When a full-blown surgery was performed, the animal was led in and "dropped" on the cold cobblestone floor for the students' edification. A large circular grate covers the central drain that collected the inevitable byproducts of the profession: blood, pus, manure and urine (the concrete grout anchoring the cobbles remains stained to this day).

As directed by the school's puritanical first Dean, the A1 "theater" was outfitted with tiered seating that rose abruptly and precipitously from the stage, so steeply in fact, that a tiny misstep in one of the narrow aisles and the fall would surely maim, possibly kill. In the old days (and still today), students sat for long hours on the fixed, unyielding, wrought-iron-framed, hardwood chairs. As a functional nod to the Almighty, nine stained-glass windows depicting the story of Noah's Ark were wrapped around the top row of seats and a simply constructed but massive chandelier was hung on a pulley system to provide light. Finally, the elegantly domed ceiling was adorned with a series of gilded animal constellations; they floated among wispy clouds on a delicate blue background. Room A1 is a hallowed relic that's still in use because it "shows well" during tours for prospective students and the more nostalgic, philanthropic types.

On this day of orientation, 85 first-year veterinary students packed the hall. Most of the flock emitted a polite, nervous chatter while thoughts like, *This is it, I finally made it!* instantly followed by, *Am I good enough?* pinballed around the room. A plain paper banner — *Welcome First Years* — hung over the heads of two professors downstage. One, a soft redhead with shimmering green eyes and in a long white lab coat, worked at the podium. A second, more perpendicular, flat-topped professor in scrubs was assisting. They were sorting boxes of manila envelopes — orientation packets. All the while, the room was accented with dappled light that filtered through the great oaks that now tower over the lecture hall. Muted shafts of sunshine, softly dyed by the multiple stained-glass panes, slanted across the gentle airspace. And, since a few of the smaller ventilation windows were canted open, small birds, mostly chickadees and nuthatches, flit freely in and out, sometimes alighting upon the massive chandelier.

In days gone by this was a young men's group (which inevitably turned into an old boys' club), but today things were different. This class, like the ten or so preceding it, was about 70% women. Smart, strong, independent women. In the very last rows, up in the nosebleed section, sat a small sequestrum of three guys and two girls — a thin moat of empty seats separated them from the masses. They weren't chatting like the rest, just observing from their perch, taking it all in.

Jack Doyle was among the group at the top of A1. He brought his closed right hand to his lips to cover an expanding grin. In this position he could smell the residue of his previous career. He'd fired his revolver at the range last night, one last time, and then turned in his sidearm and badge to his dad who also happened to be his sergeant. Jack's life, like his four brothers' (two priests, a fireman and another cop) and three sisters' (a teacher, nurse and an EMT), was preordained for honorable service. Like his siblings, Jack was driven to save souls from danger, but with less than a year on the force he'd made a switch. To animals.

It all started when he was five. It was a distraction. A form of blue-collar therapy. His dad steadied himself on the day he gave Jack a goldfish "in need of a good home." This led — as it does — to tadpoles, frogs, and salamanders. Soon, the neighbors pitched in by delivering shoeboxes filled with grass clippings and orphaned baby squirrels, rabbits and song-birds. By the time he was ten, Jack Doyle could cure the most sickly pigeon, crow or opossum (each earning the standard moniker, Lazarus #X upon release into the wild).

Outwardly, everything about Jack Doyle, down to the crucifix anchored around his neck, was traditional, urban Irish Catholic. His mother gave him that thick dark hair, those acute hazel eyes, the deep-seated guilt and, per genetic law, he could only manage a brilliant peel even after a full summer on the K-9 beat. As Jack sat in the top row of A1 on this glorious day he wondered, momentarily, if this new life would finally make his parents forgive him, if it would fill that hollow in his heart?

But rather than dwell on the unanswerable, Jack administered his own form of self-prescribed distraction. His head swiveled, making a smooth and complete left-to-right scan of the room. He tried not to stare, but his eyes paused here and there. He was a trained observer, and it was just natural. He was a guy. He was single, and there were all these women. Probably most were single, too. He realized that he'd actually been holding his breath and then suddenly remembered to breathe, starting with a nearly silent but prolonged exhale. The sound caught the attention of the guy sitting next to him. They swapped a knowing glance and Jack leaned over, "This… this is looking pretty good," slowly nodding his head up and down without breaking eye contact.

Sam Stone, raised in the isolation of a fishing village on Monhegan Island in Maine, was by any woman's definition a *tall cool drink of water*. From under the brim of his Red Sox ball cap he gathered and distilled a confluence of profound thoughts, "Ay-yuh, hot *and* wicked smaht."

Jack drew in a gallon of air and then replied, "This is gonna be a rough four years, all right." He whispered more to himself, "I want you, and you — Jesus, Mary and… twins." Jack paused, again reflexively holding his breath. The twins were composed of two averagely attractive brunettes. Individually they would be classified as "cute," but as any guy knows, it was more the twins thing that made him go anoxic.

The islander calmly metered his words, "Slow down buckaroo, you gotta remember to breathe. That's why this is a four-year degree. And then, hopefully, you'll have a year of internship, and a three-year residency — you'll have plenty of time to… *entah the rodeo*."

Jack nodded with his eyes momentarily closed, admitting he'd been too anxious, "Yeah, you're right, that makes me feel a little better, but…" He glanced to his left at a poshly dressed girl two seats over and reached out his right hand, "Hi, I'm Jack."

"I'm Kerri Feinburg." She elevated her shoulder pads and eyebrows in unison, "So, this is it?" and then paused as she relaxed, "I guess I pictured it a little different."

Even though Jack was no math whiz, he knew there had to be at least two girls for every guy so he smiled and replied, "Yeah, me too."

"Good morning, class. Good morning," the professor with flowing red hair waited to let the chatter fade. A gentle *"woof-woof"* came from the room's handicapped seating area so she added with a warm smile, "Sounds like the canine member of your class is ready to get the show on the road."

A girl with gleaming, raven-black hair seated in the front row patted her companion and then raised a finger to her lips, "*Shhh*, Petunia."

"I'm Flo Kimball, head of the Small Animal Emergency Service and a specialist in cardiology." She was outfitted as an ER vet should be, with a stethoscope, reflex hammer and dog-eared formulary poking out of the pockets of her long white lab coat. But unlike your standard-issue ER vet, a shiny gold peace sign was pinned above the red cursive script, "Florence Kimball MD, DVM, PhD," embroidered over her left breast. "Myself and Doctor Linnehan here," indicating with an outstretched arm, "Chief of Large Animal Orthopedic Surgery and NASA Shuttle Payload Specialist, are your faculty mentors." She beamed benevolently, "I'd like to welcome you all to the University of Philadelphia, School of Veterinary Medicine." Rotating her head to inspect the students, Flo Kimball revealed a sparkling crystal heart dangling from each earlobe. "I recognize many of you from the interview process last spring and am glad to have you all aboard the Class of 1992. Well," she paused, "that's when most of you will be graduating. You are our 109th class — some of your parents and even some of *their* parents sat in these very seats." She paused to take a breath, "Kind of scary, huh? I'm not going to deceive you, this can be a trying four years."

Jack Doyle inclined his head toward Sam Stone and whispered, "See, even she knows — *girls, girls, girls*."

Dr. Kimball continued, "History tells us that five from your class will not make it to year two, and unfortunately only about 65 of you will graduate. During your tenure, you'll take hundreds of tests, and most graduates will ultimately pass the state and national boards so that you will be able to practice some form of veterinary medicine."

A hand rocketed up from the front row; it swiveled frantically at the wrist. Dr. Kimball paused and nodded her head towards the student, giving him permission to speak.

"Simon JJ Harding the Third, Veterinary Class of 1992…"

"Uh, yes, JJ. I definitely remember you from the interviews." She smiled kindly, tilted her head and asked with patient inflection, "Do you have a question?"

JJ, with his arm still in the air, "Yes, thank you. I have a two-part question: first, is there a constellation of academic test results and/or standards such as college GPA, MCAT results, and Graduate Record Examination scores that will reliably predict success or failure, and, if so, what might the minimal scores predicting future success be?"

Jack couldn't help himself. Under his breath he muttered, "Holy shit…"

Dr. Linnehan interceded with a machine gun response, "Obviously, if such tests were reliably predictive you might not be here to ask that question." His flat-topped turret remained motionless while his eyes moved back and forth, Terminator style, "Any other such questions?" Days seemed to pass as he waited in silence for another victim, but even these newbies understood that elevating an arm right now would be like reaching into a bear trap. Dr. Linnehan concluded, "No? Okay."

Dr. Kimball resumed, "But please, please don't despair." She raised both arms and opened her palms to them, "Remember what you've come through to be here today. History also tells us that for each person seated in this lecture hall, there were thousands of kids that said and truly believed they wanted to be veterinarians. Then, at the final competition during your application process, there were dozens of qualified applicants per slot. So," she smiled warmly again, "you've done well to be here today and you should be proud of that. Just keep up the good work and I'm sure everything will be fine."

"Over the next four years, you will get to work with some of the most skilled veterinary clinicians in the world, establish lifelong friendships and of course, don't forget the animals. We have the largest and most diverse collection of animal patients at any veterinary school in the country. Some of you will travel the world on conservation missions while others will work with our vets to discover emerging infectious diseases." This statement seemed to jog Dr. Kimball, derailing her train of thought. She stopped, bent to retrieve a pickle jar from behind the podium and then raised it with both hands above her head like a welterweight champion. Inside was a snow-globe storm of creamy white flecks which, after a few moments, flurried to the bottom to reveal a gray fleshy organ that came to a blunt conical point. Hundreds of squiggly white strands protruded, choking every mortal orifice. Flo Kimball exclaimed, "Speaking of emerging infectious diseases…" she emphasized her point by shaking the jar which caused the lifeless mass to slosh and gobs of white squiggles to swirl, "this is the result of canine heartworm! You'll learn about its insidious pathology in coming years, but as a cardiologist I brand it Public Enemy #1." She turned to her left with the jar still held aloft, "Wouldn't you agree, Doctor Linnehan?"

Dr. Dan Linnehan, covertly known as Drill Sergeant Dan to the upper classes, nodded once, "Affirmative, a deadly menace."

Sam Stone, the rugged Mainer, interjected quietly to their little group, "All this if you act now, for the low, low price of 25 grand per year…"

Jack whispered, "Drinks not included. Some restrictions may apply. See your dealer for…"

Dr. Kimball cradled the jar in the crook of one arm and regained her focus, "This class has a diverse background like most over the past several years. As a group you've already been quite successful. There are numerous valedictorians among you." She picked up a list from the podium and began a litany, "Let's see, you have: one trial lawyer, three critical-care nurses, a pharmacist, one commercial fisherman, a standardbred trainer, two dairy farmers, a cattle rancher, a rabbi, and a professional surfer," she paused and raised her eyebrows, "a police officer, a Brooklyn beauty queen, one circus performer, and three PhD basic-science researchers. In fact, eight of you already have graduate degrees. The class ranges in age from 20 to 47. So all I can say is that with your collective broad-base of experience, if you all work together, each individual can make it to the goal." Dr. Kimball replaced the list on the podium, took a breath and leveled her head, "When you stumble," she slowed for emphasis, "*and each one of you will*, a helping hand can make the difference." She stopped.

The word "stumble" triggered something in Jack. He shifted his gaze from a voluptuous blonde to the girl with her dog in the front row.

Dr. Kimball resumed, "Please become familiar with the information in your orientation packet. On the outside of the envelope, in red, is the number of your group. You will meet with your fourth-year student advisor — two or more of you will be in each group. These advisors will help you through your first semester and, because they are successfully completing their fourth year, they will undoubtedly have numerous study tips and be able to recommend invaluable reference texts."

"Throughout the year you will 'tag along' with them on actual medical rounds in the various specialty rotations." Dr. Kimball indicated with her left hand again, "One week it may be large animal surgery with Doctor Linnehan out at the Center for Large Animal Medicine. The next it might be small animal dermatology here in the city." Dr. Kimball laughed and shook her head, "Back in the old days you wouldn't even see a live animal patient until your fourth year and that was if you were lucky! Now, you'll be asked to participate, actively." She concluded with raised eyebrows, a smile and a clap of her hands, "You start this afternoon!"

Jack Doyle sat up and leaned forward, his eyes darting from one envelope to the next as he searched for ones that matched his. He mumbled to himself, "No number twelve…" and, just as he realized that he'd only been checking the female envelopes, he felt two meaty taps on his left shoulder. He slowly turned to discover a substantial young man with a wide smile and twinkling eyes — he was holding up his packet and pointing to the big red number "12." As they shook hands, Jack's was engulfed in a calloused but gentle warmth. He muttered carefully, "I'm Jack."

The friendly bulk, capped with a cowboy hat straight from Bonanza, released his grip and replied without losing the grin, "The name's Buford Hugman, but folks just call me Hoss."

Jack blinked twice before he responded, "I bet they do," and then added what seemed most appropriate, "Pleased to make your acquaintance."

Dr. Kimball yielded the podium to Drill Sergeant Dan. This had the subtle but real effect of bringing the class to attention — instinctively, they all sat up a little straighter. "As Doctor Kimball stated, I'm Doctor Linnehan, Chief of Large Animal Orthopedic Surgery." With an efficient and precise delivery he moved into the business at hand, "Your first semester classes are as follows: Comparative Gross Anatomy — focusing on the horse, cow, pig, chicken, dog, and cat;" he didn't pause, "Physiology — function at the tissue, organ, cellular and sub-cellular levels; Comparative Microanatomy — histology of the fetal pig; Biochemistry; and finally, Veterinary Medical Ethics." He raked his head back about an eighth of an inch so that the buzz top was perfectly parallel to the floor; if you placed a carpenter's level up there, the bubble would have been exactly centered. He scanned the hall slowly again with a smooth, side-to-side sweep of his eyes. "And, since you won't have your first test until Friday, this is a good time to get your bearings."

He didn't shift his weight or alter the attitude of his turret in any way, "Your physiology and biochemistry classes are occasionally combined with those of the first-year, human medical students. As we all know, veterinarians are still well-regarded and trusted by the general public — even more than human doctors." He paused and adjusted his volume up several decibels, "And I'd like to keep it that way." His gaze locked onto the front row, "Remember, in a cursory way, now *you* will be representing *my* profession. Welcome the human medical students and help them if it is possible. Some will want to trade up at the end of their first year." He paused and then concluded, "Their class is approximately the size of yours, except the male to female ratio is reversed."

Way up in the last row, Kerri Feinburg swapped a wide-eyed glance with the girl sitting next to her and then both gradually smiled as the realization sank in. Kerri whispered to the girl, "Boys that are a little 'slower' than us but are going to make real money." Then slipping back into her native Brooklynese, "No sugalah, this is how you hold that nasty scalpel. Sweetie, use the other end or you might get a boo-boo."

Her classmate responded in mock surprise, "This weekend, visiting your mom in the Hamptons? Okay honey bunch, but remember you have to study for your quizie next week."

Kerri concluded after pursing her lips and wrinkling her brow, "Fortunately, that pesky medical ethics class of yours is an elective..."

◄ ● ►

While the first years were attending orientation, the fourth-year veterinary students were gathered nearby in a modern, windowless and more gradually-tiered lecture hall. The humming fluorescent lights were dimmed while a slide show was in progress — it was a student case presentation. On the chalkboard were the words:

Weekly Grand Rounds
Case Highlights:
– *German Shepherd, Hip Dysplasia*
– *Feline Unilateral Kidney Tumor*
– *Comminuted Fracture Repair in a Rhinoceros*

A moderator was seated at the front of the hall, while at the podium off to the right stood a male fourth-year student, the current speaker — a beanpole in scrubs with black plastic-rimmed glasses an inch wider than his head. His right lens was held in place and partially occluded by a flesh-colored Band-Aid.

Most of the senior vet students in the audience were wearing crisp white coats or jade surgical scrubs — nearly all had stethoscopes draped around their necks — but some were in field-service coveralls. Like the lab coats and scrub tops, the forest green coveralls had the veterinary caduceus and the words "Vet Med" embroidered over their left breast. Some students were flipping through tinback medical records or reference texts. Others were writing up treatment plans. Everyone multitasked while listening, but no one took notes on the presentation. And though they all looked the part, they weren't real vets yet.

One of the seniors had segregated himself way up in the last row of seats. This row, affectionately nicknamed "Death Row," can be found in every vet school classroom. Death Row is default seating for some students, while others are driven there by circumstance. Occupying a seat on Death Row is not necessarily a bad thing, nor does it give you the reputation of being a sub-par student. Usually, it just means you have "special needs" that day. Death Row is a refuge. A haven. A student on Death Row will almost never be called upon or asked to participate thus facilitating any (or all) of three critical activities:

1) Studying: But not regular studying. You cram on Death Row when you've been up all night, or more likely the last three, assisting on a run of very cool emergency colic surgeries, and the cumulative parasitology final is in two hours. You've boldly forged a solid D+ average with the wrecking-ball reasoning, "Life cycle — what is this, aerobics class? I only need to know how to kill 'em." In short, you study on Death Row when your academic life depends on it.

2) Detox: Death Row is the unofficial waiting area for the University's porcine to human liver transplantation trial. Surprisingly, the Sheep and Goat Club throws some kick ass (beef) barbeques now that their outlawed still is covertly back in operation. White lightning with a splash of formalin — billed as "liquid protection for your aging complexion" — it can take as much as it gives. Death Row tranquility is essential when you have a hammerhead hangover.

3) Sleep: The most vital reason for placing yourself on Death Row is simple, to recharge. Not to take a gratuitous, lazy type of slumber or a beauty type of sleep. Those would be downright insulting. This is quite the opposite. The Death Row slump with dried spittle on the chin, a greasy mane, and rows of half-empty caffeine containers demonstrates unambiguous resolve, dedication, and even professorial respect. The phrase, "Whatever It Takes," can be found in microscopic block lettering carved into many Death Row desktops. It's understood, if you consistently require a real, lie-down-with-a-pillow-and-blanket sleep experience, you should probably consider another career. Extreme legend has it that one student never even rented an apartment. Between his rusted out '77 Jeep Cherokee, vet teching 9 PM to 5 AM in the ES, and the luxurious Death Row accommodations, he saved about $6,200 a year. He was, of course, involuntarily celibate.

In comparison to recurrent Death Row inmates, the Front Row Geeks (or FRoGs as they were known) consistently received higher grades — on average, 3% higher. Also, FRoGs went to 82% less parties and had 96% fewer dates. With few exceptions, the sifting and sorting that naturally occurred during voluntary seating in the standard veterinary classroom was in itself an accurate prognosticator of 'future success.'

Today, Mike London was located at the top of the last tier. He was precariously balancing on the back two legs of his chair while washing down a three-pack of Twinkies with a slug of black coffee.

Mike had chosen Death Row today, but not for the usual reasons. This was not a usual class. It was a quickie, the weekly Grand Rounds presentation where the most important cases would be presented by his classmates. No one would deny the educational opportunity that Grand Rounds afforded these seniors, but it was the comic potential for a royal presentation screw-up that kept them coming back for more.

After his last coffee gulp sluiced down his last whole Twinkie, Mike discovered that he was fixated on the presenter's Dumbo-sized ears rather than the screen. He half heard, "This is Baby at five days old, third day post-surgery. She was 26 inches tall at this point and weighed 130 pounds." He added, "And she was gaining about four pounds per day."

The student flipped to the next slide which displayed a radiograph of a fracture site complete with a T-shaped piece of hardware, four loops of heavy-gauge wire, and numerous screws. "This was the first open reduction of a Salter-Harris type IV fracture in a black rhinoceros and it was accomplished by Doctor Green with her custom-designed, stainless steel internal fixator and ten #12 lag screws. With a total surgery time of 7 hours and 43 minutes, the procedure took nearly half the day."

An AV cart with a large screen TV and VCR sat about four feet to the presenter's right. After clicking the X-ray slide to a blank, the student made half a stride towards the cart when the microphone cord yanked him backwards and spun him around. The mic made a piercing, *PHFFFFFT* as it came unclipped and then a booming THUD when it hit the floor. The presenter squatted down and, raising the mic just a foot off the floor, said into it, "Uh, sorry..." before he switched on the VCR and retreated back behind the podium.

"Here is some video I shot of Doctor Green reintroducing Baby to her mom post-op." The video clip began out of focus and then zoomed to a view of the "tiny" rhino lying in straw with a white cast on her left foreleg. As you would expect, well wishes adorned the exterior: "Get well soon and watch out for those banana peels, Gordy the Gorilla; You got a horn, next time just honk! Charley the Cheetah." Initially the animal was motionless, sitting up on its sternum with only her left ear flicking at a buzzing fly. But then she must have made a decision in that five-day-old brain because suddenly she scuffled, wobbled and stood. Three or four of the seniors clapped softly.

As if talking directly to the lecture hall, Dr. Green turned to the camera and said, "You guys had better get back." On command, most people in the first few rows leaned back in their seats. Then the fourth years watched as Dr. Green unlatched a thick, tubular-steel swing gait to expose a wide, dusty corral and proceeded to usher the little rhino inside with gentle pats on its rump. The camera panned, first to the left and then to the right, revealing a circular enclosure with stout, four-foot-high by three-foot-wide, solid rock walls — clearly designed for the more powerful but vertically challenged of the animal kingdom.

The student followed inside obviously mesmerized by the unfolding events. Without turning to look back, Dr. Green asked if the gate was shut and locked. A metallic clang could be heard off camera and the videographer reported, "Yes it is," as the shot rose and fell two times in unison with an affirming head nod.

Dr. Green then yelled to a keeper on the other side of the wall, "Go ahead, let her out!" and instantly dashed to the left out of the field of view. The next image that came into auto-focus was that of a snorting, rapidly-enlarging, rhinoceros-freight-train-of-death.

A breathless, "*ooohhhh-shhhhhit…*" leaked from the cameraman as he stumbled backward, the picture frame bouncing up and down.

While an audible gasp escaped from most of the senior class, a grateful smile gained momentum and took over Mike's face. He was delighted that the beanpole didn't have the presence of mind to just drop the damned camera and run. The whole class was riveted to the presentation, when suddenly, a blonde blur streaked from left-to-right waving her arms like a professional rodeo clown. She yelled, "Get the hell out of here NOW!" as she ran, and the myopic gray mass turned deftly, redirecting its attack. Dr. Green continued her sprint across the paddock, and, performing a one-handed vault over the wall, disappeared from view.

The final image on the recording was that of the charging mom rhino skidding to a safe stop in a billowing cloud of brown chalky dust. The beanpole squawked, "Uh, the end."

The classroom burst into laughter and the lights came up.

The moderator interrupted as she took over the podium, "Okay…

good. Interesting case," and then, looking up at the clock on the back wall, said, "Unfortunately, we don't have time for questions."

She took a second or two to gather her thoughts and separate topics, then announced, "It's that time of year again — the first years have arrived." Low groans could be heard. "Now come on, I'm sure you can remember back to when you were wide-eyed and bushy-tailed. You know, nervous and excited. Well, now is your chance to give these kids the benefit of your wisdom. The advisor group assignments have been delivered to your mailboxes so please develop a list of survival tips." She paused and then added, "Just think, it's your chance to mold them in your own image or… trick them into doing your AM treatments."

The moderator concluded, "Any *quick*," knowing that she had to emphasize the word quick, "questions?"

Eight hands shot up from the first two tiers.

Mike couldn't restrain himself, "Oh God, FRoGs… Phasers on Stun." Three or four seniors in the last few rows clinched their hands in a mock pistol grip, aimed at the spindly arms and squeezed off an imaginary Star Trek beam. A light laugh followed the muffled *shhhwooo-shhhwooo-shhhwooooing* sound as the FRoGs, waving wildly for attention, were oblivious.

◄ ● ►

Back in Room A1, where Flo Kimball was wrapping up the first part of orientation, she said, "Okay class, let's break for 10 minutes and then you'll be meeting in your smaller orientation groups." She looked down at her watch and then back up, "Are there any *quick* questions?" Twelve hands from the first two rows instantly went vertical.

A 1000-watt beacon clicked on over Jack Doyle's head. He turned to face Sam, Hoss and then Kerri. He whispered, "Houston, I think we have a problem…" And then with his clenched teeth he pulled an imaginary pin from an imaginary grenade and lobbed it down front — they all imitated a low rumbling explosion in unison.

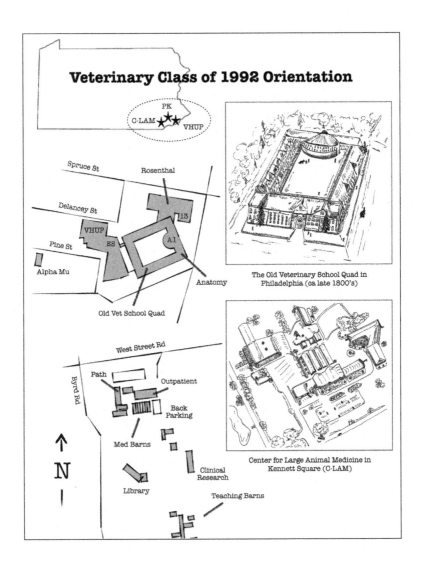

Veterinary Class of 1992 Orientation

The Old Veterinary School Quad in Philadelphia (ca late 1800's)

Center for Large Animal Medicine in Kennett Square (C-LAM)

CHAPTER THREE

The Advisors:
Part I (Mike London)

The patient waiting areas in the Veterinary Hospital at the University of Philadelphia (VHUP)

Jack and Hoss were a few minutes early. They made their way directly from Room A1 to the canine waiting bay in the small animal hospital — the meeting point for their orientation group. They observed in silence as a very Great Dane sauntered in and sat as requested. Hoss reached up to stroke the silky gray cranium and then noticed a balding man in a tight beige turtleneck shift towards the corner. He was clutching a trembling beige Chihuahua to his chest. Hoss whispered to Jack never taking his concerned eyes off the diminutive animal, "Those lap things make me nervous."

Jack snorted a quiet laugh and smiled. He'd just learned that Hoss — among other large animal pastimes — was an accomplished standard-bred harness racer. This colossus that routinely handled fire-breathing half-ton equines was anxious about a peanut with legs. For a moment he imagined a woolly mammoth wearing Hoss's voluminous checked shirt, brown suede vest, and ten-gallon hat teetering on a step stool as a mouse patrolled for crumbs. But then something shiny followed by something curvy caught Jack's eye.

Jack nudged Hoss with his elbow.

They both recognized a woman from their class slowly making her way through the hospital's revolving door. She was the only student who had a dog with her and now the reason was clear. This sturdy black lab was some sort of assistance dog.

The girl held the animal's leash in her right hand, limping slightly as she supported her weight on a slender cane using her left. She had nearly cleared the doorway when the cane's black rubber tip got lodged as the door attacked from behind. Sensing it was jammed, the drive motor disengaged but the door was still stuck. Anna Heywood, using all of her clearly compromised strength, tugged on the walking stick but it wouldn't budge.

Jack Doyle jumped into action and was at the girl's side in an instant. It was just natural for him to grab the shaft of the cane and say, "Can I give you a hand?"

Anna whipped her head around and shot the offending do-gooder without hesitation, "No, you cannot."

Jack stiffened. She'd winged him but he pushed on, "I'm in your class..."

She glared at him. All the wonderful curves had vanished, replaced by sharp, dangerous angles. "Let go," she almost growled. "I don't need you."

Jack was stunned and wondered why she wouldn't let him help. Since his only response was to flinch, she ordered, "Stand down, Superman."

The muscles in Jack's forearm acted on their own accord, relaxing their grip before his brain knew why. "Uh, sure, of course, I'm sorry, I just..."

Anna turned away from Jack and directed her attention back to the problem quite literally at hand. She gave the stick, the God-damned stick she was stuck with, another tug. Nothing. Meanwhile, her dog sat patiently by her side. Anna hunched over and spoke into the liquid brown eyes, "Okay Petunia, we need to figure this out, hon." The dog remained seated but perked her ears as she looked up at *her* faithful companion.

Pointing to a spot on the glass door, Anna Heywood gave the suggestion, "Petunia, door." The animal knew what Anna wanted; she'd helped push doors open before. Standing on her hind legs, Petunia planted her soft front paws on the glass. The weight of nearly 90 pounds nudged the glass backwards about a quarter of an inch, just enough to free the cane. Anna turned and exited the revolving trap.

Safely out of range, Anna Heywood stopped and gently patted the animal's head. She praised her pet just loudly enough to be overheard, "Good girl Petunia, *you're* my hero." Petunia sat her hind end on the cool linoleum and looked up at Anna with adoring eyes. This was the look that Anna needed, the one thing she let herself need. She thought (as she always did), *Will I ever meet a man who will love me as truly?*

Anna looked up; Jack stood there expectantly.

"Well, good job, I mean, uh, I didn't mean to presume to, uh, good…" As verbiage dribbled from his mouth, other words trickled along a parallel circuit in Jack's brain — *you're patronizing her.* Jack looked into Anna's deep chestnut eyes and watched as her attractive face — flawless, tawny and clearly of Asian descent — was beginning to retighten. Among the progressively tensing facial muscles, the orbicularis oculi drew her eyelids together slightly while the depressor labii thinned and flattened her previously sensuous lips. Jack sensed that his current trajectory would drop him squarely in a minefield, so he redirected toward the dog — maybe that could defuse the situation. "Good job, Petunia."

Anna's lips softened, "She's the best."

Jack smiled. His shoulders relaxed. But, as men in the trenches understandably forget, surviving a battle does not mean you are winning the war. He took one step further, unaware of the trip wire. "There's an automatic…" He paused, noticing the large handicap symbol embossed on the glass, "sliding door over there. Maybe that would be easier." It was too late. He knew instantly what he'd done and there was no way out, so he braced himself for the attack.

Anna's eyes narrowed into defensive slits like those in a knight's helmet. She was sure she'd jousted with guys like this before, so she proceeded with her usual strategy, "You mean the handicap entrance?"

He hesitated and then stammered, "Well, um, that door is less difficult to negotiate."

Anna picked up on the stumble so she unsheathed her sword, "So then, are you handicapped?"

This time, without hesitation, he replied, "Well, not physically but it seems I'm developing a rapidly progressive mental impairment."

Anna thought, *nice recovery*, but I'm gonna take one more stab, "Am I handicapped?"

Hoss, still quiet as a stone, now took on the physical appearance of one. He froze, hoping not to be noticed.

She had Jack in the corner, but not on the ropes. Anna's only real handicap in this circumstance was that she did not know her self-created opponent. She was unaware of his training in the law, his family's service mantra, or that his actions only served to reflect the true image of his good heart. She prejudged him — when you're alone and scared that's what you do.

After taking in and exhaling one deep breath (to give him time to gather his thoughts and rectify his tension-induced acidosis) Jack replied,

"Yes. You are handicapped, at least in the eyes of the law."

Anna was surprised by the direct response but, for some reason, the overall sensation was good.

He continued, "I would guess — and I'm sure you'll correct me if I'm wrong — that your driver's license and car plates will serve as evidence in support of this statement. And I'll add, if you'll allow, that although you may have the distinction of being labeled a handicapped person, functionally I can see that you are both as capable and as frail as us." He pointed to himself and Hoss with his thumb.

In the brief pause that followed, Hoss sensed his moment so he carefully offered up each word, "I got stuck in that door on the day of my interview…"

They both looked at Hoss, his sincerity and empathy unmistakable. Anna's combat visage melted ever so slightly and she felt a smile coming on, but fortunately was able to suppress it by turning back to Jack. He continued, "Please accept my apology. I realize that I have offended you and that was not my aim." He paused and then concluded, "I'm Jack Doyle and this is Buford Hugman."

Again sensing his chance, "Miss, just call me Hoss."

Just then a set of double doors behind them sprang wide open and in waltzed their fourth-year advisor, Mike London. He held a giggling nurse tight at the waist, their left hands clasped and held high. The pair performed a tight spin and ended with a classic Viennese bow. Mike wordlessly blew the middle-aged woman a kiss and turned to face Jack, Hoss and Anna.

After cursory introductions, their advisor stuck his head through a small sliding glass window at the Emergency Service admissions counter. To the left, on a gurney out of public view, lay a big black dog with a distended abdomen. A little girl in pink footie pajamas clutched a stuffed bunny with one arm and her mom's leg with the other. Tears streaked her flushed cheeks. Dr. Kimball and a nurse were inserting catheters, hooking up EKG leads and intubating — all in one fluid motion.

A pulsatile stream arced through the air and Mike pulled back just in time as it splattered across the inside of the window. Sticking his head back through the crimson-framed opening he asked, "You guys need some help?"

The nurse responded nonchalantly, "Nah, that's okay Mike, we're cool." And because she knew he'd want to know, she added, "Two-year-old pregnant dobie HBC. Once she's stabilized we'll take her to radiology-land and surgery is ready for us. You take a break, it was a hell of a night."

"Well then, I'm gonna take the kids on orientation over to Murph's. If anybody needs me, just holler." He held up a black walkie talkie and depressed the transmit button twice. A *click-click* reported on the ER base station. Mike then turned back to the first years who stood stock still while displaying varying degrees of saucer eye — the big one's mouth hung open about an inch.

Mike London smiled, "Have you all eaten?" They shook their heads no, slowly and in unison. "Let's fix that straight away. I missed dinner last night *and* breakfast this morning. I've been on 36 straight." The group congealed as Mike led them out through the automatic sliding doors and they slid diagonally across the street.

Their destination was an unassuming wooden doorway with peeling birch laminate and one flagstone step. A stubby, rusted neon sandwich sign with the three block letters B A R jutted out over the door. These three letters gave Mike personal and professional comfort. In veterinary parlance, BAR stood for Bright, Alert, and Responsive — the goal for every patient and the only kind of people he drank with.

Murphy's Tavern was not really a place. It was more of a vehicle with a biphasic daily life cycle driven by its clientele. To save managerial time and effort (money was not the object), its dark, dank spaces were perpetually decorated for all the major and some minor holidays. A string of outdoor Christmas lights outlined the hard liquor spectrum from "Old Grand Dad" to "Wild Turkey" kept behind the bar — three bulbs still blinked. Cheap cardboard skeletons and green four-leafed clovers were speared to the walls with three-inch nails next to hand-made, hand-shaped Thanksgiving turkey cutouts. One dust-encrusted banner proclaimed *Happy Birthday*, just in case.

From 9 AM to about 8 PM Murph's was typical of Philly's old man bars where yellowing Andy Capp cartoons were the obvious choice to patch crumbling wallpaper. This was the time of day when critics of both the mayor and the Eagles met for fluid therapy. From 10 PM onward, the place was seeded with animal types, usually second and third years. Occasionally, small invasive forces of MD's and dentists-in-training ran recon. They were usually repelled, not by the customers, but by the smell.

Mike eased through the front door — Murphy's Tavern was as much a home for him as the vet school and a lot more than any place he slept. Mike tipped his head to the bartender, "Howdy, Burt."

"Hey, Mike."

Mike gestured to the three first years, "New recruits."

"You guys should stick with Mike London," advised the bartender.

"Burt, how's Max?"

"Oh, just grand. You did a great job — he's actually bouncin' today."

They focused their attention on a graying Boston terrier curled up asleep under a stool near the door. Mike said with a wry smile, "What are you feeding him, PowerBars?" and then added, "I think we'll have a bit of lunch."

Leading his group to a 3/4 circle booth, Mike motioned for them to sit. He depressed a worn button combo on a nearby jukebox and pulled up a chair so he could sit downstage in his mini amphitheater. Johnny Cash's "Walk the Line" began in the background as he pursed his lips and silently assessed each of them in turn.

After what seemed like an hour, he finally spoke, "You ready for the time of your life?"

He checked their vitals: Jack grinned and gave a little nod yes. Hoss showed some pearly whites and settled more comfortably into the booth. Anna Heywood remained rigid, impassive.

Mike's lips curled up at both ends. "It's gonna be an absolute blast. Pretty much a continuous marathon with daily wind sprints thrown in for fun. You'll get beaten up, battered and bruised — more some times than others." He paused and then added, "I wouldn't trade it for anything."

Mike was now rolling so he shifted into second, "Hope you don't like sleep, and if you're married it had better be a strong one. If you don't drink, consider starting or take up another vice." He paused, reconsidering this statement, and then added, "A legal vice will do. Let's see, survival tips…"

He leaned back in the skeletal wood chair, stretched expansively, clasped his hands behind his head, and then looked up at the tarnished tin ceiling as he thought.

The first-year trio now had a chance to take in their randomly assigned mentor without having to process any auditory info. Somehow, the fatigue amassed during 36 hours of small animal emergencies was not appreciable on Mike's face. There was an attractive vitality here that was also a little unnerving. Mike London was tallish, 6' 2", about 24-25 years of age. Muscular, but not from pushing metal plates at the gym. With his arms raised, his advisees could see the tail of a tattoo trailing from the underside of his left scrub shirtsleeve — the body of the unidentifiable animal was safely hiding somewhere in his armpit. A neatly trimmed goatee, his one real concession to a professional appearance, added to his solid-looking countenance. Given the choice, he'd let his beard grow thick and full like his favorites in ZZ Top. But on him, for some reason, this made regular people wary as they wondered where his Hog was parked (it was in the vet school quad).

Even though the story of the previous day and a half was not evident in his demeanor, it could be deciphered from the clues left on his clothing and forearms: The four parallel, raised-red lines that ran across the inside of his right wrist were evidence that Mike had recently engaged in some form of hand-to-paw combat. One could easily imagine the exchange — "Come on nice kitty…" *Reeeoooooowwww—phhhhhhhh—Hiissssss* (This is one animal phrase that's easy to translate: *back off bud — I'll cut ya'— Back way off…*). The yellow fuzz and occasional stiff black fiber clinging to his scrub top were unmistakably animal hairs. This was certainly no surprise. Nor was the X-ray dosimeter badge clipped to a pocket. Interpretation of these clues was fairly straightforward, but then there were the brownish fluid tracks — this was where it got interesting.

Fine droplets of a randomly scattered, dark-brown fluid were likely the antiseptic Betadine, indicators of a hurried surgical prep. Larger, vertically elongated stains with a pale beige appearance, centrally located over the chest region, were presumably coffee spills — again caused by haste. A long continuous streak of reddish-brown fluid that started mid chest and trailed down and into his crotch looked like blood. There was no way to tell if this represented serious blood loss, that depended on the size of the patient. However, if this was from a Dachshund puppy or a parakeet, it was probably a goner.

Then came the real mystery stains — this was where a nose would come in handy. A large splotchy, amber stain covering his right knee could have been just about anything one would kneel in, but in this case, closer olfactory investigation would reveal the acrid presence of highly concentrated cat urine. Likewise, a whiff of the variegated patch covering most of Mike's left torso would make you think regurgitated dog food. The small but chunky flecks of orange and green vegetable matter cemented in place represented some form of high-fiber, weight-control diet — a fat dog with GI disease.

Breaking the calm and interrupting their organic analysis, Mike's beeper went off. Unfazed, he pulled out the walkie talkie and spoke, "Emergency Service, this is Mike."

"Mike? This is Sarah. Your treatment orders on Mr. Jaglum's boxer say an initial IV bolus of 2 milligrams per kilogram Lasix combined with a Dopamine CRI at 2 micrograms per kilogram per minute, then a Lasix continuous rate infusion at 0.1 microgram per kilo per hour? That's kind of unusual, is that what you wanted?"

"Yup, I ran it by Doctor Kimball and got consent from the owner. It's a new initial regimen we're working on for Boxer cardiomyopathy with signs of congestive heart failure and Sally is a good candidate."

"Okay, Mike, just making sure." The radio clicked once and then went silent.

Mike laid the walkie talkie on the table. Regaining his focus he leaned forward in his chair and faced them squarely, "The most important survival aids you should use as a vet student are: student Note Service, and Friday Night Happy Hour.

He added, "Not necessarily in that order."

"As far as student Note Service goes, it's sorta' like a co-op with your class members taking turns pulling transcription and typing duty. The volume and rate of information delivery in our lectures is huge. Taking down all the important stuff is like trying to collect the water from a fire hose with a teacup." He looked at them with as much seriousness as was possible for him and leaned forward even further, "People have tried to go it without Note Service and failed. Literally. Even if you join and memorize everything, you still have to study extra stuff just to pass. So don't be proud, use the service. It's also a form of communication, a mini class newspaper that comes out five times a day. Things are going to be said in the notes, and the transcribers will have their way with you. The only way to retaliate is when it's your turn."

Mike London leaned back and smiled again, "As for Happy Hour," his hands went up, "if I have to explain the importance of that, I don't think I can help you. Just go, religiously, and take Communion."

CHAPTER FOUR

The Advisors:
Part II (Trisha Maxwell)

1:15 PM — TUESDAY, SEPTEMBER 6, 1988

*The Field Service bay at the Center for Large Animal
Medicine (C-LAM) in Kennett Square, Pennsylvania*

You will never see tumbleweeds or tridents of lime-green saguaro in Kennett Square. You'll never hear a player piano or locomotive whistle over the farrier's clang. And you won't run into a coarsely mustached sheriff toting his trusty Colt six-shooter. You won't ever encounter any of these things at the Center for Large Animal Medicine, but you wouldn't be surprised if you did.

No one knows why, but the large animal hospital has a curious effect on people — an arousing, liberating, often intoxicating hormonal effect. This may be due, in part, to its western position separating this campus from the one in Philadelphia. Or perhaps it's the lush pastures with craggy stone barns. More likely, it's due to the animals. Even with centuries of domestication, horses, cattle, and their kin remain stubbornly part Wild West. Willfully unpredictable and thankfully dangerous. There's something elemental and even romantic about 1,500 pounds of rippling muscle with a hair trigger.

Trisha Maxwell and Dr. Green returned to Kennett Square to restock the Rover and pick up Trisha's recommended yearly allowance of first-year advisees. The zebra-striped truck glided around behind the clinic and into its usual "stall" between the all-white, 4x4 Field Service unit and the Swine Team's van. Stenciled in sharp black letters over the left front wheel well, "The Other White Truck" stood out against the oxidized finish of the Swine Team's ride while the moniker "Good Old Becky" was hand-painted on the Field Service's bug deflector.

Dr. Green turned off the ignition and released the clutch, "Trisha, thanks for your help this morning, you did a great job castrating those wildebeest — fast and effective with minimal trauma." Violet knew Trisha would make a fine vet. Smart and technically capable, she was just lacking the experience to know it herself. Dr. Green added, "Have you ever considered an internship in large animal surgery?"

"Not really, but thanks, Doctor Green, I was nervous with the keepers hovering."

"Yeah, I know. Nothing like an outwardly supportive but obviously cynical audience to give your adrenals an extra squeeze. That's Primate Behavior 101. The keepers at the Philly Zoo did the same thing when I was a fourth year. But they wouldn't have let you work on their animals if they didn't have confidence in you."

Trisha smiled with a blush, "They have confidence in you."

"It was a good job done." As far as Dr. Green was concerned, the subject was closed. "Can you do me a favor and check the fridge to see if we've got enough Ceftiofur?"

Trisha moved along the starboard side of the vehicle's bed and opened one of the larger securely-latched doors. The bottles clinked as she counted the stock in the shimmering, almost-fall sun. "According to the inventory list we need another eight vials."

Dr. Green replied, "Okay, I'll get them now while we're thinking about it."

Trisha nodded and turned to begin the fourth-year student ritual of sorting half-used supplies and cleaning instruments on the folded down tailgate while Violet disappeared into the pharmacy.

The back parking lot at the Center was reserved for large animal clients and the zoo and wildlife crowd. A variety of animal transport was parked here and there, coming and going. Huge, 18-wheel cattle and swine carriers (the kind you smell on the highway) were uncommon because cows and pigs are not transported to the vet in herds; vets usually go to them. But the situation with horses was different. Horses and horsey people are different. The University's large animal center is nationally known for having one of the finest and most comprehensive teams of equine specialists and amazing facilities to back them up. Horses are routinely referred here from Kentucky, Upstate New York, and even Florida — pretty much anywhere east of the Mississippi.

Today, parked across the lot from Trisha was a huge 12-horse carrier with Ohio plates. The dark, satiny-purple behemoth with tasteful gray and black accents was pulled as a semi-tractor trailer rig. The whole thing could have doubled as a touring vehicle for an upper crust country band. With large tinted windows, AC units poking from the top, and soft country music spilling out the boarding ramp, you might have expected Reba McEntire to poke her head out and meow "Howdy, ya'll. I hope you enjoyed the show." But there was one thing that identified the vehicle's true occupants: the large block lettering of "HORSES" on the side.

Trisha looked back over her shoulder as a creaky pickup towing a two-horse trailer pulled up next to the purple monster. She marveled at the contrast. The truck and trailer were dwarfed and in fact could have fit inside their mountainous neighbor. The rusty Ford F150 was perfectly battered and scraped; it made Trisha smile. The trailer was newer but not new, and so clean it actually sparkled. Squinting through the glint and four point shine, Trisha could see two big, docile eyes looking out the side window at her.

She watched as the animal shifted its attention to the guy jumping out of the pickup's cab. Through the open window of the horse trailer Trisha heard a deep, gentle nicker and followed the equine gaze to the object of the animal's affection. The driver unlatched the back trailer door and laid it down to form a ramp and then moved in alongside the horse. Trisha couldn't help but overhear the tender conversation between man and animal.

"How you doin' hon, I didn't go too fast did I?" Another guttural purr. "Good. You did so well today sweetheart, a blue ribbon and not a bad paycheck for us." He must have offered up a treat because she heard some crunching followed by, "Why don't you munch on this while I go find a doctor to take a look see? I'll be right back."

Not wanting to intrude, or even worse, be caught in the act, Trisha quickly turned back to what she was supposed to be doing. She had just plunged her hands into the tub of warm, soapy water when she heard a soft, rhythmic *cling… clang… cling…* approaching from behind. Her pupils spontaneously dilated and her lips flushed ever so slightly. She thought, *spurs…*

"Excuse me ma'am?" She turned to face the voice. "Howdy. I'm real sorry to disturb you but I'm afraid that my horse is injured and I was hoping to have someone take a look at her."

Trisha swallowed. She had difficulty breathing but managed a whisper, "Is it an emergency?"

"No, something happened to her left, front leg while we were competing at the fair. Hopefully it's just a strain." He paused and then continued apologetically, "We don't have an appointment or anything, I just withdrew and came straight over."

Without thinking — in other words, without her usual fear — Trisha's heart said, "Can I take a look?"

"I'd be much obliged. Thank you, ma'am."

She started to follow the driver back toward the trailer when it hit her: this man, the man directly in front of her, close enough to touch, was a real live cowboy. She couldn't help but scan him from head to toe because, she reasoned, practicing her physical examination skills was a professional responsibility.

> Recording her PE findings on the medical record in her mind —
> X Head: Off-white Stetson mounted on a thick stock of short brown hair.
> X Neck: Deeply tanned with a warm pink hue (likely from today's outdoor activities).
> X Back and Torso: An inverted triangle, tapering to his waist covered with a forest green, western-cut, short sleeved shirt and the competition number "1325" safety pinned in the center.
> X Waist *and Associated Structures*: A stout, brown leather belt was threaded through the loops of his tight, functionally-faded jeans; a second, slung an inch lower on his hips, supported a plain leather pair of batwing chaps.
> X Legs: Thick, fusiform limbs; with each flexing stride she could see his thighs expand significantly, the denim stretch, and then relax.
> X Feet: His boots were constructed with a plain coffee-brown leather, not the flashy lizard skin worn by wannabe urban cow dudes.

And finally, there were those spurs: substantial tools for animal persuasion — or at least they were when they came out of the box. Trisha could see that the sharp points of each star had been filed off. Only a smooth, blunt disc remained to make animal contact. She thought, *they wouldn't make a fly budge.*

That was it for the clothes. They were simple, a little dusty, but functional and pleasantly snug in certain very important places.

And the body? Plain and simple, Trisha could tell that this body was where he worked. Its strength, endurance, and agility were essential to his job as a rodeo cowboy. As such, this man was lean and solid — well muscled, but not overly so. It was just natural that his back, arms and hands had to be strong to hang onto 2000 pounds of fire-breathing bull. Other than the back of his neck, the only exposed parts of his anatomy were his forearms and hands. Initially, the only "subjective" descriptor that came to her mind was *powerful*. Then another word rose from the depths: *rivers*. This man's arms were like rivers. The power flowed downward, smoothly and uninterrupted, from the broad plateau of his shoulders to his fingertips.

Just then, a wonderful thing happened, a simple thing. This man that was leading her forward — this man who was close enough to touch — reached up with his left hand to scratch the back of his neck. The repeated action of flexing fingers caused a series of muscular and tendinous ripples. Like water flowing over submerged boulders, she could imagine what lay beneath the surface. Trisha knew anatomy, or at least she thought she did, but in that instant, she recognized a man's arms for the first time. They were real, hard-working, and, she imagined, a safe place to be.

Trisha stopped in her tracks. She shook her head slightly and thought, *You gotta focus*. And, since no physical exam is complete without a TPR, she placed two fingers lightly on her wrist: her pulse galloped, her respirations were shallow and she felt mildly flushed. After taking a deep breath she thought, *isn't it amazing how thorough you can be in a five-second physical exam when properly motivated?*

They entered the trailer to the left of the animal.

"This is Suzie." Suzie turned her head at the sound of her name. "She's my one and only. A natural cutter horse. I've had her since she was a pup and she's been pretty much injury free 'til now. We were cutting a calf and she snagged the outside edge of a hoof during a left turn. She was trying to fake the little guy out and give me that extra split second for the perfect angle to throw." The man tickled Suzie's warm, soft lips and then ran his hand tenderly along her neck to the point of her left shoulder and then down her leg. "She's favoring this one a bit. I know it bothers her, but she'd never admit it."

Trisha noticed Suzie shifting her weight to the right. "Can I examine her?" she asked.

"Sure thing." The man began to move aside to let Trisha in. She thought that the close quarters would require them to brush against one another but the man respectfully turned his back towards her and leaned away to let her slip past. Although Trisha did not touch him, the closeness allowed her to feel his passing warmth and draw in his scent. Her nostrils flared slightly. It was her brain's primordial attempt to use olfactory clues to assess this man's potential. His scent was altogether new to her, a pheromonal blend of leather, sweat and humble confidence. Even though she did not formulate the words in her mind, he smelled sweet, like vanilla. She shook her head again and thought: *okay, refocus. Horse. Horse hurt. Something with the leg.* All this thinking turned over the fear engine in her mind. *What do I know about equine lameness? I'm not even a real vet. And this guy is trusting me to look at his one and only.* Trisha mumbled under her breath, "Okay, calm down. Just start with a systematic exam and remember — above all, do no harm." Just as the man had done, she placed her hand on the point of Suzie's shoulder. As Trisha worked her way distally on the limb, Suzie leaned slightly to her right and folded the injured foot back to present it. Trisha cooed, "Good girl, sweetie, I won't hurt you," and cradled the hoof in her hands.

The warmth and weight of the hoof triggered a cascade. It all started to click. The distal equine forelimb — incredibly modified as compared to other animals and man. Essentially, this animal carried all her weight and that of her rider on the equivalent of the tip of our middle finger. The hoof, just a highly specialized fingernail, is the part that has working contact with the ground. It's the critical link between this half-ton beast and its job — to move over the Earth like the wind.

The wall of the hoof and horseshoe looked clean, no rocks or bits of foreign metal. Trisha did notice a shiny chip in the outer edge of the shoe. Maybe this was where Suzie got hung up. She would need nippers and a lot more room to do a thorough evaluation of the hoof wall, so for now she just palpated, pressing gently with her fingertips. The frog, the fleshy central cushion of the hoof, similar to the pads on a dog's foot, felt normal. She imagined the navicular bone lying deep to the frog and pressed a little harder. Suzie did not seem to mind this. Okay Trisha thought, *work your way back up.* Cupping the distal limb above the hoof with both of her hands, she used her thumbs to palpate the flexor tendons that run along the back side of the leg. She could feel the nubs of the splint bones on either side and pressed on them a bit. Suzie winced ever so slightly but did not attempt to pull the hoof from Trisha. Maybe this was the spot, but to be thorough she continued upwards. Nothing else seemed to bother her patient, so Trisha refocused on the area over the splint bones. Squeezing the medial bone produced no response, but gentle pressure on the outside one (MC4) made Suzie tug just a bit. The animal had been gazing out the window, almost disinterested during the exam, but now turned to look back and down at Trisha as if to say, *Yeah, that's the spot.* Trisha didn't have to tell the man that she'd discovered something, he knew his friend well. "Looks like you found the problem."

"She may have injured one of her splint bones. It may be fractured and if that's the case, just a few weeks of rest and it should mend on its own." She concluded, "But a real, umm, an orthopod should have a look at her. I'm sure that they'll want to do a more complete lameness exam and take radiographs."

The man nodded, "Sure, whatever is necessary."

Trisha gently placed Suzie's foot down and stood up. Facing the man she said, "Let me show you to the reception desk, they'll get you all set up." The man, at first still focused on the animal, absently nodded okay but then remembered his manners. He withdrew a neatly-folded, brilliant-white handkerchief monogrammed with the letters BR from his back pocket. He gave it to Trisha to wipe her hands.

As they exited the trailer, Trisha noticed a folded up bunk attached to the left trailer wall and a couple snap shots taped above. She thought, *so this is where he sleeps.* One of the photos must have been of the man as a child riding a pony. The animal was being led by a woman in black horn-rimmed glasses that Trisha guessed was his mom. The little cowboy riding bareback was all of four — decked out in shiny boots, a sweet little Stetson and the biggest, brightest smile. A smile born of unconstrained satisfaction, complete absorption in life, without worry of self presentation. Trisha thought, *Wow, to feel that safe, again.*

Outside the trailer, Trisha pointed across the lot, "See those red double doors?"

The man responded, "Yes, I do."

"Just go straight through them and you'll be at the reception desk. Tell them the situation and they'll take care of Suzie for you."

The man paused, extended his hand and said, "The name's Buck Riley. I really appreciate your help. I feel less worried now," and then added, "Thanks, Doc." Trisha was taken aback, but not just by the kind words. This was the first time she had been called "Doc." She thought, *I should correct him, I'm not a vet yet. It's true that I did what a real vet would do, but... I really like the way this feels. And I wouldn't want to make this kind man feel foolish.* She placed her hand in his and managed to respond, "My pleasure," and then added with particular emphasis, "Don't mention it." It wasn't until after the man had tipped his Stetson, turned and started walking away, that Trisha felt the soft handkerchief still in her left palm. She brought it to her nose, drew in the sweet vanilla and then, without a second thought, stuffed it into her back pocket and returned to the Rover.

In addition to the surprising promotion to "doctor," there was another more important part of the exchange with this cowboy that left Trisha feeling off balance. As far as she could remember, this was Trisha's first interaction with a man of dating age that carried absolutely no romantic insinuations. What a relief, what freedom. Trisha's widely-spaced, disarming, crystalline blue eyes, Ivory-girl skin and ideally proportioned breasts had fueled much unwanted attention over the years and even shaped her childhood nickname. Since high school, she'd been known as "Sex Kitten." Not because of promiscuity — she was now 25 and had had exactly one serious boyfriend — but because of all those irresistible wholesome curves, those sparkling eyes and her thick dirty blonde hair. In truth, even though she appeared at ease with men buzzing all around, she never really felt comfortable. They always seemed to want something from her, something physical, something wet. For her, life was a perpetual summer's evening walk: wherever she went, a swarm of tiny man flies — annoying gnats and thirsty mosquitoes — hovered about. But now, in this moment, she felt a surge of warmth and security. This man had just given her a tremendous gift. She felt safe.

Within minutes, the sounds all around Trisha softened and became supportive of her peaceful mood. She plunged her hands back in the soapy water and continued to remove debris from the instruments before their final cleaning and ultimate resterilization in the hospital. A little dried blood here, a little fur there, some chunks of unidentified organ tissue. She fell into the contemplative rhythm that can often be found when washing dishes solo. The gentle clinking of the metallic tools and soft intermittent mooing mixed with the distant clip-clop of hoof on pavement. What a comfort it is, on those rare occasions, when the world decides to tune into your frequency and adjusts its broadcast to nurture your thoughts. But, as with all good things, we don't fully appreciate them until they're gone.

"Excuse me, EXCUSE MEEEE, hey hon, my name is Rick Larson and I'm looking for Doctor Green. Know where I can find him?" It was as if someone came along, reached through the open window of her perfect day and screwed with the dials. She thought, *What the hell station is this?* Trisha tensed. She was inclined to inform the intruder that he'd left out the "babe" suffix. As in, *Know where I can find him, babe?*

Trisha blinked her way into this harsh reality, "Huh?"

"Look," continued Rick, this time slowing his delivery, "we are vet-er-in-ary students at this school and we're supposed to meet with a vet for orientation. Is there anyone else on the nursing staff that can go find Doctor Green for me?"

Trisha thought, *Oh-my-God, is this guy for real? He needs orienting — and fast.* Beyond Rick she noticed two more students, Sam Stone and Kerri Feinburg standing about ten feet back. Sam, obviously embarrassed, averted his eyes and acted as if there was something interesting in the dirt at his feet. He even went so far as to start scratching the ground with the toe of his right boot. Kerri, on the other hand, was so incensed it looked as if her head might pop. She bored into the base of Rick's cranium with her eyes, presumably trying to estimate if it was 80, 90 or 100% filled with pus.

Trisha nodded, "Okaaaay, let's go see if we can find someone to help you out." She motioned to Sam and Kerri, "You two will want to come along for this."

Trisha gave Rick Larson a glance and thought *this place is gonna kick your butt if you keep up this crap so let's see if we can rub your nose in it right now to save you a world of hurt.* She headed toward the Field Service pharmacy and found just the right person in the outpatient exam area.

"Oh nurse, *Nurse Linda*, this vet—er—in—ary student would like someone else on the nursing staff to go find Doctor Green. He has some or—E—en—TAA—shun or something." Violet Marie Green was in plain sight a few feet away at the pharmacy service window with her back to them counting out pills. She heard Trisha say her name but didn't acknowledge it, instead she stayed focused on the task at hand. Nurse Linda was in the middle of cleaning a horse's hoof so she took three more skillful flicks with her pick and set the hoof down. She stood up ever so slowly, wiped off the pick on her leg and planted her hands on her hips. Kerri and Sam widened the buffer between themselves and Rick to 15 feet — as if to show they were only accidentally associated with him.

All Nurse Linda said was "Hmm," as she stared. "So you need a nurse to go find somebody for you."

Rick was clearly frustrated, "Look, it doesn't have to be a nurse, it could be a janitor or anything, *whatever*."

Linda repeated herself, "Hmm," paused and then said, "Your orientation starts here and now, so listen up bucko."

"Lesson #1: Veterinary nurses don't go find people for vet students. They don't even do that for the doctors unless they like them or it helps the patient in some way.

"Lesson #2: Veterinary students go find people, get medications, collect urine samples, and clean up crap or ANY-thing else the nurses tell them to do. You have been granted the privilege to be here, to learn from us and to help us do our jobs." She added, "We also grade your work.

"Lesson #3: My husband is in charge of maintenance for this campus — a janitor, if you will — and he works real hard. He works for the school, our family, our patients, but not for you. So, I hope this impromptu lecture will help you fit more snugly into the food chain here at the Center for Large Animal Medicine."

She paused and then smiled, "This one's on the house." She pointed to Violet Marie Green, "That's Doctor Green and this is Trisha Maxwell, her senior student and I'm guessing your fourth-year advisor. You should be all set."

Rick Larson did a red-faced, ping-pong from Dr. Green to Trisha to Linda-the-Nurse and back around again. All he could muster was a weak cough to clear his throat followed by a mumbled, "Thanks much."

Violet waited with her back turned until the carnage was over. She had overheard it all and, truth be told, had heard it all before. She walked over and said to Trisha, "So are these your advisees?"

"Yes, I believe they are."

CHAPTER FIVE

Note Service

Class intermission, Room 13 in the Rosenthal Building, Philadelphia

Jack Doyle fidgeted imperceptibly as he switched on the microphone in Room 13, "Hi, guys." It was Wednesday afternoon, smack dab in the middle of their first full day of classes.

He tapped lightly on the mic to get their attention, "Hey guys, sorry to interrupt your break." The class settled quickly as they focused on their classmate at the podium.

"Well, I guess that this is our first official class meeting and we need to keep it short because our next lecture starts in 10 minutes." He took a breath and then proceeded, "Uh, this feels kinda' awkward, but we need to talk about our class elections. Yesterday, Doctor Kimball told us that we had to have a Class President selected by Friday — that's in two days. She and Doctor Linnehan posted a sign up sheet for those who wanted to run but no one signed up. Well, somebody wrote in my name — five times — so that's why I'm up here, I guess. It sounds like we need to make some decisions pretty quick." He paused and asked the obvious, "So, does anyone want to be Class President, Vice-President, Secretary or Treasurer?" Jack scanned the class from left to right and back again. Likewise the class scanned itself, heads turning left to right and right to left, like a stadium of tennis fans watching 50 different matches. Not a hand raised.

Finally a disembodied voice emanated from Death Row, "Why don't *you* just do it?" Two or three mumbled agreements could be heard. "Yeah—yeah, you do it."

Jack squinted and cocked his head eight millimeters to the left. His eyes moved from side to side as he watched Sam Stone and Hoss quietly scurry from Death Row. They flanked the class and moved up a couple of rows. He thought about the proposition for a second or two before responding, "You just want me to do it?"

"Yup," came from Hoss now seated to his left.

"Yes, we do," originated from Kerri Feinburg at the back of the room.

And, "Ay-yuh, just do 'er," came from Sam, now on his right. The surround sound activated a bleating agreement from the flock. *Baaa, yeahh, be President.*

Jack stammered, "Uh, well, okay. I guess I'll do it, but does that mean that I can pick people to fill the other positions?" Lots of heads nodded up and down. Sure, they seemed to say, *what the hell, what could go wrong with that?*

This time a Brooklyn twang from Death Row said, "All those in fava of Jack Doyle for Class President raise their hands." A bunch of hands, probably two-thirds of the class, went up quickly, followed by more over the next four or five seconds. To Jack it appeared that everybody raised their hands. Everybody except Anna Heywood that is. She was hard to miss because the podium was directly in front of the handicap seating. She sat there with her arms folded tightly across her chest. She wasn't exactly scowling but appeared immovable, Easter Island-ish.

Again, from the back came, "Those opposed?" There wasn't even a pause before three hands shot vertically. Three hands that were connected to three arms that were attached to three bodies seated in the very front row of the class. Anna sat sternly with her arms still crossed. Jack turned his attention to the three conscientious objectors and thought, you didn't want to do it, no one else wants to do it, but for some reason *you don't want me.* He blinked twice.

All in all, it was as unceremonious as an election can be.

Jack concluded, "I guess that's it then. If you are interested in any of the other positions, see me at the end of lecture today or first thing to-morrow in Anatomy Lab." The scattered denizens of Death Row clapped heartily, their plot to gain political control already in full swing.

Jack continued, "Uh, the reason Doctors Linnehan and Kimball recommended that we get our act together was so we can organize the class's Note Service. I assume that your fourth-year advisors told you about Note Service." As he looked around, most everyone nodded. "I've only got five minutes, so I'll quickly go through what I know about it so far. According to our fourth-year advisor, Mike London," Jack felt the need to clarify, "our orientation group is me, Buford Hugman," Hoss slowly waved a friendly, thick arm now back in Death Row, "and Anna Heywood." Anna had been scribbling on a pad, looking down at her desk when Jack announced her name. She raised her head just far enough to give Jack a look through the edges of her eyebrows. She did not even consider raising her arm. She was not a puppet on a string. Jack paused, waiting for some reason to acknowledge her, then said, "Yeah, anyway, our advisor told us that using the Note Service is critical to passing the tests," this got everyone's attention. "Here's how they've done it in the past."

He turned to the blackboard and started an outline. In another situation it might seem odd for a classmate to step up so quickly, but Jack Doyle was both blessed with considerable experience in front of a crowd, and at the same time cursed with a compulsive drive to serve. As a former Philly cop, he had a background in making points for a jury. This situation, as he would soon learn, was not all that different. Except in this case, he was both prosecution and defense.

Jack wrote as he talked.

1) Each lecture is tape-recorded.
2) The Transcriber takes complete notes during lectures and reproduces all important diagrams.

"Then, that evening, the transcriber types up the notes and delivers them to the Copy Center by midnight." He wrote this on the board too, the chalk rapidly clicked and hissed.

A hand went up from the first row, "Why?"

Jack responded, "They're open 24/7, but they want the original by midnight so they can get the copies done by the morning for us. Each morning there will be one person responsible for collecting the duplicate notes and distributing copies to our mailboxes in the lounge." Jack dropped the chalk in the tray and clapped his hands once. "That's it. And I have to say that it sounds pretty good to me. Are there any questions?"

Inevitably — we all do it — we look back over our lives, examining the times we've really stepped in it. This will mark the event of John Fitzgerald Doyle's first major blunder as Class President/Defendant. Axiom #1: Never (under any circumstances) ask a full class of vet students, *"Are there are any questions?"* Unless, of course, you don't care about getting things accomplished, eating again that day, or getting home before midnight.

Hands instantly went up, "How many pages are in each lecture?" "Are the notes verbatim?" "Do we have to type out everything that is said?"

Jack held out his hand as if he were back on the street directing traffic, "Whoa. No. Mike London said the transcriber has to use some discretion and common sense. If a concept is complicated, I guess they may need to go word-for-word, but condensing the lecture into a concise outline is what we should shoot for." He repeated, "Discretion and common sense are the key."

Rick Larson's hand slinked upward and Jack pointed to him with one finger, "Yup?"

Rick talked slowly so as to emphasize his suspicion, "How much is *all this* gonna cost? *Who's* going to pay for it *AND* who will be accountable for the money?" Rick made it sound like Note Service was some kind of scam for someone, *somewhere* to rake in a sizable profit.

Jack scratched the side of his head, "We do the work ourselves, for our benefit, and we only pay for the photo copying. Last year the other classes had a deal with the Copy Center for 2 cents per page — each person kicked in 40 bucks a semester to cover expenses." There was a pause, no one said anything. Jack sensed that the high point of his Presidency had occurred approximately two seconds after the election. He wanted to terminate the bizarre insinuation that anyone was getting coerced, used or scammed. "Look, it's a voluntary co-op. If you don't want to do it — if you don't want the notes — you don't have to participate. But the more people involved, the less work for each individual. Everybody wins." Jack paused momentarily, turned to Rick Larson and added what he assumed was a good idea, "And Rick, you can be our class treasurer, just to make sure everything is on the up and up." The flock sat quietly bleating, mulling it over, chewing their cud.

Seeing the real potential for things to go sideways, Jack added, "Just to give you some perspective, the human med students pay a professional secretarial service to type up the recorded lectures and it costs them each about $250 per semester." He continued, "They don't get the notes for three days, there are tons of extra pages, and no diagrams. Our Note Service — the one I'm proposing — has a faster turnaround time, costs less, and will yield better notes."

Death Row became impatient. This was obviously a great deal. Sam Stone whispered to Kerri Feinburg, "Includin' room and boahd, I'm on the hook for $35,000 a year to go to this school. God-dammah, what's the big deal about 40 bucks?" He spoke up, "Sounds GREAT: let's do it!" It had the tone and punch of those Miller Lite ads, *Great Taste, Less Filling!* Again, a little prodding was just what the class needed. Most of the sheep heads nodded affirmatively.

Jack continued, "Great, I'll get a class list and assume that everybody is in. But if you don't want to participate, just see me and I'll remove your name." Jack noticed that the next lecturer, Dr. Linnehan, had entered the room and was waiting in the back for him to finish so he concluded, "Okay. Thanks," and began to swiftly make his way off the stage when two hands went up in the front row. They were two of the three hands that had voted against him. Jack reluctantly inquired, "Uh, yeah?" He glanced at the clock, his time was nearly gone but he pointed to one guy anyway.

"Don't you think we should make use of the library's computers? It seems irresponsible to use that much paper, to kill that many trees." The other chimed in without lowering her arm, "Yes and then the notes could be distributed by floppy disk and would be immediately available."

Jack was perplexed, he stammered, "Yeah, hmmm, that's a suggestion. Look, I'm sorry but we're out of time, the next lecture has to begin now. How about we talk after class?"

This sensible plea just ricocheted off the hardheaded FRoGs. The first one kept on going, "And then it wouldn't cost us *40 dollars a semester*." His intonation made the cost sound outrageous.

Jack realized that he had to manhandle the situation, "Okay, those are great ideas but there are three reasons why we're gonna table this discussion: First and foremost, our break is over and Doctor Linnehan needs to get the lecture going. Second, we should probably stick with what has worked well over the past few years, we can make changes as we go. And third, we need to start this by tomorrow because we have tests *this week*."

FRoG #1 re-elevated his spindly tendril, arm-like appendage, "Yes, however, the point my colleague was making..." Jack was incredulous; he was so surprised that he couldn't even hear the rest of what was said. He thought *colleague*, what colleague? You're a freaking first-year, first-semester vet student. He tuned back into Station WFRG to hear the end of the suggestion or criticism or whatever it was, "...and so you see, and therefore must agree, that this approach makes infinitely more sense."

Jack was astounded, "Yeah. Great. Good idea. Catch me later and we'll talk." He severed eye contact, jumped off the stage and sprinted back to Death Row.

Sam received him with a sturdy handshake, "Discretion and common sense. We-ah so full of it." He added with a wide grin and a slap on Jack's back, "Nice job, Mr. President."

Unbelievably, FRoG #1 re-elevated his appendage. FRoGs are not known for their physical prowess. Their spindly necks can barely hold up their massive craniums and this FRoG's arm was weakening so he used the other as support. There was no teacher, so he just sat there and waited while the professor walked down the aisle, installed himself behind the podium and slowly clipped on the microphone.

Dr. Linnehan took in the FRoG and asked, "*What?*" The male FRoG croaked, "I wondered if…" and then fell silent because the look on Drill Sergeant Dan's face warned even the most oblivious that they were treading on dangerous ground. "Son, if you've got a question about the anatomy of the equine forelimb, then ask away. But, if you want to discuss the finer points of your class's Note Service, you are," he paused briefly between each letter, "S. O. L." And then raising both thin eyebrows, "You read me, private?"

The arm snapped down and as it reached the end of its rapid descent, it caught the edge of the folding desktop causing the surface to rotate and spring up. FRoG #1's notebook catapulted into the side of FRoG #2's head. This caused a FRoG chain reaction, a domino effect that was instantly transmitted down the front row — a series of ouches, flying pens, protractors (why have a protractor?), and paper ensued. When the mini train wreck was finally concluded, Dr. Linnehan did what only he could do — safely that is — "Now, are there any *other* questions before we get started?" All metabolism halted; the class's collective trillions of mitochondria held their breath. All thoracic excursions that normally lead to the inspiration or expiration of air were momentarily suspended. The sheep fell silent as Drill Sergeant Dan scanned the room again with Terminator precision. Nobody moved.

"Wonderful. Innervation of the equine extensor radialis muscle is effected by…"

CHAPTER SIX

That Smell

Comparative Anatomy Laboratory in the old veterinary school building, Philadelphia

Youth. As summarized by a searing line from "It's a Wonderful Life," *Youth is wasted on the young.* This truth accompanied other unsolicited advice to George Bailey, "Why don't you just kiss her instead of talking her to death?" Sound advice. Why waste time especially considering Donna Reed's wholesome but ephemeral beauty?

We never ask, *Why are we young?* Youth makes intuitive sense. Continuing the condition is an aspiration of most. We only lament — *Why do we grow old?* — while even the best of modern molecular science can't fully answer that question. Cellular membranes pucker and fail, lysosomes prematurely lyse, DNA mutations fatally accumulate. Creases appear, blood vessels harden, organs sag and follicles dry up. In youth, our bodies grow vigorously and heal rapidly — so, why not through time?

First-year veterinary students don't ponder such questions. It's not that they are impetuous, brash or arrogant. They don't worry about aging because they aren't. They have stumbled upon what Ponce de Leon exhausted his life searching for — the Fountain of Youth. Lo and behold, it's filled with formalin.

Formalin, a product of pure formaldehyde, is a curious and deadly substance. Its central purpose on this planet, its occupation — its raison d'etre — is to snuff out life, and death... or more accurately, decomposition. Formalin has an impressive *Curriculum non-Vitae*. Its skills include: rapid penetration of biological tissues, strangulating ribosomes, denatur-

ing proteins, and mummifying microbes — essentially killing and preserving all in its path. And first-year veterinary students, these novice
protectors of animal life, nearly bathe in the stuff. The first three to four
hours of each and every day is spent carving up (dissecting) horses, cows,
pigs, dogs, cats and the occasional chicken that have been injected with
and even soaked in poisonous vats of formalin. Thousands of pounds of
formalin-drenched meat, this is Comparative Anatomy Lab.

Since dissection is a vigorous, physical type of work, it's nearly impossible to avoid the spray as fluids fly when chunks of pickled sinew are
severed, splatting in puddles on the floor. Likewise, aerosolized formalin
is inhaled with each breath, coating the nose, throat and lungs. And finally, bits of dissected debris — veins, arteries, nerves, and muscle — are
sprinkled in shirts, shoes and hair. Students like Jack, Hoss and the others
were of course issued "protective" gear. They wore their Latex gloves, lab
coats and goggles. But formalin will not be so simply deterred. Formalin
is unthinking, uncaring, unbiased and unrelenting. It will always find a
way to permeate and preserve the tissue it craves.

If you were able to look closely enough, you'd notice that first-year,
first-semester veterinary students have an unnaturally smooth complexion. Smiles are fixed, wrinkled brows relieved. And their hands… their
hands are encased in a thick, yellowing layer of lifeless epidermis. They
are, at least temporarily, young. Preserved. The other day Jack kidded
with Hoss, saying, "I like you just the way you are you big lug, and thanks
to 10% neutral-buffered formalin, that's the way you'll stay."

But getting sufficiently close to first-year veterinary students to
witness these miraculous anti-aging effects is an olfactory endeavor requiring significant fortitude. In short, first years *reek*. Obnoxiously. But
not to each other. Formalin has an initial sharp, metallic, nose-crinkling
smell but that sensation fades rapidly as intranasal neurons choke and die.
And, owing to another occupational skill, formaldehyde is insidiously
volatile — it escapes saturated tissues (including vet students), effortlessly
wafting into the surrounding air. Probing, seeping, hoping to find a more
permanent home. As such, groups of three or more first years represent
a formidable gaseous force, the effects of which are evident when a pack
cruises down Spruce Street. In their wake: flowers prematurely wilt, pick-
pockets are mysteriously deterred, and winos take on an unexpected air of
superiority — for once, relatively speaking, they smell pretty darn good.

The University of Philadelphia's Comparative Anatomy Lab is
housed in an ancient, rectangular, brick and mortar garrison called the

Old Vet School Quad. The semi-circular A1 amphitheater, where Jack and the others sat for orientation, is an adherent and much-loved curve attached to the larger superstructure — it bulges out into the central, open-air courtyard. This hidden university square is an artifact with stone cobble pavement and gargoyle sculptures of animals ornamenting the rain spouts. In the early days, colonists herded their ailing beasts (usually draft horses, dairy cows, sheep and goats) out from the wilds, through the massive wrought-iron gates and into this secure, high-walled fortress for veterinary attention. There remains a grassy central island bounded by granite curbstone around which the one-way, patient parade flowed. It had essentially been a "hoof thru" clinic with various medical specialties located in sheltered bays — Bay 1: horseshoeing and foot-rot maladies; Bay 2: mastitis, teat and mammary issues; Bay 3: tooth floating, eye cankers and ear bots; And, if all else failed, Bay 4: butcher shop and postmortem exam. It was Bay 4 that was ultimately converted into the Comparative Anatomy Lab.

This morning, like every other weekday morning for the last 22 years, Big Moe, the head anatomy technician, arrived early to help the class turn out the "herd." Big Moe was a full-sized, ex-lumberjack (do undersized lumberjacks exist?) with a graying, close-shaved cut and a barrel chest. Massive tree trunks protrude from his ever-present, aquamarine scrub shirt. And although he worked all day, every day, with these stinking animals, he somehow never smells like a first year. There's a fine art to everything — very Zen — and Big Moe knows dissection.

A litter of Front Row Geeks assembled in the quad outside the lab 10 minutes early. The FRoGs squeaked like mice as Mountain Man Moe unlocked Bay 4, "good morning moe — 'morning moe — hi moe."

In his booming baritone, Big Moe replied, "GOOOOD MORNING LITTLE MOES." All first year students were "Moes" to Moe. It was just easier that way. He did, on rare occasion, add a prefix to the Moes he liked. There had been, for example, "Pretty Smart Moe" and "Not Too Annoying Moe" from last year's class.

"Time to make the dog-nuts," said one FRoG trying to parody a Dunkin' Donuts commercial. Big Moe paused, squinted at the murine form and shrugged, "Okay, if you say so little moe."

The Anatomy Lab is a cavernous, 6,000 square foot, open work space with rolling stainless steel dissection tables and a massive biohazard containment locker at one end. A greasy, steel I-beam runs overhead as an oval monorail around the lab. Spurs protrude from the loop at the individual dissection stations while the main supply tracks converge and penetrate the huge doors of a containment locker — affectionately known as "The Barn." This locker was where the formalin-soaked animals "bedded down" each night. Just like a real barn, a horseshoe was mounted over the entrance. But unlike a barn, with peacefully respiring equines and ruminants, this shoe pointed straight down — these poor guys were definitely outta luck. The inside of The Barn was packed with ex-racehorses, dairy cows, farrowing sows, and the occasional Great Dane dangling from meat hooks in more or less "natural" positions — in suspended animation. Sharp, steel gaffs pierced shoulders, withers and rumps and were suspended by rusty chains from metal trolleys. This way the entire stiff-legged herd could be moved around the lab for dissection by even the most diminutive of the little moes.

Big Moe took a burly grasp of the levered handle and unlatched the freezer type doors. As they swung open wide, a wall of supersaturated formalin fog spilled out causing a wisp of an oily female FRoG to sputter, gasp and cough. It was like opening a toxic Egyptian tomb — statues of horses, cats and other animals frozen in time, staring blankly ahead. Big Moe made one loud clap with his hands and bellowed, "GET ALONG LITTLE DOGGIES." He slapped the first horse on the rump as its trolleys clinked and clattered on the way out to the lab.

This class, like those in recent history, was segregated into dissection groups composed of two or three students each. It was a free-choice situation that was worked out on the first day of lab. At that point, the students knew as much about animal anatomy as they did about each other. Fortunately, there was some natural selection at work and like usually ended up with like. In this vein, it was quite biological for Sam, Hoss, and Jack to ally. But Kerri Feinburg's choice for a partner was more challenging. On advice from Jack, Kerri asked Anna if she was interested; she accepted with a flat-sounding, "Fine."

By about 8:05 AM most of the class had arrived and began to work on their charges. It was like an animal assembly line. Or, more precisely, a dis-assembly line, and as the semester progressed each animal took on a nickname and developed a unique personality to replace the physical parts that were meticulously stripped away.

"Whoa, Nelly. Come on Daisy Mae, come on moo-cow. Sooie! Here pig, pig, pig." Jack usually regaled something to this effect each morning as they rounded up their animals. "Sit Spot! Stay boy — staaaay." He paused and then added, "Good boy. Who's the best boy, who's the best dog? Hmm, very stoic this morning." Sam shook his head slowly and laughed lightly. Hoss chuckled as they maneuvered their dissection subjects into position, the tips of their feet swaying inches above the concrete floor.

Today Jack was unencumbered, available to call the strategic plays and interject semi-clever commentary, because today was his day to stay clean. Every day one student in each group was the designated reader. This person's main job was to flip through the texts and dissection manuals to help guide the process while the others cut, probed, identified and ultimately removed parts. Since the first two weeks of lab were devoted to the comparative anatomy of the limb — starting with the front and working to the hind leg — the animals were still essentially intact. The skin was removed from all four legs of their horse making it look as if he wasn't completely dressed, as if he'd forgotten his pants in a hurry to leave the barn. Jack remarked, "I'm late for work honey, gotta gallop. Sweetie, can you pick up my saddle at the cleaners on your way home?" Since one side of each animal was just a mirror image of the other, the left legs were used to learn veins, arteries and nerves, while the rights were for bones and musculature; bilateral symmetry had its didactic advantages.

Jack cheered, "Okay boys, gimme an Ulnaris Lateralis!"

Hoss replied, "Ulnaris Lateralis," while pointing to the muscle.

"Gimme an Interosseus." The same call and response happened. "Gimme a Flexor Carpi Radialis," this time they just pointed, already tiring of the game. Jack checked their work against the text and nodded affirmatively. "And where does it originate?"

"The caudomedial aspect of the humerus."

"Go team!"

With his slow Maine drawl, Sam asked, "Are yah gonnah put on a skirt and cheerlead, or just tell us what we're suppostah find next?"

"Today, team," Jack continued, "we're gonna be the first to isolate all of the components of the equine stay apparatus." Jack said this knowing that Kerri would overhear.

"Yeah right. Do you guys even know which one the horse is?" She kidded warmly.

Jack asked with a grin, "The pink one?"

"No."

He pointed to Hoss, "The big one?"

"Nooo," repeated Kerri with a wide smile.

"Okay, well crap, this advanced veterinary stuff is too much for me. I give up."

Anna looked down, she couldn't help but smile and yet would not share it with the others. She muttered, "Hoss, you know where the horse's ass is, don't you?"

Jack tipped his head back and laughed, "You sunk my battleship!" It wasn't really a defeat. He just wanted to encourage Anna's integration.

Kerri refocused and rattled off the list from memory, "The major components of the hind leg stay apparatus are — from proximal to distal — the medial, intermediate and lateral patellar ligaments; the superficial digital flexor; and, to a lesser degree, the peroneus tertius."

Jack looked up from his manual, faking shock, "What the..? You cheated."

"No, we just worked ahead yesterday while you boys were discussing the finer aspects — if there are any — of largemouth bass fishing." Kerri playfully sang the first line of "Sittin' on the Dock of the Bay," then added, "You boys surely do waste time," and started whistling the tune. They all joined in (except Anna) and were nearly finished with the song when Big Moe walked up. He was carrying the whole hind leg of a draft horse. It was fresh off the animal, not formalinized. Part of Big Moe's job was to create demonstration dissections. He was an expert and his demos always seemed to clear up any misunderstandings the students had.

The manhole-sized horseshoe clanked as he planted the leg on the concrete floor. A puddle of blood formed around the massive, fringed hoof. Big Moe rested a hand on the shiny white, knob-like protrusion exposed at the top of the femur. This round knob, the ball part of the ball-and-socket hip joint, previously fit into the horse's acetabulum. Moe leaned on the leg as he spoke, "Okay, do you little moes have any questions about the stay apparatus?" No one said anything. "Well then, let me ask a few." He waved his two-foot machete-style knife up and down the leg, "Can anyone tell me what this system is used for?"

Jack piped up, "It locks the leg and doesn't let it bend, essentially allowing the horse to sleep standing up."

"That's right, moe. And boy are you going to wish you moes had two of these during 10-hour large animal orthopedic surgeries." He continued, "Okay, now for biomechanics. *How does it work?*"

Hoss took the question, "Uh, sir, the patella is pulled medially, looping the medial patellar ligament over that tubercle thing of the medial trochlear ridge. It locks the joint."

"Excellent. Now name another species that can do this?"

"Uh, zebra?" Hoss added.

"Good job, Large Moe." Because Hoss was the only person in the class as big as Big Moe, they had a connection. "On to identification. What components on this fresh leg would you cut *last* if you wanted to keep the stay apparatus intact — if you did not want the horse to come crashing to the ground in agony?" This was just an interesting way to look at the anatomy because you'd never cut any of the parts if you didn't have to. To emphasize his point and really get their attention, Moe pulled over a chair and stood up on it. He turned, locked and then sat on the horse's leg, placing most of his weight on the top of the femur. "Who's brave enough to start cutting?" With that, he extended his right arm and offered the group his very big knife. They looked at each other wide-eyed. "I'm done with this demo, so let's see who really understands this thing." This game was a veterinary cross between Russian roulette and Milton Bradley's "Operation."

"Come on, little moes." At that, Hoss stepped up, accepted the knife and extended a slightly shaking hand to make the first cut. Nothing happened. The leg stayed locked and Big Moe was still balanced on his perch.

"Nice pick, Large Moe. You're a good moe." By now the rest of the class was aware that something fun was going on so most began to gather around. "There are four more sites to choose from. Next?"

Sam asked for the knife from Hoss. He placed both hands on the large wooden grip and made a steady incision. The leg stayed rock solid.

"Nice job, Yankee Moe. Can you tell me the name of the structure you just cut?"

Sam replied, "The gastrocnemius."

"Who's gonna be next?" The group gradually realized that as the game progressed, their odds got worse. "How about you, City Moe?" Big Moe was referring of course to Kerri Feinburg. Sam handed over the knife. Kerri thought, *Maureen, her closest friend from Queens, was never going to believe this one.* As she wrapped her fingers carefully around the handle, everyone could see her manicured, blood-red nails poking through the Latex glove. She reached over, in a fencing stance, looked up at Big Moe and cut. There was a slight tremor, but she'd made a good choice. The class gave a collective sigh and Kerri was spent. The blade hung from her hand like she'd just committed a stabbing. So now it was the last choice, one ligament was safe and one was the trigger. Big Moe boomed, "WHO'S GONNA BE LAST? WHO'S BRAVE ENOUGH?" Silence blanketed the lab rapidly accumulating like snow in a blizzard. Jack looked to Sam, but before he could act, Anna limped forward, pushing her way between them. She briskly took the blade from Kerri and didn't even hesitate before she sliced deeply into the leg. Big Moe jolted, bounced up and down an inch, but did not fall. The class instantly erupted in applause and Big Moe nearly smiled, "Good job, Confident Moe. Well done."

Jack Doyle, the Philadelphia street cop with a scrappy prizefighter's build turned to face Sam Stone, the handsome, weatherworn commercial fisherman who'd battled half-ton behemoths while braving the high seas. The two looked at each other in silence as their classmates cheered all around.

Jack finally spoke with a nod, "That girl's alright."

Noting the faded scar over Jack's right eye and flat, long broken nose, Sam winked, "Wicked tough-ah than you, that's for sure."

Jack grinned and then replied, "Could well be. But damned if I don't like it."

NOTE SERVICE- Anatomy Lecture   TR: Sam Stone
09/12/88   (1:00-2:00pm)   DD: Hoss
Dr. Linnehan   Page 9 of9

Hindlimb Passive Stay Apparatus (the end of his discussion)

     The point is, when the muscles of the equine
quadraceps, peroinius, and the vastas medialis contract to
pull the patella medially and prximally, the MPL hooks over
the medial trochlear ridge thus locking the stifle (it can't
flex).   Then the "reciprocal mechanism: consisting of the
peroneus tertius (anterior) and superficial digital flexor
(caudally) link the hock. See figure below

Transcriber (TR) note- Folks, I tried to reproduce the most
important diagrams Dr. Linnehan presented but, if I were
you, I;d also refer to the figures in Dyce Sack and
Wensing.   Sam.

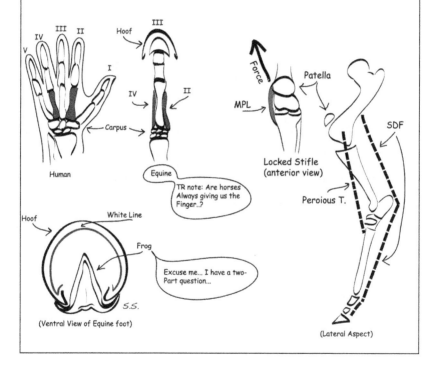

III II
IV
V
I
Hoof
III
IV   II
Carpus

Human   Equine

TR note: Are horses
Always giving us the
Finger..?

Force
MPL   Patella

Locked Stifle
(anterior view)

SDF

Peroious T.

Hoof   White Line

Frog

Excuse me... I have a two-
Part question...

S.S.

(Ventral View of Equine foot)

(Lateral Aspect)

CHAPTER SEVEN

Mentoring 601

9:26 PM — TUESDAY, SEPTEMBER 13, 1988

Room A1 in the old veterinary school building, Philadelphia

Τ he photocopied note in their mailboxes read:

Dear First Years: Jack/Hoss/Sam/Anna/Kerri/and Rick

    You are cordially invited (actually, it's mandatory) to meet with us tonight at exactly 9:23PM in Room A1. We have a surprise for you. (dress is casual)

Signed, Your Advisors: Mike London and Trisha Maxwell

The chandelier's low-wattage, incandescent bulbs cast a dim glow that barely lit the cobbled center stage of A1 while complete darkness engulfed the uppermost seats. The first years sat in the semicircular first row while Mike London, with Trisha Maxwell at his side, faced them from the podium.

Mike began in a hushed tone, "We are gathered here tonight, in this hallowed hall that has witnessed 104 years of veterinary schooling — to relive the *Legend of the Harvard Grad…*" He squinted, staring eerily at each of their charges in turn. He was sure they had all heard the legend, the horror. It was the story of a brilliant and popular first-year student (who would remain nameless and, in their minds, headless) who failed out of this school even though he had graduated from Harvard, Summa Cum Laude, with a 4.0 GPA. That's 100% straight A's. Just a mention of *the Legend* raised goose bumps on the first years' arms. Mike boosted his voice to mimic Andre the Giant in the *Princess Bride*, "I am here to tell you — THE LEGEND IS TRUE!" He punctuated the sentence by slamming his palm on the podium top.

Hoss jumped.

Rick Larson stammered, "No, no way."

Mike replied casually, "Yes, way." Trisha nodded her head in silence. Mike confirmed, "He was in our class." This nightmare, the failing of the Harvard Grad, had the power to launch the most confident, routinely sound-sleeping veterinary student bolt upright in bed, drenched in rivers of clammy sweat. "He was no freak, no loser. He was kind, crazy smart, and often funny."

Rick shrugged, "So, how did he fail? How did they catch him?" Mike noticed Rick's right eyelid twitch.

"He didn't know what to study. He was used to learning everything in college so he tried the same approach here. But the medical onslaught just swamped him. Sadly, he spun to the ground in flames."

Rick Larson was getting nervous. This was hitting a little too close to home, "Okay, so how do we know what to study?"

Mike feigned a covert glance over his left shoulder and then his right. It was almost as if this was a secret arms deal, and in some ways it was: a promise in exchange for the armaments to combat numerical failure. "There are methods," he paused for effect, "There are ways." He waited again before adding, "Everybody has a slightly different approach, but it all boils down to one basic tactic: study humans, not animals."

Hoss screwed up his face, "Human medicine?"

"No, human nature. You need to know the teachers." The first years looked confused so Mike said, "I'll bottom line it for you — study old tests. Even though the questions will change, the new tests tend to focus on the same topics and take a similar approach." He added, "Past performance is the best predictor of future behavior. You're gonna get surprised from time to time, but I'd bet the farm that if you study old tests, and memorize your Note Service notes, and do lots of group studying, you'll have a good chance of getting 7 out of 10 questions correct."

"That's a 70." Rick moaned, "That's just barely a C and a C is just passing."

"Yup, that's right. And with some tests you'll be thankful to get that."

Rick asked slyly, "But isn't studying the tests sort of like cheating?"

Trisha spoke up, "Nope. The profs return the tests to be used as study guides. They want you to learn the material."

Mike shook his head, "Shit, you can still fail quite decisively. Lots of times you can't even answer the old test questions with your notes and books in front of you. You need to get inside their heads." He looked at Rick, "You have to think like a thief to catch one."

Jack cleared his throat, "What about anatomy? We have the lab practical and lecture tests this Friday."

Mike smiled, "That hurdle is exactly why we're here tonight." He paused and then added, "You've had a few warm-up tests but this one, this will separate the women from the girls. And, since you've been really good," he reflexively looked back at Rick, "these presents are for you." Trisha produced two gift-wrapped items from behind the podium and then languidly drew her hands over the boxes as if she was a "Price Is Right" girl. One container was a three-foot-long cylinder, the other shoebox-sized. Rick Larson tried to snatch the biggest gift. Mike instantly slapped his wrist causing Rick to blurt, "Ouch," even though it obviously couldn't have hurt. Mike wagged his finger, "There's one condition. You all need to raise your right hand and repeat the Real Veterinary Oath."

Rick whimpered, mainly in response to the slap, "We recite the Veterinary Oath when we graduate. It's not valid until we complete all requirements…"

Interrupting Rick and surprising everyone, Hoss stood, put his hand over his heart and began to recite, "At the time of being admitted as a member of the veterinary medical profession: I solemnly pledge myself to consecrate my life to the service of humanity; I will give to my teachers the respect and gratitude which is their due…"

Now Mike cut in, "Yeah, yeah — hold on. This isn't the Geneva Oath, this is the Oath of the Real Vet. This oath was developed by *our* fourth-year advisor, Violet Marie Green. Doctor Green is the Gold Standard. Sit back and just listen." They tried to sit back although Sam Stone could hardly relax more; as always he was nearly prone in his seat.

Mike paused, raised his eyebrows for added effect and said, "I solemnly swear that I Will Do The Right Thing and *Primum non nocere.*" Hoss squinted while Jack frowned. They were confused by the Latin so Mike clarified, "and above all, do no harm." He paused again, they waited for more. In their experience you always got more of everything except what you wanted. Mike asked, "Is that agreeable?"

Rick inquired suspiciously through his nearly permanent scowl, "That's it?"

"Yeah, that's it. That covers pretty much everything you'll ever need. You all know in your hearts what the Right Thing is. You don't have to look too deep to know what you should always try to do. The key is following through." Mike paused and then resumed the ceremony, "Raise your right hand and repeat after me."

"I…" said Mike.

The group followed with, "I…"

"Say your name…"

A conglomeration of "KerriJackSamHossAnna" was followed a second later by, "Rick…"

"Will Do the Right Thing…"

In unison, and now with noticeable enthusiasm, the little group of first years chanted, "WILL DO THE RIGHT THING AND, ABOVE ALL, DO NO HARM."

Mike and Trisha clapped their hands, "Congratulations, that's it! The rest is up to you." Then Mike remembered, "Oh yeah, by the powers vested in me by the city of Las Vegas and the state of Nevada. I gotta say that to make it binding and legal."

Trisha asked, "So, who shall open the blessed gifts that have been passed down from generation to generation?" Now there was no hesitation, Rick's arm sprang up like a catapult. "Okay Rick, you open the big one and Kerri, here, you can open this."

Rick tore into the wrapping as if it was his birthday — with gusto and absolute self-absorption. He forgot where he was, his age, or even to notice the wrapping paper.

"Nice wrap job, Mike," Trisha smirked. He'd used Playboy wrapping paper, a flat-black background with a sparse and almost elegant pattern of little silver bunny heads.

She glared at him in mock disapproval. He shrugged his shoulders, "What, mine fits the animal theme doesn't it? Laurna wrapped it for me right after we were through playing 'Jedi Knight gets Princess Leia.'"

With a deep level of sister-like affection, Trisha said, "Yeah, speaking of animals, I almost forgot — you're a fetal pig."

Laurna was a cocktail waitress at the local Hooters and one of Mike's rotating gallery of girl-type friends. Mike would happily inform anyone who had the guts to ask, *so, what does she do?* "Pretty much any—thing—you—want." This was one of his two standard answers. If the inquisitor was a guy, he usually revealed her job title with an emphasis on the *tail* syllable. He found this generally magnified the average male fantasy — mix the words cock, tail, and waitress with a tall serving of alcohol and voila, it must yield hot sex. Guilt-free, porno-quality sex. But Mike knew something the drooling males didn't: aside from her night job at Hooters, Laurna was just finishing up her Ph.D. in astrophysics. Yes, *astrophysics.*

Mike generally created a stir whenever he invited one of his "friends" to a Friday Night Happy Hour. The question on most minds preceding his fashionably late arrival, was, *So who's it gonna be this time?* Mike London had a reputation as a man's man who was at ease with women. But his close friends knew he was just at ease with himself. This attracted women, and friends. Even animals could sense it. In reality, Mike didn't date all that frequently or repeatedly, much to any individual girl's chagrin. And he didn't date loose or easy women at all. It was just that most had an occupation that *suggested* looseness. So cocktail waitresses and stewardesses were the stereotypical norm. Every now and then he'd pitch a curveball. The novice Geisha was, and still is, his most fondly remembered escort.

Rick got enough paper off one end to open the tube and slide out the contents. It was a plastic sword, a replica of a Star Wars Lightsaber. He grasped the handle with both hands, and with a combination of reverence and defiance of tyranny, he held it out rigidly in front of him. His transformation from boy-man back to just plain boy was almost instantaneous. His eyes glazed over when he clicked the switch at the butt end of the toy. The "blade" glowed a vibrant fluorescent green and a speaker in the handle emitted the low, but reassuringly familiar *humm-humm-hmmmm.* He made two sweeping arcs and was rewarded for his abandon. A reed switch sensed the movement and triggered the now universally known sound effect that real live Star Wars Lightsabers made — *Vooooosssh… Vooooosh…*

When Rick meekly whispered, "Obi-Wan… Can you hear me?" Mike knew it was time to bring him back to Earth.

Mike snapped his fingers like a hypnotist, "I'm sure Obi-Wan Kenobi would agree: The Force can have a strong influence on a weak mind."

The intrusion into his fantasy world startled Rick and, with a hint of shame for his childlike play, he tried to distance himself, "What's *this* for..? I mean, it's just a toy."

"No. It is not a toy. It's a reminder." Mike paused and then said, "The key to The Force is in your hands."

Just then Rick felt a sharp edge under his right palm. He uncurled his fingers to reveal a tiny key held in place with a band of scotch tape.

Holding the mock saber vertically with this part of the handle visible to all, he asked, "What's this for?"

"Oh that. It's the key to a locker containing 10 years of old tests."

Trisha grinned, "Mike, you're a goof."

"You think so?"

"Yeah, I really do. *The Key to the Force is in your hands.*"

Kerri's attention had been diverted by the gripping portrayal of the 1970's Star Wars melodrama. Her unwrapping had ceased until Jack prompted her, "What's in the other box?"

"Oh, yeah." She opened the gift like the refined young woman she was, breaking the tape at the seams. It was a battered shoe box.

Rick rolled his eyes as he applied some pressure, "Just open it, will you. I got some real studying to do."

Kerri peeled away the top to reveal hundreds of 3x5 cards bound in bundles. She lifted out one of the blocks and flipped it over. The card on one end had a picture drawn on it. On the other end of the stack was a title card: *Physiology- First Semester, Test #1.*

Mike explained, "That's the vet school version of Pictionary. The first edition. The only edition. The rest are in the locker with the old tests." With this cue, Rick held up the saber with a *vooooshh.*

Mike continued, "These flash cards have been used by several graduating classes. No one knows the inventor of the game but each class adds their own new cards and updates old ones. It's the ideal study aid because you can play individually or in groups." He nodded to Trisha, "Come on, let's show 'em." He paused and then added sarcastically, "Of course, no money is *ever* involved."

Trisha responded, "'Cause you know I'm gonna kick your butt." She shuffled the deck, and then fanned the cards so Mike could choose.

"Let's see," was all he said as he read. Mike returned the card, walked to the blackboard and without even pausing exclaimed, "GO!"

Trisha checked her watch and then read the instructions aloud, "Please, if you will, diagram the working parts (at the molecular level) of a skeletal muscle myomere. You have 60 seconds."

Mike moved swiftly, fluidly. While he drew with his right, he grabbed for a second piece of chalk with his left. The image pouring from his right hand took shape rapidly. As he finished each section, he drew a line away from it and then began the labeling process *with his left hand.* It came out a letter at a time M Y O S I N. Astonishingly, he kept this going, simultaneously drawing shapes with his right and labeling with his left.

Hoss' mouth hung open. Anna's eyebrows raised and her eyes widened. Trisha just smiled. She'd witnessed it all before: wham, bam — and without a lot of fuss or muss — thank you Ma'am. Mike dropped both pieces of chalk in the tray simultaneously and asked, "Time?"

Trisha rechecked her watch, "47 seconds. Nice. Now to check your work."

"There's really no need but if you feel you must, go right ahead," sublimed Mike.

She flipped the card over and compared the answer to the board. She looked at Mike, "Perfect. 100%." He smiled and clapped once to remove the chalk dust from his hands.

Trisha turned to the first years, "Well, there you have it. It's Monday and your anatomy tests are on Friday."

Jack interjected, "We only have one night of open lab, then they close it up like a drum to set out the pieces and parts. And we have a physiology test on Thursday morning."

Anna added in a monotone, "And the Biochem test that afternoon."

"Great, we got to you just in time. Now you have The Force." Mike turned to his classmate, "Trish, remember our first semester?" They both smiled.

Trisha responded, "The Good Old Days. I hate to say it was the easy part, but — in retrospect — it really was." A light bulb flickered on over her head and she reached for the box of 3x5's. Trisha found a small bundle of blanks and wrote out a question, then flipped the card over and quickly sketched the answer, pursing her lips as she added the final touches.

Trisha looked up to Mike and read, "Please, if you don't mind — but do it anyway — graph the life of a typical vet student over the four years of school. Please chart all major stressors and positive factors. You have two minutes." She laughed adding, "Do not include this question as a major stressor."

A grin of admiration spread across Mike's face. He loved the way his friend thought. Nodding his acceptance of the challenge, he lined up several pieces of colored chalk, grabbed two and exclaimed, "Let's rock!"

This time Mike decided to lecture as he drew. "Ok, axes first." He drew a big "L" on the board and said, "The X-axis is time, and time zero is the start of life as we know it — the beginning of vet school." He ticked off hash marks with the numbers 1, 2, 3, 4. "This is first through fourth year. Then after that, just for grins, let's add an internship, followed by a residency.

"This is the Y-axis, as in, wh"Y" the Hell am I doing this?" Without pausing for a breath, "And here is the maximum for all factors." He wrote MAX and drew a dashed line two feet above and parallel to the X-axis. "Now, going to vet school, at least in my humble opinion, both greatly simplifies and complicates your life. Your life will boil down to two main negative elements and two main positive factors. First, we'll start with test stress since that's what brought us together today. Right now, you are about here on the relative test stress scale." He put a dot on the Y-axis about five inches above the baseline. "And your first year will go something like this..." He drew a line that trailed off with a downward curve. "Basically you'll get better — less stressed — with each passing test. Then comes second year and they crank up the heat — ten times more tests and more difficult material to boot." The line jumped up dramatically, "But again you acclimate and your stress drops. By third year, you get a double benefit, the testing frequency slackens and you hit your stride: *The Force is with you and you know it.*" Then in the fourth year he drew a sharp peak that went vertical and actually pierced the MAX level and then dropped precipitously toward zero. "That's the National Board Exam. You'll make it, but since everything rides on that one big-assed test, some people feel the stress."

Trisha interjected, "But not Mike. Mike's test stress is not portrayed here. Just for kicks during third-year spring break he took Boards early and, of course, crushed them."

Mike proceeded, "After National Boards, test stress is a thing of the past unless you go into a residency, and then the specialty board exams make this line look like Pinocchio lying about his hardwood attraction to Sleeping Beauty." The last peak Mike drew shot to the top of the blackboard. "So that's it for test stress.

"The other negative element is the sleep factor. In summary, you've had as much as you are ever gonna get, and it only gets worse." He drew a decreasing, stair-step line that actually dipped below zero during the years after vet school.

"And now on the positive side, you've got RVS. Starting with junior surgery in third year, you get to do Real Vet Stuff." He drew and labeled an arrow that sliced through the National Boards' peak and curved upward. "And of course from fourth year on, you're in it up to your eyeballs. Now, these three factors all add up to form the fourth element. I like to call it F-U-N. The FUN curve basically just goes up." He drew a squiggly line with a peak near the middle and end of each year and another just after the National Boards. "Anybody care to guess what the smaller peaks represent?"

This was an easy one for Jack, "Friday Night Happy Hours?"

"Yup," Mike said and then pointed to the larger, semiannual FUN peaks, "And these semester-end bashes are called Skits Nights." He concluded, "What the graph looks like after graduation is entirely up to you. But for now, this is your life."

Trisha said, "Excellent job, Mikie. Accurate and complete."

"Well…" Mike responded with a strained look on his face, "there is one more element, one more variable that can dramatically affect all the others." Trisha looked confused. "This is just my opinion I guess, but there is one major element missing from the graph."

Trisha was curious, really curious; she'd missed something that Mike thought was major. She lowered her head and focused her thoughts. How did her life differ so much from his? Mike followed the Eagles and the Phillies — that was the only thing she could come up with. She raised her head and quizzically said, "Sports?"

He shook his head no, "The graph is supposed to apply to *everyone*."

Anna thought she knew what Mike was getting at but there was no way she was going to say it out loud. Not to this group. Not to anyone but Petunia.

Mike turned to the blackboard, "Even if I do say so myself, this is beautiful work but…" he took a piece of chalk and turned it on its side so it would leave a thick, broad mark and then drew a vertical line with arrows at both ends next to the wh"Y"-axis. "It makes the X-axis go up and down. It changes how we feel about all these other things." Nearly everyone in Room A1 was puzzled.

Then he wrote out the letters T R U E L O V E .

Trisha was confused. She asked rhetorically, "Love, what's love got to do with it? It's just a secondhand emotion." The guys chuckled.

"Well, *Tina*, it's quite simple," Mike paused, looking at each one in turn, "True Love has the power *to shift your baseline*." He let the concept sink in, "Love changes everything. If you have True Love, the baseline soars — test stress is obliterated." He proceeded to demonstrate the effects of True Love by mimicking the movement of the X-axis with his left arm. "If all goes well, you get even less sleep. You'll enjoy the Real Vet Stuff even more. And ultimately, the FUN curve goes through the roof."

Mike polled his audience by checking expressions. Kerri had a comprehending grin. Trisha smiled softly, recalling her recent encounter with

Buck Riley, that sweet rodeo cowboy. The boys (Jack, Hoss, Sam, and Rick) displayed looks ranging from *What the heck are you talking about?* to *Whatever*. And then there was Anna. What Mike saw in Anna's face confused him at first. Anna's jaw tone slacked, her eyes became liquid and full. And then in a half-completed, slow-motion, stuttering blink, Mike recognized the collision of hope and despair. His heart skipped a beat.

Mike London concluded, first looking directly at Anna and then settling on Trisha, "Trust me. True Love's got everything to do with it."

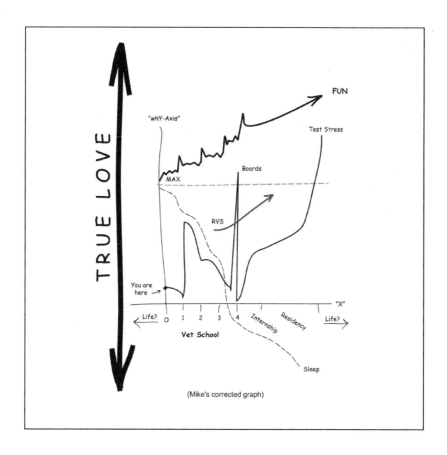

(Mike's corrected graph)

CHAPTER EIGHT

Trust

The Peaceable Kingdom's large animal surgical suite, Chadds Ford

William Digby, the Peaceable Kingdom's lead keeper, was Mount Augustus with a golden sheen. On anyone else, his park uniform of khaki shirt (conveniently missing the top two buttons), cargo shorts, stout hiking boots and side-snapped bush hat might have appeared a costume. But William's brawny Australian thighs and Popeye forearms were bronzed in such a way that most women, and even some men, lapped up his image without so much as a second clean thought. His face matched his chest. Both were sturdy, broad and appeared honest, but one part of his facade was designed specifically to disguise: dense, bilaterally symmetrical sideburns ran to earlobe level and then used their sharp anterior points to direct an admirer's attention away from the defects and toward his brilliant smile. Hidden beneath each sideburn was a scar. Scars that most guys would not have concealed because the biologically welded arcs of fibrous connective tissue would only have enhanced a rugged aura and were connected to the perfect story. They had been acquired during the rescue of a baby koala from the jaws of an eight-foot croc. But William Digby didn't need the scars or the story. With his other bulging assets, they were overkill. His fair-haired looks combined with that accent from Down Under, did to women (his target audience) what direct sunlight does so easily to butter.

William joked with Violet Marie Green as she unrolled a latex finger cot over the shaft of an ice-frosted test tube. It was the kind small animal vets don for single-digit rectal exams, "Safety first, Luv." He smirked and then concluded, "Blimey, that looks the size of a British condom. Poor buggars."

She smiled but didn't look up at him.

He added, "It's not even 'Ribbed for her pleasure.'"

"Yeah, I suppose that could be a disappointment but it'll work just fine to protect the tube in the warming bath. A gentle, controlled thaw is critical to sperm viability." This was yet another of Dr. Green's clinical reproduction trials. She was testing a new formula for big cat semen cryopreservation. Her novel surfactant had the potential to dramatically extend the "shelf life" of male seed stored for the propagation of endangered species. "It'll be interesting to see how this compares to the fresh stuff we collect today."

Violet turned her head to check in with her two veterinary technicians. She asked, "How do the girls look?"

William grinned and responded first, "I'd say the ladies are right lovely."

The techs blushed, beamed and then replied in harmony, "Thank you, Sir William." Feeling it was his innate Aussie responsibility to buoy their shared fantasy, William Digby winked but really wasn't interested. At this stage in the game of life, he only stalked trophies. He didn't waste time on domestic species — the rare, wild and perfect specimen was his quest.

The girls to which Dr. Green had referred were identical twin snow leopards, hormonally induced to synchronize their estrous cycles. Violet stopped for a moment to take in the peaceful, rhythmic EKG pulse. As a surprise for Violet's last birthday, and with the hope of finally getting her in bed, William had rigged the monitors to report each heart beat with a soft chirp, like that of a small bird. It gave her all the same information without the numbing penetration of that monotone beep.

Violet eased the frozen tube into the warm water bath and turned her attention to the oversized surgery table. The Peaceable Kingdom's surgical suite was state-of-the-art. That is, state of the medical art as practiced at topflight hospitals like Sloan-Kettering or the Mayo Clinic. As compared with the average veterinary hospital, it was downright opulent. In fact, Violet could barely assuage her pangs of guilt whenever she thought of human medical facilities in places like Uganda or Belize. If she so desired, and if the case required, all she had to do was turn to her left for a full complement of video endoscopes, reach to her right to retrieve a YAG laser, or just open a cabinet to grab a portable ultrasound. And, if an essential tool was not on hand, she had only to accomplish two steps:

1) hail Mr. Davaris on the radio, and 2) warn the techs to expect a next-day shipment. Sometimes, though it had to be her imagination, it seemed all she had to do was make a wish out loud in the lab and supplies would magically appear. The relative ease of this situation would have made most vets giddy, but for Dr. Violet Marie Green it set off a gastric reflux cascade that she'd been secretly self-medicating for months.

The two all-white cats lay side-by-side, each in right lateral recumbency on closed-cell padding. Violet dimmed the ambient lighting by wireless remote and watched the first cat's rib cage rhythmically rise and fall. This female was named Peeka and her identically gorgeous sister was Boo. Their parents had abandoned them hours after birth and that's when Dr. Green stepped in. She raised the pair single-handedly with Q 3hr feedings of warm Esbilac, shuttling them to her apartment every night until they were too big, too noisy and too dangerous for the neighbors. Her success rate in rearing orphans was legendary. To date, with dozens of ungulates (including gemsbok), big cats, and even a temperamental honey badger or two, she'd only failed once. Even seasoned zookeepers, the kind skeptical of an average veterinarian's husbandry skills, deferred to Dr. Green when a neonate posed a real challenge.

Violet Green elevated Peeka's left hind leg and palpated her femoral artery. A steady throb raised the tip of her index finger and naturally triggered Violet's maternal warmth. After checking the animal's palpebral reflex, she stroked the silky fur and then moved to Boo. "Boo, you sure are your sister's twin, your pulse is identical in quality and character." Violet paused as her eyes smiled and she added, "I miss you around the house, little girl. If the Swenson's Corgi hadn't mysteriously disappeared, you might have been able to stay a little longer." She sighed and, after applying a protective lube to the wide amber eyes, she patted Boo's head. "Today you become a lady."

She looked up at William, "Boo will serve as the control. She'll receive the fresh-collected sample and Peeka gets the previously frozen trial." Violet did another quick visual of the animals, the monitors, insemination tools and announced, "I think we're ready to collect Jam."

Jam was a young adult snow leopard on loan from the Cincinnati Zoo. He was a proven breeder, or more accurately, a proven donor — his sperm had been used in Cincinnati to father three healthy cubs on three consecutive tries. Jam had one problem though. He couldn't quite figure out the mechanics of mating. He seemed confused by the subtleties of the dance. When presented with a twitching tail and arched back, he would pad up to the receptive female, sniff the right spots and then proceed to mount the wrong end. This approach usually sparked snarls that culminated with Jam cowering in the corner, licking a bruised ego and his more delicate male parts. Since his genetics were great and the risk of mating-induced injury high, Jam had to be collected by hand.

Violet and William entered the adjoining hallway that connected surgery to a series of rooms designed for anesthesia induction. Jam paced rapidly back and forth in his concrete pen, a wall of slender metal bars separating him from them. Not wishing to further increase his obvious anxiety, Violet quickly raised a three-foot long aluminum tube and drew the mouthpiece to her lips. She tracked him for two passes and then with a sharp puff, delivered the dart. Jam didn't flinch. He never growled or altered his pattern. Violet thought, *so this is what your love life has come to; I guess you accept it. I know how you feel.* She motioned to William to retreat from the animal's view and then whispered, "He should be completely out in three minutes." She twisted the bezel of her watch and then looked into William's broad face, a face she thought was professionally a little too close to hers. "So where'd you guys move my gemsbok?"

William blinked and shifted his gaze down and away from Violet's sky-blue irises. He knew she wasn't going to like this and thought fast, "Didn't you get the memo?" She just squinted, and then cocked her head in confusion, so William was forced to continue, "We shipped three to Cincinnati and the rest to North Carolina and Texas last night."

Violet Marie Green was a consistently stoic, even-keeled force for nature. She was not known for being overly expressive but right now her face registered obvious surprise. "Are you kidding me?"

William Digby shook his head no, he wasn't kidding.

"International Zoo and Aquarium regulations state that prior to shipment, all mammals need a clean exit exam and a signed health certificate at the very least." She paused, bit her lower lip, then proceeded, "Not to mention, I raised those little guys."

"Vi, what was I gonna do?" William actually shrugged his shoulders. "Davaris ordered me. It was supposed to be a gesture of goodwill in exchange for old Jammer here," he paused but not long enough for her to respond, "*and*, we're stuffed to the gills with gemsbok, other hoofstock and even big cats thanks to your good repro work."

Violet noticed a flicker in William's eyes when he said the words *even big cats* so she pressed further, "You shipped some cats, too?"

"No, not some, just one," he hesitated but then added, "Mya." Violet Green was so shocked she couldn't even respond. Mya had been a gravely ill female African lion cub Violet raised, and was her first true clinical success at the park. There were a hundred reasons why Mya should have died, but she never gave up. Although Violet would barely admit it to herself, that scrappy independent little lion was deeply important to her — a kindred spirit. William continued after another quick shrug, "Besides, we're not IZA accredited yet so we don't have to follow the rules." He returned her penetrating stare and added, "It was all perfectly legal."

Violet's pupils narrowed as if she were preparing to excise a tumor with the YAG laser, "It may have been legal, William, but that doesn't make it right." The thought flickered that she should also tell him she was hurt, but just then her Timex began to beep. Violet poked her head around the corner and saw that Jam, the romantically clueless snow leopard, was splayed out peacefully snoozing. They quietly unlocked the gate, entered the pen and rolled the striking 120-pound cat onto his side.

Dr. Violet Marie Green was back, focused as per usual on the case at hand. She squeezed a packet of KY onto a curved stainless-steel probe and gingerly introduced it into the sleeping cat's rectum. She probed William in terse staccato "He goes at 80 millivolts, right?"

William responded with a smirk, "Yeah, none of that silly foreplay required. A sequence of three pulses followed by a probe twist crescendo should produce a happy ending, I reckon."

Violet didn't respond as she positioned a collection vial and depressed a red button to apply the first stimulus.

"Vi, come on, don't be mad at me. Let me make it up to you. Let's go to dinner."

She didn't reply or look up.

He tried again, "You have to eat."

She didn't acknowledge his prodding while she applied the second pulse, but then after seeing no response she replied, "I'm thinking about it."

"You've been thinking about it for six bloody months, sweetheart. I'm not going to bite."

She applied the third and final stimulus and seeing no result, William reached over and wrapped his powerful fingers around her hand. Guiding her, he rotated and redirected the probe; the effect was immediate. Jam's body tensed and the tube nearly overflowed.

"Trust me Luv, I know what I'm doing."

CHAPTER NINE

Cramming

*Comparative Anatomy Laboratory in the old veterinary
school building, Philadelphia*

Anatomy Lab is no less toxic after dark. In reality, the atmospheric concentration of formaldehyde goes up. This is because the main lab's ventilation system is on a timer to save electricity. To formalin-sensitive students it was painfully obvious that the nighttime air stung more intensely on inspiration and that eyes watered more copiously. But most of these supersensitive individuals did not work in the main lab with their classmates. These students, the ones claiming an allergy to formalin, were impounded in an adjoining room, one with continuous wind-tunnel-like ventilation. They wore puffy white biohazard moon suits with full gas masks, *and* received fresh, non-formalinized specimens to dissect whenever possible.

The Sissy Box or "Area 51" — as it was known by the more hardy — would easily receive an OSHA stamp of approval. But like elsewhere in life, there was a tradeoff for comfort and safety. The reduced concentration of formalin was osmotically offset by an influx of FRoGs. They were drawn to the space by the hair-raising ventilation induced by the nearly constant swirling tornado of flailing arms — and Area 51, in a strange way, provided protection for the remainder of the class. It partially contained an F5 question vortex.

Since Area 51's quarantine required physical separation from the main dissection lab, Big Moe had installed a two-way intercom system and small viewing window. That way the occupants could signal their inevitable question barrage and the formalin-contaminated instructors did not invade the secure air space. A FRoG — or, more usually, FRoGs — would, after raising their hands, request attention by depressing a big red, mushroom-shaped *asking plunger*. This action triggered a domino effect: first, a pulsing red strobe over the viewing port began piercing the formalin fog of the main lab (after a couple weeks' use, the beacon took on the air of a demonic lighthouse of sorts, the kind that draws you closer to danger); second, a droning "bong" was sounded (it was exactly the same "bong" you heard when signaling a stewardess) and this kept repeating —*bong—bong—bong*— until; third, the nearest instructor sprinted to end it all by pressing the intercom reply button.

Unfortunately, two groups of regular, formalin-infused students (Jack, Sam, Hoss and Kerri and Anna) had chosen dissection stations adjacent to Area 51. They picked their work stations while still naïve. They could not have foreseen the horror. At that point there was just one student, JJ, in the Sissy Box, but after the first week or so, the more delicate students gravitated towards the relative safety and familiar seclusion. In the laboratory setting, it was the closest thing to the front row. Jack reasoned out loud, "They're just in there because they love that damned *asking plunger*." Area 51, he imagined, was a FRoG's dream come true.

◅ • ▻

This was the last night the lab would be open before the test. Big Moe, as he did for each exam, had instructed the security guards to stand down, to let the students study all night if they wanted, and the lab was full up. The first anatomy test was a big event. And thanks to people like Rick Larson, the tension of this trial was amplified by his repeated telling of *The Legend of the Harvard Grad*. The entire class was fidgety and on alert, all except the two groups nearest Area 51. Theirs was an island of calm in the vast, smelly sea of apprehension. Their relaxed approach was primarily due to the personalities in the mix: there was some cool, some confidence, some brains, some warmth, and some fun. At the beginning of the evening, Jack said to his friends with a level stare, "Others have done this and survived, so can we."

Kerri replied, "But we have to make a pact. Above all else, no matter what happens tonight, *THAT*," she pointed with her forceps to the viewing window of Area 51, "That cannot happen to us..." She added, almost pleading, "*No matter what happens*. Okay?"

Anna and Jack said, "Agreed," in unison.

Hoss said, "Yup." And Sam Stone nodded.

Jack shuddered as he thought, *there but by the grace of God go I.* He knew something the others did not. He was allergic to formalin. He knew it coming into vet school, he knew it as early as middle school biology's dissection of the leopard frog. His throat went raw, his eyes burned, but nothing short of a loaded syringe (he was deathly afraid of needles) or an anaphylactic reaction would get him in *there.*

He ruminated, "It has to be downright volatile in 51 tonight — a real pressure cooker. All those FRoGs, all that information to learn, and all those questions with no outlet." There were no teachers in the lab at night, so the pot just bubbled and boiled with the lid clamped tight. Jack could envision the spray of orphaned questions blindly ricocheting off the walls and a wild, arm-waving slap-fest as they simultaneously clambered for help. "They might kill each other," he blurted out.

Sam replied, "We can only hope so."

Kerri shivered, "Turn away. You can't save them. And don't look directly into their eyes, they might try to communicate with us…"

Paradoxically, this was the other reason for their self-imposed island of peace; they were front row center to witness the carnage, the self-destruction — the alternative to sanity.

⌐ ● ⌐

Since this was just the first few weeks of school, pretty much everyone treated each other with excessive civility — but still, no one had warmed-up to Rick. He made liking him a challenge. Although he had dissection partners, they wisely kept him at a distance. He must have felt an affinity for his orientation group because tonight he kept coming over to Sam, Jack and the others as they studied. "How the hell are we supposed to know all this stuff? It's way too much. Too much. The head and limbs of the dog, cow, pig and horse — all at once!"

Sam thought, *Are you talkin' to me?* and then replied without looking at Rick, "Ay-yuh, it's a lot I guess."

"You guess?? You had better do more than just guess." He continued to rant to no one in particular because no one wanted to hear it. "Every origin, insertion and action for every muscle. All innervations. And get this, all major veins and arteries!"

Jack Doyle needed to quell the mounting hysteria. He wanted to slap Rick but held back. "Yeah, we know. We all got the syllabus. Just remember what Mike and Trisha told us: focus on what's important and have fun with it."

"Have fun?" Rick repeated, "Have fun..? How's that supposed to happen? It's impossible to learn all this. Impossible I tell you." He trailed off with a mumble, "How the hell are you gonna have fun with this?"

"Look," Jack jumped in, "you're just psyching yourself out. The time you spend worrying is time lost. Focus. We have fun because we make a game out of it. You know, quiz each other. You should do that with your group."

"MY group? They aren't *my* group, I don't take any responsibility for them. You think *I'm* paranoid, *they're* totally freaked out."

Sam looked to the other end of the lab, to the table whence Rick came. The girl and guy were working intensively, studying quietly. Natural human behavior. In fact, it appeared as if the girl was flirting with the guy. Sam could recognize flirtation from a considerable distance; it was one of his talents. "Yeah, they do look wicked freaked."

Rick continued, "Um, since we're all in the same orientation group," Jack thought, *Damn, here it comes,* "do you think I could study with you guys?" Kerri looked at Sam and thought, *Shit, how do we get rid of him?* Rick's the kind of guy who is perfect for a crisis. More accurately, Rick's the kind of guy who incites a crisis. They all looked at each other, eyes blinking Morse code for: *Hell No!* All except Hoss. He was, as always, an amiable mountain. You'd have to pop him a good one in the lip to get him riled, and even then he might construe it as a friendly gesture.

Hoss spoke up, "Sure, Rick. The more the merrier." The four of them glared. Hoss smiled, not knowing that he'd done anything wrong.

Rick looked relieved and a smirk crawled onto his face but Anna cut his exuberance short, exclaiming, "You can stay but only if you keep your mouth shut!" Jack's eyes bulged as he thought, *She's got balls.*

Rick stared at her, "Are you serious?"

"I'm always serious. You want to stay, you have to focus — no freaking out. If you can't relax, hit the road."

Jack choked back a laugh. Rick reluctantly nodded okay, then searching for a foothold he said, "But how will I answer questions in your quiz games?"

"You will speak only when spoken to."

There was a tense silence, but then Rick swallowed his pride for two reasons: first, he was terrified he'd fail without their help, and second, he did not want to get into a metaphorical boxing match with Anna Heywood because then, it would be fact — he would have been bested by a woman, and this time in public. He acquiesced with a sulky, "Okay..." and then pantomimed locking his lips with a key.

But of course, he couldn't leave it at that. He was Rick Larson. He had to do something moronic, something to try to degrade his female opponent. He sucked in his prodigious gut, pulled out his pants at the waistline and pretended to drop the make believe key into his crotch. His waist band snapped back and he gave Anna a smirk with his tightly clamped lips.

Anna laid him out, "Perfect, you may never talk again."

The two dissection groups, plus the lone mute, made progress in fits and starts, then settled into a rhythm of hunt, point and query. Each group had their own horse, dog, cow and pig, and at this initial stage of dissection, these animals kept their heads and two left legs. The right limbs were disarticulated where they normally attached to the trunk and then further dissected to reveal details of the neuro and vascular systems. The dissection plan was simple: right side — veins, arteries and nerves; left side — bones and musculature. This system of dismemberment uncovered freakish, even devilish looking beasts from within these once warm and furry mammals. The heads — especially the heads — were ghoulish, the things of which nightmares were made. Stripped of their skin except for eyelids and ears, the exposed web of red and blue latex-injected blood vessels intertwining with the off-white bands of innervation was almost, well, unnerving. On one side, chunky windows were carved in overlying muscles that could be flipped open to expose important landmarks. The other side was completely denuded, laying bare the gleaming ivory of jaw, tooth and eye socket.

Somehow, as a vet student, you get used to things that would make civilians cringe. Things like a skinless horse head "looking" at you, with half of one eye dangling via the optic nerve, and the other eyeball hastily stuffed in its socket, backwards.

After a long hour of review, Jack said to Kerri, "We need a break. How about a race?" She didn't reply. "Come on, it'll only take ten minutes."

Kerri looked up from the dissection manual and said, "Stop nagging. In fact, your nag couldn't beat our stud even if it did have four legs."

Jack teased, "Are you chicken?" He flapped his elbows a couple times while asking the same question in chickenese, "*Bauk-bauk?*" He was hoping to goad her into a quick match of dead-horse steeplechase. It was a timed, one-lap event where their formalinized horses were pushed around the monorail system while attempting to negotiate the standard obstacles of water hazards (formalin puddles on the floor) and jumps (broomsticks supported between overturned garbage cans).

"Nope, chicken is next week's lab." She pursed her lips and then smushed them slowly left to right as she considered the challenge. Jack was right she thought, they could use a study break, "Okay, you're on. But let's make this interesting. How about the loser — obviously you — buys a round at Friday Night Happy Hour."

Jack grinned, reached out, shook her gloved hand and said, "Let's make it two!"

The trick to winning at dead-horse steeplechase, as any casual observer could discern, was to have the appropriate rider. The horse was really secondary to the effort. It was vital to have someone agile enough to hang onto a wildly careening, formalin-saturated horse and light enough not to cause the meat hooks to pull out. Jack summoned the ideal jockey, José Rizal. Phenotypically, José was indistinguishable from a prepubescent Filipino girl — he was small and light and Jack figured that his appendicular hairlessness would reduce aerodynamic drag. And, having been born into a well-known Filipino circus family, he had valuable high-wire experience.

Kerri, on the other hand, surprised Jack and the guys by asking JJ to ride for her. He was so flattered, he downed three times the maximum allowable dose of Benadryl and came scurrying out of quarantine. Kerri bent over, clasped her fingers and gave him a hand up as he clambered aboard Old Paint in his white Tyvek space suit. The slippery material only made brief contact with the cold, greasy animal's back as JJ skidded right off the other side, his arms still locked around the horse's neck. The second mount was the charm.

Jack and Sam maneuvered Nellie (their horse) and José (their jockey) onto the mainline monorail. A medieval series of manual track switches clanged left then right as Jack pulled on dangling cords while Sam pushed on the horse's rump. Meanwhile, Hoss set up an obstacle on the far side of the track. They were ready.

Anna raised her wristwatch, waited for the second hand to hit 12, and then proclaimed in a surprisingly heady voice, "AND THEY'RE OFF!" Sam sprang out of his runner's crouch and into action as if he'd been tagged by a riding crop. For the first instant, his legs pumped wildly but suddenly the laces of his worn hiking boots came undone. Just as quickly as it had all begun, Sam found himself face down on the slick concrete floor. Jack laughed and jumped in to push. At the first obstacle he swung Nellie left so they'd miss the broad lake of formalin. Then, picking up speed, they reached the curve at the far end of the lab. The centrifugal force of rounding the tight curve caused the animal's two remaining legs to swing out widely; all the while, José performed an amazing impression of a sequined circus entertainer. He lay back, pointed one leg in the air and arched an arm gracefully back over the horse's rump. Through the curve and now in the home stretch, Team Nellie gracefully vaulted the horizontal mop handle as the jockey slung down to raise the animal's legs. They crossed the finish line just as Anna pronounced, "37 seconds. Not bad — for a loser."

Glancing back over her shoulder and seeing her team in position, Anna rechecked her watch and casually, lazily announced, "Go." Kerri and JJ had previously agreed on their strategy. It consisted primarily of his hanging on for dear life while she pushed — nothing fancy. There really wasn't much else he could do since his gas mask had completely fogged in the excitement.

After a tentative start, they barreled forward over the lake and around the far turn until JJ started to lose his grip. He swung down under the bare belly with his legs and arms still tightly clamped, but he managed to hang on as they plowed through the "jump" scattering the mop and upturned garbage cans.

Jack laughed out loud and began chugging imaginary beers with both hands until he noticed something odd. Anna was smiling at him. He thought, *Why would she be smiling?* That's when he noticed the brown piece of horse flesh. She tossed it up and caught it in her right hand. Anna's smile broadened as she nonchalantly extended her arm across the finish line announcing, "35 seconds! Old Paint, the winner by a nose!"

The class responded with immediate applause partially muffled by latex gloves and as the muted clapping trailed off, they heard a soft metal clicking and the motorized hum of the nearby freight elevator. They had only seen this elevator used once during lab, and that was by Big Moe.

After dismounting, as it were, JJ said, "Big Moe must be coming up to check on us."

Jack shook his head, "This late? Nah, it's almost 2 AM…"

They looked at one another in confused silence. The elevator was ultra slow, it clanked and creaked. Its job was to lift heavy, messy loads — speed was unimportant. But in this case, the slowness only served to magnify the tension. After what seemed like an hour the hum became louder. As the inner cage reached the laboratory level it slammed to a halt with a bang. By now, everyone in the hangar-sized lab was focused on the enormous elevator doors. The top and bottom portions had interlocking tines that gave the appearance of a toothy maw. Then, the doors (too heavy to be lifted by hand) slowly ground automatically open. Normally a naked bulb illuminated the interior but now, for some reason, it was out. A dozen stout, flickering candles were scattered on the elevator floor, and in the center stood a metal gurney with a stainless steel domed cover.

No one moved. The lab was dead silent. Even the FRoGs quietly let go of their test-induced panic and filled the void with a fear of another kind. Their faces pushed together and completely occluded the viewing port.

Then it happened. The stillness was shattered: BONG! Followed by *Bong-Bong-Bong*. 93% of the students in the main lab shot vertically at least three inches while 6% jumped two inches. Less than 1%, Sam Stone, just responded with, "Hmmm."

A request squawked from the Area 51 intercom, "What is it? Is it more material for the exam?"

Although still fogged, from under JJ's gas mask came a muffed voice, "Damned FRoGs."

Jack Doyle thought, *Well I guess it's my job as Class President to sort this out*, so he moved carefully towards the elevator followed by Hoss and Sam. Together they stared at a large orange note taped to the metal cover. It said, "Open Me."

Then it happened again. BONG!! And this time Jack, Hoss and even Sam jumped. Jack looked fiercely towards Area 51 as the intercom whined, "What does it say? What does it say? *What does it say?*" Jack turned, and then without a sound wheeled the gurney out into the center of the lab where some of the braver students moved in to surround it. It was obviously a dissection table of some sort with a steel basin underneath and a domed metal, roll top lid that could be rotated down and out of the way.

Hoss spoke up, "Looks like a barbecue we'd use for a pig roast."

Jack grabbed the lid's handle and said, "Oh, what the hell..." and proceeded to roll back the cover. There, enshrouded inside a semitransparent plastic body bag was the unmistakable form of a nude man. A second, smaller note was stuck to the plastic just over his forehead. The note said, "Good luck on your testes, with love, Mr. Cadaver."

Jack turned to the class and announced, "It's a body. *Freaking human med students*... Very funny." Jack reached above Mr. Cadaver's head, grasped the bag's zipper and pulled — when the corpse was exposed to the level of his bellybutton, it sat bolt up! A clear, snot-like gel spurted violently from its nose and mouth as the body coughed and gasped for breath. The students who had moved in for a closer look yelled in horror. The FRoGs in Area 51 repeatedly pressed the asking plunger as they shrieked into the intercom. Kerri stumbled backwards. Hoss fell over a stool, landing solidly on his butt, while Jack and Sam were still frozen in place when "Mr. Cadaver" started to laugh.

Jack shook his head and smiled in appreciation, "You fucker..."

"Gotcha!" replied Mr. Cadaver. It was a time-honored prank that had been performed every year since there were cadavers. The med students somehow, someway, would slip a body into the Comparative Anatomy Lab, and this was a new and highly effective variation on the theme.

Mr. Cadaver lifted his right hand which was operating a small camcorder and panned the room of stupefied faces. "This'll be great for our skits night at the end of the year." And with that, he turned the camera toward himself, flashed a dripping smile, and jumped off the table. Clutching the body bag around his midsection, he ran into the elevator bidding farewell, "Good luck little vets. Top that!"

As the jaws of the elevator devoured the professional prankster, Jack vowed quietly to their group, "Oh, we will. Don't you worry. We will top that."

CHAPTER TEN

Testing 1, 2, 3...

7:56 AM — THURSDAY, SEPTEMBER 15, 1988

*The physiology exam in Room 13 of the Rosenthal
Building, Philadelphia*

Anna Heywood eased herself as steadily as she could into her usual
seat in front of the podium. She closed her eyes and sighed. No one needed
to remind her, her doctor didn't have to scold. The subtle erratic movements and muted screams from her every muscle drove the point home.
Last night she'd pushed well beyond the limits that her "situation" would
allow. Those three hours of sleep, followed by a Wawa corn muffin didn't
come close to recharging ATP stores, restocking glycogen, or compen-
sating for the harsh realities of diminishing motor control. At this point
in the progression, her physical capabilities waxed and waned. It was true
that she could strengthen her endurance if she ate right and got a monkish
ten hours. But what was she supposed to do? It wasn't as if her coandition
would improve — completely the opposite. These weren't the Olympic trials again. This time she needed to maintain her balance, and now vet school
was the beam. The ironic thing was that she knew this stuff. She didn't have
to gut it out last night like the rest. So why did she punish her body to work
with the group when she knew the toll it would take?

Slowly, arduously, Anna bent at her waist to retrieve a pencil and fat
eraser from her backpack. Now everything about the process of writing
irritated her. First, she was forced to use lead instead of ink, how juvenile
was that? And second, she could barely maintain a grip long enough to
answer a complete essay. Usually about two-thirds of the way through
she'd notice her "L's" widening. When they began bowing into O's, she'd

swear under her breath, erase and rest. This morning she was already swearing like a sailor denied shore leave after twelve months at sea. Right off the bat, her index finger wouldn't clamp and the pencil pivoted and fell. Petunia, who was as usual lying at her feet, didn't need a command. Anna patted her head, wiped the saliva from the yellow No. 2, took a deep breath and began.

◄ • ►

The night before (at about 3 AM), despite vociferous objection, Jack had escorted Anna safely to her doorstep. He knew better than the rest that darkened Philly streets were no place for a lone woman, even with a dog. Jack waited to hear the second heavy deadbolt clack into place and then headed back to Room A1 where he rejoined Hoss, Sam and Kerri as they switched gears from anatomy to prep for physio.

Now, during the test, Jack raised his eyes skyward offering up a short prayer, "Thank You for our advisors and thank You for Vet Pictionary." Although the questions weren't verbatim, he was able to whip off the correct answers with detail and even a little flare.

◄ • ►

Kerri Feinburg had told a lie during her veterinary school interview. The one she had chosen to tell was odd, especially considering the truths she decided to reveal. But when questioned about her absolutely perfect grades from high school through college, she shook her head "no" to the speculation she might have a photographic memory. This response was technically untrue. Kerri Feinburg held, tightly coiled in her temporal lobes, a continuous ribbon, a video diary that could be accessed at any time. Diagrams, graphs, the never-ending strings of text she'd skimmed, and numbers (especially the phone numbers of cute guys) were instantly available from her magical mental Rolodex. As a result, Kerri flowed effortlessly in and out of test questions like a giant slalom skier. She rarely studied in the traditional sense and last night, after the cadaver caper was pulled by that med student, Kerri packed up so quickly she'd actually forgotten her text and two notebooks (in this case, they would have only slowed her pursuit of knowledge). Kerri accurately reasoned that the study of anatomy was only "comparative" if you included *all* major species and it was that glimpse of Mr. Cadaver's well-proportioned attributes that spurred her real desire to learn. And now, with a half-angled grin, and only so much as a cat nap between a series of intimate "form and function" tutorials, Kerri plowed through the testing process by accessing that ribbon when and where she needed.

—◄ ● ►—

Sam Stone was not as covertly fortunate as Kerri. He had to study for good grades. In fact Sam had to study hard. But like Kerri, Sam kept a secret: he didn't see letters, words and numbers the way others did. For him, they didn't really register in coherent clumps. So Sam Stone dismantled run-on blocks of text in much the same way he broke down the massive diesel engine on his dad's trawler or the one in his own 1950 forest-green Chevy pickup. He dissected the written words on his Note Service pages and medical texts, and converted the parts into images, either by circling and highlighting related clusters or sketching out the concepts. When he was done he'd have pictures he could process, remember and access. Once the machine was in pieces — dissected, cleaned and oiled — he could launch into the reassembly with an ease and confidence that yielded no orphaned parts.

—◄ ● ►—

Well into the second half of the second full day of continuous testing, Hoss still wore a beatific smile under that ten-gallon hat. While many of his classmates withered under the strain, a serene atmosphere enveloped his colossal mass. Sure, he should have been worn and eroded, frayed and frazzled. He'd studied with his friends again last night (highlighting, condensing and quizzing until 4 AM), but Hoss was a young man largely unaffected by time. He didn't internalize stress because he rarely considered the future. Thunder rolled off his back like rain off an oilskin. Hoss lived now. He smiled now. Hoss was Buddha in a vest and checked flannel shirt, and his indestructible calm had the power to unnerve those who needed to worry.

Although Rick Larson sat in the same row directly next to Hoss during the test, attempting to insinuate the illusion of association, mentally they were worlds apart. While relative peace and earnest endeavor brewed and perked throughout Death Row, even Hoss could recognize the waves of chaos rippling from Rick. He shifted and strained. Sighed and whirred. His head whipped on its swivel. If Hoss were a stoic panda casually munching stalks of bamboo, then Rick was a rabid squirrel stealing furtive glances from nearby feeders. When Rick's twitching finally reached an epileptic buzz, Hoss reached out with a muscular paw to steady his classmate. He whispered, "It'll be okay buddy. Just close your eyes and breathe. You know the Right Thing." Rick repulsed the gesture, instantly flicking Hoss' hand away with a disdain that was congenital. Rick was blind to the warmhearted concern and caring displayed on Hoss' soft round face. He couldn't see such qualities in another because they were alien to his experience. And besides, he was looking for something else.

Physiology Lecture Exam #1   (on all pages) NAME: *Anna Heywood*
9/15/1988

#1) Please describe and diagram all pertinent components of the normal Action
Potential (AP) and its saltatory conduction (propagation) along a normally
myelinated neuronal axon. Assume, for this question, that dendritic
receptors are stimulated to Threshold Potential and the signal is relayed to
skeletal muscle (4pts). And, why are some axons myelinated (1pt)

The Resting Membrane Potential (RMP) of the average neuron is approx. -70mv. This differential is generated by a conc. gradient of Na+ and K+ (inc. [Na+] outside and inc. [K+] inside). When dendrites are stimulated (pushing MP above threshold), voltage-gated Na+ channels are triggered to open thus allowing a massive Na+ influx down the conc. gradient (depolarization). During depolarization, the neuron cannot be re-excited regardless of further stimulus application (Refractory Period). Repolarization occurs when the MP increases above 0 mv and triggers the opening of the voltage-gated K+ channels. Then K+ rapidly exits the cell and re-establishes the RMP. The combined events of depolarization and repolarization constitute an Action Potential.

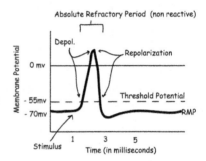

Certain axons are ensheathed in a fatty material called Myelin (it acts like insulation on an electrical wire) which is produced by Schwann cells. Gaps, called nodes of Ranvier, occur between adjacent Schwann cells and the AP jumps from node to node (saltatory conduction) transmitting the signal to the target cell (a muscle fiber in this case). Myelin helps to increase the speed of signal transmission to near the speed of light so that when an animal feels fear/pain, etc. it can signal the appropriate response (fight or flight) rapidly.

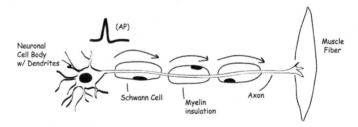

Physiology Lecture Exam #1   (on all pages) NAME: *John Fitzgerald Doyle*
9/15/1988

#23) Sensory function is critical for any organism. Please list the
predominant anatomical distribution and primary function(s) of the following
specific or general sensory receptor types. (1pt ea)

Ex: Pacinian Corpuscle: General cutaneous distribution within the dermis;
Transduce deep pressure and fast vibrations.

Chemoreceptor for Blood CO2 concentration: *Found mainly in the Aortic Arch, Carotid Arteries, and Medulla Oblongata. They detect elevated [CO2] in the blood and stimulate the SA Node to inc. heart rate (also increase respiratory rate).*

Ampullae of Lorenzini: *Located in the skin of the face/head; Sense electrical fields/salinity in sharks and other fishes.*

Proprioceptor (muscle spindle fiber): *They are found nearly everywhere, muscles, joints, skin. They sense "body awareness," orientation and position.*

Meissner's Corpuscle: *eyelids, lips, fingertips, nipples and external genitalia; sense fine touch, pressure, texture and slow vibrations*

Merkel's Disc: *Cutaneous (digits, groin and elsewhere). sustained touch and pressure.*

Vomeronasal Receptors (organ): *Located in the nasal passageway, the VMO detects airborne neurotransmitters, pheromones (helps males sense female estrous or "heat").*

#24) Briefly describe the process of image projection onto the mammalian
retina. What processing occurs within the occipital lobes? (2pts)

Light Reflects off the object of an animal's attention, then passes through the cornea, the pupil and ultimately is focused by the lens onto the retina which lines the back of the eye. The convex shape of the lens flips the image backwards and upside down.

The occipital lobes receive the electrical signals via the optic nerve, then invert the image (back to right side up) and fill in any unconscious defects or missing information.

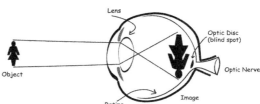

Lens

Object

Retina

Image

Optic Disc
(blind spot)

Optic Nerve

CHAPTER ELEVEN

The Testicle Festival

Friday Night Happy Hour at the Center for Large Animal Medicine in Kennett Square

Kersplat…

Plop, splat — *whump*.

The overhead speakers clicked twice and then hissed to life in the warm night air. Fireflies blinked all around. With the cordless microphone brushing against his bristled goatee, Mike cautiously proclaimed, "Umm, B-12. That's vitamin B12, cyanocobalamin." The crowd in the bleachers grumbled politely but Jack, ready for some fun, spoke up. It was probably the beer in front of him combined with the long week behind him that was talking. "It sounds like he's not sure and she was still moo-ving!" The last two syllables drew a sizable laugh from the crowd. "MOO-ving, good one," somebody said. Jack continued the friendly heckle, "By definition that's a crap call and it's on the line. Get the REF!" Play continued as the referee nimbled her way across the playing field to the point of contention. The ambulatory paddock next to the outpatient clinic had been transformed into a limed grid-work of labeled squares. First there was pointing, then the outline of impact determined, followed by up and down head motions. The ref reached to her hip: click, *hissss*, "B-12, definitely B-12." There was no questioning Dr. Green's ruling, she knew manure. Besides, it was all in good fun. Proceeds from cow pie bingo supported the Bovine Club's MAD COW lecture series — ultimately, everyone was a winner.

During the ruling process, two other "plays" had happened and flags marking their locations were already on the field. The next call was easier for Mike. It was well-formed, as firm as cow manure gets, and completely within the box, "I-2. Incision 2!" He turned to the audience half-expecting dissension, but only muted giggling and low-level party talk trickled from the stands. Mike pushed on to the next flag with two first years close on his heels. His helpers, Hoss and Kerri Feinburg, were a study in extremes. Hoss appeared a mesa rooted in steel-toed work boots, overalls and a John Deere cap, while Kerri's petite and refined form was clad in spiked, calf-high leather boots, matching black leather mini and white angora sweater. Hoss toted the bucket and Kerri, reluctantly, brandished the shovel. Regardless of how she soldiered on, Kerri's taut lips telegraphed displeasure, while Hoss wore a comfortable grin. He was literally in his element — and his element was smeared on both pant legs where the bucket made contact with each stride.

"Somebody should have hit by now," Jack was simultaneously amused and frustrated by the glacial progress.

Mike inspected the latest play, straightened up, took a sip of beer and declared, "O-4, that's Ovine 4." There was a two-second pause and then Jack yelled out, "BINGO! Sam, you got Bingo!" which was followed by the requisite mix of "Damn's," and "Oh-crap's!" The crowd felt obliged to at least feign disappointment, that was part of the fun. Nobody took the game too seriously, nobody except for the FRoGs. Holding true to form, the first-year FRoGs were piled on the bleacher's front row like pond turtles on a log. Somewhere in the recesses of their hard-wired craniums, BINGO must have gotten transposed into the ubiquitous end-of-class re-mark, *"Any questions?"* Three arms sprang up instantaneously.

"Excuse me, Doctor Green, I have a question and then I'd like a follow-up, if I may?"

If you closed your eyes (and held your nose), the intensity of the rapid-fire interrogation made you think of a State Department press briefing. That was, of course, unless you took the subject matter into ac-count. "First, how exactly would you rate the consistency of bovine #6's fecal matter? Does it fall within the range of normal limits or would you consider it diarrheic? And, as a follow up, if it is an abnormally runny stool, what are your top differential diagnoses?"

Jack Doyle turned to his new friend Sam Stone, "Jesus, Mary, and Joseph... We don't have to stand — or even sit — for this. This is a party." He paused and then jumped down from the risers, "I'm hungry. Wanna' get something to eat?"

Sam let his long, lean body stretch over three rows. He remained "seat-ed," clad in a white tee, faded Levi straight legs and ostrich-hide pointers.

Jack looked back, confused, "You're staying for *this*?"

Sam Stone gave a molasses nod then motioned with the brim of his cap toward the bingo field.

Jack replied, "Yeah we know... Doctor Green's gonna be there dealing with FRoGs 'til the cows come home. Let's get outta' here."

Eyes still trained on the action, Sam rotated his head from side to side, "Look closah." Jack surveyed the field. He saw Dr. Green on the microphone discussing Bovine Viral Diarrhea, 20 Guernseys with massive swinging udders chewing their cud while continuously making "pies," and their two friends cleaning up after them. Hoss and Kerri were currently scooping up the *number two* that produced the O-4 winner. Jack noticed, over Dr. Green's left shoulder, that somehow Kerri managed what appeared to be a Vogue-quality runway performance. While keeping her weight forward, so her spiked heels didn't spear the muddy turf, she was simultaneously operating the steaming, manure-loaded shovel with only the thumb and first two fingers of each hand. Her pinkies pointed delicately up and away from the offensive instrument of manual labor. It was almost as if she were holding a teacup and saucer.

And then Jack saw what held Sam's attention.

Betsy, the O-4 generator, had moved about three feet away from the site of her last deposit and had assumed the most logical next position. She planted all four hooves, stood stock-still like a sawhorse, and fixed her gaze on somewhere far away. It was obvious from the animal's unblinking stare that she was deep in cow thought, or, perhaps just taking aim.

"Oh—my—God," said Jack.

"Ain't it great," added Sam.

Jack nodded once, smiled and then made the sign of the cross to make up for the pleasure he was about to receive.

Betsy arched her back ever so slightly, giving her midsection that characteristic saddle-like appearance. Unfortunately — or fortunately, depending on your point of view — Hoss was too busy positioning the bucket to notice as the animal's manure-tipped tail began to slowly rise.

Jack reported in a NASA monotone, "All systems go," then turned his head slowly and added, "Shit..."

"Naw, I don't think so," whispered Sam.

The stream was a perfect golden arc. The rope of hot, sticky fluid hit the back of Kerri's knee, 2 inches above the top of her left boot and because she was leaning forward, a nice gap enabled instantaneous filling. Her shock was expected, but the events of the next few seconds were not.

Kerri responded reflexively (that's the ancient cow-pee response reflex) by taking weight off her warm, soggy left leg and then spinning on her right to face the bovine assailant. Unfortunately, this rotation drilled her right heel deeply into the ground and lurched her center of gravity backward. As Kerri staggered, snapping off the heel, her arms sprang up shooting the fresh-baked meadow muffins vertically. Just like a fallen water skier who can't seem to let go of the rope, Kerri still gripped the shovel now with all ten brightly painted fingers as she landed flat on her back in the soft turf. The projectiles rocketed straight up and were lost in the thick night air.

Sensing the trajectory, Jack stated with admiration, "Nice, very nice." *Splat-Plop-Squish.*

Luckily, or so it would seem, Kerri was only pelted by two of the chunks — one impacted her left thigh and one grazed her right shoulder. But then Kerri's luck ran out. As if the splatter and spray from the torrential urine downpour wasn't bad enough, Betsy shifted her stance directing the last few gallons for the final coup. The garden-hose flow caught Kerri squarely in the Angora and then trailed off, dribbling across her previously unaffected miniskirt. It was over. Apparently satisfied and relieved, Betsy blinked twice, chewed once, and moseyed away. She and the FRoGs were oblivious to the laughter pouring from the two first years in the stands.

In between gasps for breath, Jack said, "Okay, my stomach hurts, no more laughing for a week."

"Ay-yuh," Sam chimed in, "I think I pulled my spleen." Then he added, "Now, I am hungry. Wondah what they have?"

Jack replied, "The guy in the toga from Alpha Mu gave me a flyer." He produced the simple photocopied sheet which was filled to the brim with hyperbole.

Sam skimmed the flyer, "Looks like the major food groups are represented. Why don't we just wander the Midway?"

"THE TESTICLE FESTIVAL: First Years, you got Balls!"
(sponsored by your friends at Alpha Mu)

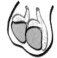

Congratulations on surviving your tests!!!

  FREE BEER.
  FREE BEER *(did we mention? Free Beer!)*

Club Booths—

The Feline Club
The Bovine Club
The Sheep and Goat Club
The Colic Team
The Equine Club
SCAVA *(Student Chapter of the American Veterinary
  Association)*
Theriogenology Club *(Come on over to our Kissing Booth and
  then See who's going down in the Dunking Booth)*
The Swine Club
The Zoo and Wildlife Clubs
AAVV (American Association of Veterinary Vegetarians)
Vets for God Club

Rides—

Back by popular demand: "The Bullinator" (Alpha Mu)
Hay Rides (Equine Club)

Competitions—

Model Yacht Races on the Cesspool (Swine Club)
Build a Better Artificial Vagina (Therio Club)
Rocky Mountain Oyster Eating Contest (Therio Club)
Cow Pie Bingo (Bovine Club)
Horse Shoes (Equine Club)
Dart your Favorite Professor (Zoo and Wildlife Clubs)
Meat Judging (US Department of Agriculture)

Great Food at every Booth!!!!

Including: Funnel Cakes / Elephant Ears; Pig Roast; Hot
Dogs / Hamburgers / Corn Dogs; Cotton Candy and much, much
more!

At the University of Philadelphia's School of Veterinary Medicine, Friday Night Happy Hour events are more than just parties. More than pressure relief. They form an elemental agar. Just as animal cells require glucose, water and lipids, at a molecular level, vet students require beer, laughter and each other. You couldn't survive vet school alone nor would you ever want to try.

Many Happy Hours were subtle affairs held in the lounge outside of Room 13, but special events, such as the Testicle Festival, required the expanse and ease of the large animal campus. Where else could you put on a full-fledged country fair with a veterinary flare? And although hundreds of first through fourth years, faculty, interns and residents milled, joked and drank, the large animal hospital was still very much in operation. In between party announcements, pages could be heard, "Doctor Linnehan, please report to the NIC-U. Code blue." Nurses and seniors in scrubs on duty, scurried from surgery to post-op, glancing longingly at the party and then their watches.

Booths lined the space between two of the long, low hospital barns. Barn A housed the general, non-critical equine cases, and Barn B was reserved for sheep, goats and an occasional sow. Jack purchased a funnel cake from the Feline Club and the pure-white powdered sugar must have tickled his nose, because he coughed and sputtered after the first bite. Sam bought a corn dog and then won a stuffed cobra at the Zoo and Wildlife's blow-dart shoot. He popped the balloon adorned with a caricature of Dr. Green on his second shot.

The duo had been strolling the Midway, laughing and wisecracking, when Jack was stopped dead in his tracks. "Well, would you look at that." He paused and then added in awe, "What are the odds..?" As luck would have it, the American Association of Veterinary Vegetarians' booth (co-sponsored by the Animal Liberty Militia) was sandwiched smack dab between the Swine Club's pig roast and the USDA meat judging contest. Jack concluded, "Oh, that is rich..."

"Step right up little lady, step right up." The "carnie" behind the counter hocked his wares. "Correctly identify the cut and grade and win a canned ham!" An attractive female second year fanned her cheek with her hand, batted her eyelids coyly and replied in her best southern belle, "Why thank you kind sir, how could a lady refuse such a gentlemanly offer?" She turned to face Sam and batted her eyelashes some more. He smiled, plunked down fifty cents, and they waited for the challenge.

The beefy USDA vet wore a spotless below-the-knee lab coat, white plastic hardhat and gleaming shop goggles. He bawled over his shoulder, "FRESH MEAT, I need FRESH MEAT." His assistant in identical garb pulled a shiny, marbled mass from a cooler and slapped it down on a glistening white cutting board. The girl hesitated, pretending to think, and then answered, "Rump Roast, Grade A, Choice?"

"We have a WIENER!" The lab coat trumpeted, "We have a wiener. See folks, fifty cents can win you a canned ham. Step right up and judge that meat!"

Jack noticed that every time the guy yelled the word "meat," the lead veganarian's face briefly flushed with color. He watched as she cupped her pale, nearly lifeless hands to form a megaphone and counter the carnivorous assault, "Tofu, uh, it can lower your cholesterol by three to seven points, umm, if you eat at least 25 grams per day, for a year… And uh, soy milk, it's not just for breakfast anymore." The fish-belly white slabs of frigid, wet tofu was so repulsive, it parted the sea of fair goers. The crowd was evenly bifurcated by, and uniformly disinterested in, the pasty white booth staffed by pasty white people with their pasty white product. She continued, "Research shows that soy is chock full of isoflavones and daily drinkers can extend their life expectancy by up to 1.2 years."

Sam muttered under his breath, "I'd be a *daily drinkah* if I looked like them."

Jack noticed Anna at the back of the booth carving a tofurkey so he sauntered up to the counter and warmly called out, "Hey, Anna."

She spun around and paused. He wondered if she didn't look a little lost. "What do you want?"

He shrugged his shoulders, "I just thought I'd say hi," and then added, "Nice, err, nice booth you guys got here."

She wasn't convinced, it was weak. "Very funny, pig boy. Why aren't you over there swilling beer with the Swine Club for Men?" He looked to his left at the 300-pound porker with an apple in its mouth rotating on a spit. He couldn't help but grin at the boisterous, rib-munching, beer drinkers. They wore bib "overalls" without shirts, stubby plastic pig noses and curly pink pipe cleaners protruded from their butts. He thought, in their defense, they weren't all guzzling beer. Some sipped clear fluid from Mason jars — the club's proprietary distillate, "swine shine." Just then a thick cloud of fat-laden smoke wafted over Anna. She coughed and leaned on her cane. Jack was about to fire back that Anna was being sexist, but realized that she was at least partially correct. There wasn't a girl in the bunch. It was indeed a boars-only, Swine Club for Men. In fact, the scene could have doubled for a Hee Haw rerun, with one exception. Rick Larson, in starched shirt and tie, was passing plates of steaming pork to a throng of customers. Jack watched their class treasurer making change from his pocket with one hand, and stuffing the proceeds into a big, fat piggy bank with the other.

The overhead speakers hissed back to life, "Attention-Attention. The rodeo is about to begin!" Mike sounded as if he was announcing a monster truck rally, "Annnnnd, the first event is BULLLLL Riding." He paused then added, "The ONLY event is BULLLLL Riding."

Jack looked back at Anna who eyed him defiantly. He shook his head slowly and said, "Okay, sorry I bothered," and set off towards the bullring with Sam.

In addition to orchestrating the annual festival, Alpha Mu, the School's resident veterinary fraternity, had also rented a mechanical bull. Since Mike had just relocated from bingo to the bullring, he was still warming up at the pneumatic controls. With a joystick and two buttons, he put the "Bullinator" through its paces. The rider-less, leather-bound pommel beast was a life-sized mockup of a real bull. Mike started it low to the ground then gradually raised it up, gently bucking its hind end. He spun it to the left and then to the right, eventually throwing in fits of rabid bucking, cuts, jumps, and stalls. Satisfied, Mike brought the mechanical beast to rest just as the first rider approached. It was Mike's date du jour, Miss Colorado, 1987.

Mike tipped his imaginary hat, "Howdy Ma'am," as she smiled her greeting and strode confidently into the ring. After giving the machine a playful slap on its rump, Miss Colorado took in the crowd while chalking her left hand. A moment later, she raised her right and delivered the classic beauty queen wave into the charged night air.

Mike announced, "Miss Colorado, Nancy-Sue Gatlin, is ready to RUM—BLE!" The crowd responded with applause, whistles and cat calls. Two rodeo clowns ran in with mock sections of fence — one for each side of the "bull." The beauty queen sprang, catlike, to the top rails and stood completely erect, straddling the ride.

Jack noticed that Miss Colorado's leather chaps and faded jeans framed an amazing sight. Mesmerized, he poked Hoss in the ribs with his elbow then turned to Sam and said, "Absolutely spectacular…"

The cover girl lifted her pure white Stetson, slowly shook out her long platinum mane and waved to the crowd again. Mike reacted by playfully rocking the "bull" left and then the right into the fence. Miss Colorado tipped her head back, laughed, flashed a brilliant smile and then blithely mounted the machine. After lashing her chalked palm to its back, she raised her right hand and nodded to signal that she was ready. The horn blared, the clock started, and the gates were whipped away.

Mike showed no mercy. He took the mechanical bull out of the imaginary box and went instantly into a fast right spin, bucking roughly several times and then slammed on the brakes. He then cut hard to the left dipping the front end down and in. Miss Colorado was unfazed. Her head remained a stable center of control while her body flowed and sparkled like mercury. The clock on the scoreboard ticked away: 3 seconds, 4 seconds, 5 seconds… and then Mike took the bull into its final rhythmic, high-kicking sequence. Miss Colorado synched easily with the rhythm, laying back and into each rise and fall. Her smile morphed, reflecting something more intense as she closed her eyes and wrapped her legs tightly around the hot leather for the last 3 seconds. She climaxed the perfect ride at the buzzer with a long, exclamatory, "Yesss!" and then, just like a real rodeo, with a real bull, Mike kept the power on. The machine pounded ahead like a locomotive. At the end of one dazzling spin the beauty untied her left hand. On the upstroke of the next mechanical kick, she swung her leg over its back and dismounted by spinning 180 degrees, landing solidly on both feet. Miss Colorado sprang back on the soft mats, extending both hands in the air like a gymnast.

There was a noticeable lag before the audience exploded in applause. A refractory period was required for nearly every guy there to scoop his jaw off the floor. Jack put his left arm around Sam's shoulder and his right around Hoss. He turned his head, looking at each of them, and then declared, "I don't know about you boys, but I *love* vet school."

Mike shouted into the microphone, "A perfect ride. Come folks, give it up for this cowgirl extraordinaire!" They clapped and whistled as the woman sauntered out of the limelight.

"Now folks," Mike strode into the ring with microphone in hand, "it's time to recognize the top two first years!" The crowd clapped some more. "They have finished their first major round of testing and I'm happy to report that the top-ranked, male *and* female newbies are in my very own orientation group. The grades were posted and you've all been to the Wailing Wall, so the rest of you know where you stand."

"Will Jack Doyle," he hesitated, "and Anna Heywood please come forward?"

"Whooo-hoooo," whooped Sam and Hoss. They were proud of Jack's Death Row representation. Jack grinned as he was more or less propelled forward via back slaps and attaboys. Ultimately, he stood next to Mike and waited, but Anna was nowhere to be seen.

"Anna, Anna Heywood, are you out there?" Everyone looked around, until finally some movement was seen.

Petunia, Anna's guide dog, pushed her way forward, "Come on hon, let's get this over with." Anna, steadied by her cane, moved with a difficulty that contrasted sharply with the supple display the crowd had just witnessed.

When she finally reached the center of the ring, Mike announced, "Let's hear it for the King and Queen!" Applause went up as he placed the paper Burger King crowns on their heads. Then, almost naturally, members of the Swine Club started clinking their mason jars with greasy plastic knives, *tink-tink-tink*, *tink-tink-tink*, the universal signal for the "happy couple" to smooch.

The proprietor of the kissing booth chimed in, "Come on, one kiss for charity! Who will give a buck to see these two kids kiss?" A dozen hands sprang up, then dozens more, until finally, over a hundred hands were waving, everyone chanting: "*KISS—KISS—KISS...*"

Anna lanced Jack with her eyes. With all the whooo-hoooing and clapping filling the gaps between the stars of that summer night, he had to practically yell for her to hear him. "WHAT?? DON'T LOOK AT ME THAT WAY, I didn't plan this." Then he added what he thought would help, "I DON'T EVEN *WANT* TO KISS YOU!"

His words produced the opposite of their desired effect. Anna hissed, "I could just spit."

Jack countered, "Kiss now, spit later" and then leaned into her, put his hands on her hips and pressed his lips gently to hers. For an instant, her eyes met his and they saw where they were and Jack couldn't believe what he was feeling — Anna wasn't resisting. Her lips pursed and then parted subtly; the effect on Jack was atomic. The noisy crowd faded into the background and he felt a surge in his parasympathetic core. He couldn't help himself. He started to pull her hips toward him but then noticed her eyes widening. The next feeling for him was a new one — a swirling mixture of intense pleasure and sharp pain. Anna pulled her right hand back, made a tight fist, hauled off and slugged him hard in the chest, right where the big red "S" would have been. Jack dropped like a sack of potatoes and the crowd exploded with laughter.

"Did you see that?" blinked Hoss.

Sam replied, "Now, *that* was christly spectacular... She cold-cocked him!" The crowd shifted into a TKO count down: "one thousand one— one thousand two—one thousand three..."

Jack coughed and sputtered. He shook the stars out of his head and then looked up at Anna.

Placing her cane on his chest, pinning him in place like a bug she warned, *"Next time, ask first."*

Jack nodded, whispering to himself, "Next time…"

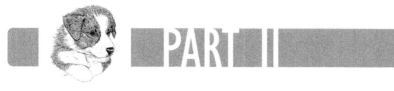

PART I

Veterinary School Interviews (continued)

Two adjacent rooms in the old veterinary school building at the University of Philadelphia, School of Veterinary Medicine

Interviewer, Room 1: "In your opinion, what makes a great veterinarian?"

Applicant: Sam Stone didn't have to think about his answer but he did rein in his Mainer accent, "The same things that make any human great: compassion, kindness, mastery of elemental skills, intelligence and a sense of humor. I believe that a veterinarian should aspire to be well-rounded, as versed in medicine and surgery as art and great literature." He paused as he remembered his grandfather's words, a man should be complete. An understandable goal when you subsist on an island five miles out in the Gulf of Maine.

Interviewer, Room 1: "Speaking of literature, what was the last book you read?"

Applicant: Though the interviewer couldn't appreciate the herculean struggle this represented for Sam, he responded, "I'm working on three projects right now. The Odyssey by Homer, Zen and the Art of Motorcycle Maintenance, and transcripts of Steve Mahtin's standup work."

Interviewer, Room 1: The interviewer smiled and noted, "Likes Steve Martin" followed by a check mark in Sam's file.

◄ • ►

Interviewer, Room 2: "Can you describe your animal experience in more detail?"

Applicant: Without hesitation the young woman replied, "I have no animal experience."

Interviewer, Room 2: "But, you indicated on your application that you've assisted at the Uptown Feline Clinic for the past six years. And, you have glowing letters of recommendation from three of the practice's veterinarians?"

Applicant: This time, Kerri Feinburg thought for a moment before she responded, "Oh, I see what you're getting at. But you don't really believe that cats are just animals, do you?"

Interviewer, Room 2: The interviewer eyed Kerri's chinchilla stole, trying to decide if it was faux or real, and checked a box next to the words, "Minimal Animal Experience."

CHAPTER TWELVE

Mrs. Oliver

1:10 PM — MONDAY, OCTOBER 10, 1988

Examination Room #2, the small animal Emergency Service at VHUP in Philadelphia

Veterinarians are taught that over 70% of all meaningful diagnostic information can be found within a patient's oral history. This is true. Sometimes, even more can be learned if we listen.

Recounting her companion's most recent history, Mrs. Irene Oliver patted the ancient retriever's silky smooth head. And, even though she had pinned her mother's Elgin broach on her left lapel to draw attention away from the fraying hemline of her deep purple and black hound's-tooth dress, she still fingered the fibers with the other trembling hand.

"Doctor, he bumps into things. Especially when we're outside during the day." Mrs. Oliver paused to catch her breath and then continued, "Nothing major mind you, he still knows when it's safe to cross the street, but when he bumps into little things, so do I…" She started a light chuckle which turned into a cough. After raising a gray hankie to cover her nose and mouth she added, "He's just not as sharp as he used to be. I'm feeling pretty dull myself." Mrs. Oliver gingerly placed the handkerchief on her lap and then drew a shaky hand across her forehead, "It's early for flu season, isn't it?"

Flo Kimball replied warmly, "You're right, Mrs. Oliver, it does seem a little early for flu season." Dr. Kimball brushed back her cascading red hair and continued, "You've owned Clancy for how long now?"

"You mean, how long has he *owned me?* I'm very much in his care. It'll be ten years next month. He's my golden oldie." She paused to think and then added, "He still eats well, but wants to tinkle more than usual."

Dr. Kimball reached down and cradled Clancy's soft, graying muzzle in the palm of her hand and said, "I think I should perform a thorough eye exam, would that be okay?"

Mrs. Oliver used her right hand to adjust her dark glasses — they covered nearly a third of her still-beautiful face — and then offered up the harness handle. Mrs. Oliver knew that this was why they were at the vet school, but the implication still took some time to sink in. "Of course, we'd greatly appreciate it."

A quiet knock came at the door. Mike London and his first-year advisees entered the room. "Mrs. Oliver, it's wonderful to see you again," he took her hand, gave her a peck on the cheek and patted Clancy. The dog's soft face smiled up at Mike with a lolling tongue while the long, feathery tail swooshed from side to side, fanning the linoleum behind him.

"Doctor Mike, it's good to hear you," She coughed again and turned in Florence Kimball's direction. "Doctor Mike saved Clancy's life last year. I'm so thankful he was in your emergency room that night."

"You're too generous Mrs. Oliver, I just helped a bit. You were never in any danger of losing him."

She shook her head, "No, we owe you a lot."

Mike grinned, "You mean you haven't paid the bill yet..?" They both laughed and then he continued, "Mrs. Oliver, I'd like you to meet some first-year students. This is Mr. Hugman, Mr. Doyle, and Ms. Heywood."

Jack stepped up without hesitation, offered his hand and said, "Hello, Mrs. Oliver." The woman stuck out her right hand and Jack automatically closed the gap, "I'm Jack Doyle. It's nice to meet you."

The elderly woman nodded her head silently, gathering her thoughts, "Nice firm grip. I think you've already been established doing something to help others." Jack blinked, he wasn't sure how to respond so he looked to Mike who dipped his head urging Jack to follow his instincts.

"Yes, Ma'am, I was a K-9 cop before this. I did try to help people."

"Ah, that explains it, yes," she kept his hand in hers. "Mr. Oliver, my Henry, he was a police officer, too. Thank you for taking care of us dear," she concluded, "then and now."

Hoss followed suit, "Pleasure, Ma'am."

"Lots of gentle strength and kindness here."

Then Anna stepped up. Drawn to the woman, she did something she'd never done before. She cupped Mrs. Oliver's unseeing hand in both of hers. Anna winced protectively — it was one thing to presume that others saw her as a cold, distant fish, it was quite another to hear it straight up. "Oh dear," Mrs. Oliver smiled warmly, "what confidence and intelligence." Anna relaxed almost imperceptibly. "And, underneath it all, compassion. You are going to make a fine veterinarian, dear."

Jack choked back a laugh that was ignored as a cough by everyone but Anna. Not relinquishing the warm grip, her head whipped around and the centrifugal force launched daggers at him. She wanted to hurt Jack again, but refocused her attention. "Thank you, Mrs. Oliver," and she squeezed the kind woman's hand in both of hers.

Dr. Kimball interrupted clinically, "Well folks, how about we examine this very *patient* patient." Mike gently scooped Clancy up, placing him on the exam table while Dr. Kimball dimmed the lights and retrieved the ophthalmoscope from a charger nearby.

Flo asked, "Can you steady his head for me?" So Mike wrapped an arm around Clancy and then placed one hand behind his head and the other gently under his muzzle. He inclined the dog's nose upward slightly. Turning to the first years, the professor instructed, "It's important to always conduct a systematic evaluation of the eye. I suggest that you start outside, work your way inward and then back to the retina." She used the small light beam projecting from the ophthalmoscope to highlight the fur around one eye. "I look for signs of discharge or swelling first. Then we check the white part of the globe, the sclera, and it should be just that — white. Cue ball white in young animals. If the eye is *bloodshot*, or the more appropriate clinical term *injected*, this is where you'll see it best. Or, if the sclera appears yellowish this could indicate a systemic problem such as liver disease." Dr. Kimball redirected, "Mike, what's your assessment of these?"

Mike didn't hesitate, "They look great." He added, "Good boy, Clancy." The animal's unrestrained tail swooshed across the table top in response.

"Everybody take a look. This is how normal sclera should appear."

Mrs. Oliver smiled and said, "That's nice to hear."

Patient examinations in a veterinary teaching hospital can be lengthy affairs. The client trades speed for thoroughness and expertise. Three primary variables control an exam's duration: the complexity of the case; the level of patient cooperation; and the type of students involved — fortunately for Clancy and Mrs. Oliver, there wasn't a FRoG in the bunch today.

Flo Kimball went on to explain that the cornea should be crystal clear and the iris should rapidly respond to light. She flicked the beam across Clancy's right eye to demonstrate the pupillary reflex, "Mr. Doyle, when exposed to bright light, is the pupil's response active or passive?"

Jack wrinkled his brow and thought for a moment; the gap was just long enough for Anna to jump in. "It's active," she interjected, "in both directions. In bright light, concentric smooth muscle contracts to decrease the aperture of the pupil. In dim light, the radial muscles contract pulling the iris back to let more light in," she added, "like Venetian blinds."

Mrs. Oliver said with a nod, "Confident and smart."

Dr. Kimball examined the deeper structures then murmured, "Uh-huh," and handed the instrument to Mike. "Just behind the iris is the lens and this is where you should all be able to visualize the problem."

Mrs. Oliver readjusted her dark glasses, cleared her throat, and then asked with a waver in her voice, "Is the problem, is it the glaucoma?"

"Oh no, Mrs. Oliver, it's not serious, just small lenticular cataracts." She added for clarification, "A little clouding in the center of the lens, nothing we can't deal with. When Clancy is in dim light, his pupils dilate letting more light around these opacities. That's why he sees better indoors and at night."

Mike handed the scope to Hoss. The first year engulfed the silver-handled, black plastic lollipop in his right hand and did exactly what 95% of all novices do — he positioned the keyhole in front of his dominant eye, flicked the switch and *whamo*, Hoss saw stars. He had the ophthalmoscope flipped exactly backwards, the piercing white beam lit up *his* retina and at point-blank range. Jack chuckled as Mike led Hoss shuffling to a chair and sat him down. "Just keep your eyes closed, it happens to everyone."

Jack, learning from his sidelined friend, clicked on the light, aimed it into his palm and then with the correct orientation put the instrument up to his eye. But his capable start quickly bumbled and stalled. Peering through the tiny lens, Jack could barely find the entire dog let alone the animal's eye. The circular light beam scanned and panned blindly across Clancy's golden fur as if a flea had attempted a prison break. The little round disk of light circled Clancy's head, paused briefly on his right ear then went downward, finally landing on the table. Anna smirked in silence as Mike clamped Jack's head with both of his hands and guided the searchlight towards the medial canthus of the left eye. Jack said, "Thanks," and then after a moment of fumbling he did what every good newbie should, he said, "Oh, okay, I see it," even though he didn't have a clue. Rather than stressing this sweet dog or wasting even more time, he instinctively knew that his time was up.

Mike said, "Don't worry, it'll come," and handed off the instrument to Anna who proceeded to describe the small blobs with a precision that demonstrated she was actually looking at the lesion.

"I see three cloudy wisps, probably a millimeter across, in the center of the right lens and one in the left."

Dr. Kimball nodded, "Well done," and turned to face the client. "Mrs. Oliver, I'd like to draw a small sample of blood if that's okay. We should probably rule out diabetes and we will double check for glaucoma, but I doubt that's an issue." She reached over and flipped on the room lights. The jump in intensity caused everyone but Mrs. Oliver to squint and blink.

"Of course, I just want to make sure he's okay." Mrs. Oliver coughed twice and again covering her mouth with her handkerchief added, "I was going to the doctor's myself today, but I'd like to wait for Clancy's results."

Mike interceded, "No Mrs. Oliver, you should keep your appointment. I'll call you when we know the outcome. And, please don't worry about Clancy's eyes, if necessary the cataracts can easily be removed."

Mike and his students watched as her shoulders relaxed. "I was starting to wonder if we'd have to find a seeing-eye animal for him. He does love kittens. But then I'd probably spend most of my day chasing mice!"

Mike added with a smile, "Or worse, scratching in the litter box…"

CHAPTER THIRTEEN

Dead Animal Medicine: Part I (Stan the Path Man)

The large animal necropsy room at the Center for Large Animal Medicine in Kennett Square

"Crows? We're working on *crows*?" Simon JJ Harding III was incredulous. He didn't even try to mask his feelings. Like most prejudice, his was a parentally amplified predilection.

At Harding's Dog and Cat Hospital, the focus was clear. Occasionally a loss leader was endured, for example a beloved budgie disposal for a burgeoning borzoi breeder. But wildlife medicine? That was fringe. As JJ Senior counseled his teary-eyed, five-year-old boy holding a cracked-shell reptilian (with a wag of his finger and a mixed metaphor to boot), "Remember son, like tie dye or exceeding the posted speed limit, the Harding's do not treat turtles! Who pays the bill?"

Dr. Violet Green was physiologically unable to comprehend such distinctions, and since she was unaware of JJ's impersonal history, she reached another conclusion, "I'm sorry, I know you guys wanted to tag along on rounds at the zoo but," her biceps bulged as she lifted the two heavy-gauge, black plastic bags filled with avian bodies, "this situation takes precedence. Let's get suited up."

Suiting up to work in the vet school's necropsy room was not dissimilar to preparing for a search and recovery mission in a contaminated nuclear power plant. Necropsy was a dangerous place — a biohazard-impregnated hot zone where the sickest of the sick patients ended up. The dead ones. You can't get much sicker than dead. And even though the nonporous walls, stainless steel tables and implements of investigation (cleavers, hack saws, pruning shears and knives) were routinely decontaminated, at any given moment you were likely to be up to your elbows in animal juice laced with botulism, tetanus, or even rabies.

Dr. Green and her students began by donning a base layer of scrubs. Unlike the hallowed jade surgical scrubs, these robin's-egg icons of medicine would never see the life of day. Sporting a skull and crossbones and the words "NECROPSY ONLY" scrawled in black permanent marker across the front, they were confined to the darker side of veterinary practice. After duct taping knee-high plastic booties over her sneakers, tying on a surgical mask, and pulling on a full-length face shield, Dr. Green got JJ prepped. She tied the strings of his yellow vinyl apron in a neat bow behind him at his waist and then strung a thin, elastic cord around the back of his neck — suspenders for a pair of evening-gown length, clear plastic rectal gloves.

JJ's classmate, a female first year, snickered to their senior advisor, "I'll be the belle of the ball." The fourth year replied, "Yeah, the Monster Ball," then added with a smile, "and here comes the prince."

Dr. Stan Oblitzski — Stan the Path Man — exclaimed, "Violet! What'd you bring today? Anything cool?" Without waiting for a response, he turned to the students and spluttered with an infectious passion only a pathologist could display, "Violet always has the coolest cases! Vi, Violet, remember the day you brought in the humpback head, three poison dart frogs and a bison..? Remember that Vi? And remember — remember vertebrae day?" He turned back to face JJ, his eyebrows raised so high they were almost mid-forehead, "A twenty foot python and an adult giraffe. It was SO cool."

"Yes, Stan, I do remember. That was last week..." Violet Green laughed and shook her head. If Stan Oblitzski were a puppy, he'd be wagging his entire hind end and piddling with excitement.

The necropsy room — in fact the whole subspecialty of animal pathology — was a repository for veterinarians who were different. Irregular. Just this side of eccentric. Pathologists can't be shoehorned, even with copious amounts of K-Y, into the usual animal-lover form of the regular vet. Of course they care immensely about animal life, and are arguably as smart or even smarter than their brethren in other demanding specialties like soft-tissue surgery and internal medicine. But guys like ACVP board-certified, Dr. Stan Oblitzski are missing a gene or two. Specifically, the genes that code for social enzymes. Enzymes that catalyze the production of empathetic dialogue between animal doctors and pet owners. For instance, a sentence that should sound like: "Mrs. Smith, I am so sorry to tell you that Fifi has cancer," comes out of a pathologist as, "Oh my God, Fifi has the coolest, most invasive hemangiosarcoma I've seen in a looong time… She's absolutely riddled with it. *You wanna' see?*" So, it's a win-win situation that well-meaning, brilliant guys like Stan Oblitzski are cloistered in necropsy, out of general veterinary circulation.

The pathologically-clad first years splashed through a disinfectant foot bath and entered gross necropsy. The students shivered as they drew the chilled air into their lungs. A fat, hairy housefly sputtered slowly like a World War I biplane around their heads in a big, looping circle, *buzzzz—buzz—buzzzz.* The female first year watched as the hypothermic bug got distracted by a three-foot-long cluster of ice-blue fluorescent tubes mounted high on the wall. She whispered, "Don't go to the light…" just before a sharp electrical *ZZITTT* and phosphorescent burst made her flinch.

The three students waddled along in tow like baby ducklings following their mom to one of the massive hydraulic lift tables. Dr. Green dumped out the contents of the first bag — 14 crows, three scarlet ibis and two Chilean flamingoes. Before she could sort the pile, Stan dashed over from the opposite corner of the room, his plastic booties allowing him to slide sideways to a wavering stop just like Tom Cruise in *Risky Business*. But very much unlike Tom Cruise, with a fake microphone in his hand and stylish Ray-Bans on his boyish face, Stan the Path Man's beady eyes peered out though a pair of blood splattered, wood shop safety goggles. He pointed to the birds with an ungloved hand as tomato-tinged mayonnaise dripped from his BLT, "Flamingoes and ibis and crows, Oh my…" He looked to Violet, "Follow the yellow brick road. It's a gold mine!"

Violet Green smiled at her former classmate. She adored Stan Oblitzski because what you saw was what you got. He was entirely without pretense, 99.9% ego-free. The asylum of pathology and the relative biosecurity of the necropsy room fostered the perfect environment for him to thrive. He was free to flex his special kind of veterinary muscle, to become a topnotch forensic sleuth. One might think that when a patient died the pressure was off, but in fact the opposite was usually true. It was then that you knew you had a proven killer on your hands. And, especially in herd health cases, other lives were now at risk.

"Vi, let me know what you need: aerobic, anaerobic or fungal cultures, fluorescent antibody or tox screens. Whatever I can do to help." Stan paused because the option of tox screens reminded him of Violet's favorite case, "How's our friend Mya the lady lion doing? She's got to be getting pretty big by now."

Violet let out a low sigh, "Honestly Stan, I don't know how she's doing, she's gone. The park shipped her to someplace in Texas." She shook her head, "I can't talk about it just yet."

Stan was surprised by the news. He knew how much this one animal life meant to Violet, but figured she'd tell him more when she was ready. So he just replied, "Hmmm, 10-4," then flat-palmed the rest of the BLT into his mouth and pointed towards the remnants of a once-massive milker. Sputtering flecks of bread he said, "I'll be over there helping the kids finish that Holstein."

The cow to which Stan was referring was split from stem to stern and the floor around it ran with a mixture of clotted blood, grassy rumen contents and streaks of blue-white fluid. Violet, Stan and the first years watched as two fourth-year students stood back to back and then sloshed, high-stepping away from each other. After counting out ten paces, they spun around for an impromptu duel. Each hugged a quarter of the udder under an arm like bagpipes and gripping the teat squeezed out long jets of milk. One parodied Bob Hope singing, "Thanks… for the mammaries," but then in true, budding pathologist style, she stopped in mid squirt to pool a sample in her hand and remarked, "Hey, this is pretty thick, I bet it's hyper-cellular… I wonder what her IgG profile looks like?"

Stan swallowed the sandwich wad and JJ stared as the mass slid behind the pathologist's pointy Adam's apple, down his pencil neck and disappeared into his thoracic inlet. Stan the Path Man burped and then with a shoulder shrug concluded, "All work and no play…" broke away from their group and skidded over to the cow.

"Okay," Violet Green refocused and emptied the other body bag on a second nearby table for the students to examine. "Let's divide and conquer. This is the perfect opportunity to learn because we've got multiple individuals from three species." She paused and then added, "JJ, why don't you work with me over here."

She plunged in, "So where should we start?"

JJ squinted, "Well, everybody hates crows. I would guess they were poisoned, so let's look in their stomachs."

Violet held up a gloved hand, "Whoa, hold on, poisoning is a possibility, but we need to back up. Let's start with the history. You're good at asking questions, correct?"

JJ's female classmate looked up to their senior advisor and muttered grimly, "If good at asking questions equals blindingly annoying, then he's incredible." The girl thought that prompting JJ to ask *more* questions was like encouraging the little Dutch boy to give complicated directions that required lots of pointing... If the dike broke loose, they were all in deep trouble.

Dr. Green took a deep breath, "As the veterinarian, what do you want to know?"

JJ blinked and stepped up to the plate, "Uh, where were they found?"

"Excellent. These guys were found over the last three days and all were in or around the Lagoons' exhibit." She paused and then added, "Other information you'd want to know is that we have some clinically affected birds still alive. Two flamingoes are ADR and mildly ataxic."

JJ asked in a skeptical tone, "The zoo has a crow exhibit?"

"No, they're wild but were found on park grounds," replied Dr. Green.

"Wild? Who's gonna pay for them? The zoo can't be happy with this."

"That is an excellent observation and to tell you the truth it's a situation that every administrator will ask you to defend." She continued to teach as she dipped a black bird in a tub of water to keep the feathers from flying. "They'll probably say something like, 'Why do we care about crows and other wildlife? We're a zoo, we need to take care of our own.'"

JJ nodded and blinked again, he was glad that he'd asked another good question.

"The answer is simple. It's because we're all connected. None of us — not the animals in the zoo, nor the people in this community — lives in a vacuum. What affects one, affects us all. When crows die like this, we know that something is wrong. You almost never find one dead corvid let alone a dozen." She could tell he was still confused. She shook her head, "Look, the administrator's job is to save money, but your job," she paused, "you're going to be a vet so your job is to try do the right thing even if people get upset. You're the animals' advocate. Who else can speak for them?"

JJ thought for a moment and then raised his right arm. Dr. Green stopped, took in the student standing before her and made a knee-jerk but accurate diagnosis.

"Where do you sit in class?" JJ's arm retracted. "From now on, avoid the front rows." She reiterated for clarity, "No sitting in the front row."

JJ practically swooned — he was rapidly spiraling into the first stages of shock. Not expecting this kind of information, the words hit him like a physical blow. He had to try to reject this prescription somehow. The front row was and would always be his home. From the first time that alphabetized seating was no longer required in school, he naturally floated to the front row of every class. The forward pull of the front row was as real as the gravity that kept his butt in his chair after the bell rang. He was accomplished at pushing the subconscious facts that he was geeky, nerdy, and unpopular to the back of his mind. He shoved those thoughts behind him like the students in every class. If he sat up there, and they weren't in his peripheral vision, he felt safe. Just being under the nose of the teacher afforded him a measure of comfort but it had the added benefits (or so he thought) of showing the teacher how much he cared about the subject, how much he liked the teacher, and, he deduced that it shortened the distance information had to travel from the teacher's mouth to his brain. In the long run, he calculated, this would save time and he would learn more than all the cool kids goofing off in the back.

JJ, lost in the classroom of his mind, unconsciously raised his right hand again. Violet Green crinkled her nose under her mask, "Do you have a question, JJ?"

"Uh, yes, what if a good student had a vision disorder?"

Dr. Green responded without ambiguity, "Corrective glasses or contact lenses are preferable." She added, "Even the use of binoculars is an acceptable alternative to front row seating."

At this point, JJ could not be expected to recognize that this bit of advice, this pearl of wisdom, had the potential to change his life for the better — if only he could let it. He countered with, "What about auditory dysfunction?"

Now fully comprehending the extent and severity of the presenting "disease," Violet quickly prescribed a treatment, "External hearing aid or even cochlear implant. Enough said?"

JJ didn't reply. He just stood there bewildered, motionless although not emotionless. Violet tried again to close the topic and effect the best outcome for her "patient." She stepped up the volume, "ENOUGH SAID?" JJ blindly nodded yes. "Okay. Good. No closer than the third row for you." Then, clearing her throat, she concluded, "We'd better get cutting or we'll be here until midnight."

CHAPTER FOURTEEN

Dead Animal Medicine: Part II (Dumpster Diving)

The large animal necropsy room at the Center for Large Animal Medicine in Kennett Square

Stan the Path Man helped as the two, previously dueling fourth years cleaned up the remains of Bessie the milk cow. Stan pushed a broad, deep shovel across the necropsy floor like he was clearing slush from a driveway. He scooped up his tenth shovel full of gastrointestinal contents and heaved the slurry up and over the lip of a bright yellow dumpster. The container on the necropsy loading dock was labeled "Parts is Parts" in black electrical tape and was emptied by a rendering company in the wee hours of every weekday morning. The parts were destined for cans and bags of pet food brandishing the claim, "Select cuts of real meat." Stan joined forces with one of the students as they both bent to the floor and dug their fingers deep into the bovine's forty-pound liver. Stan, always the consummate teacher, said, "This is what you'd call friable hepatic tissue, see how it fractures so easily in our hands." With a tenuous grip they hoisted the tissue up to the dumpster's lip, which was level with the top of Stan's shoulders, and then let gravity take over. The slippery, greenish-brown organ slithered from their grasp and splashed heavily into a stew of pig's intestines, horse heads and goat legs. "Fabulous!" he turned to the students, "Great work. You guys go get cleaned up, write a draft of the gross report and pop it in my mailbox. I'll grade it and get it back to you in the morning."

But before he could add *today was pretty quiet*, Stan felt a rumbling from within the concrete floor. The vibration passed through his boots, into his tibia, up his spine and made his goggles hum. He swiveled to face the necropsy room's gigantic cooler doors because he knew exactly what this meant. Someone was making a deposit. And it was something big.

Stan skated across the room with undiminished *Risky Business* enthusiasm and yanked on the handles to open the twin, 12-foot tall doors. An icy fog spilled into the room causing Dr. Green's students, who were still working on the birds from the zoo, to shiver.

The forklift growled as it squeezed through the outside entrance into the holding cooler. Draped across its metal tines was a roan-colored draft horse. Stan nodded to the driver, pointed to the center of the cooler and then felt a light tap on his shoulder. It was Trisha Maxwell. "Hey, Doctor O. I'm really sorry about this, I know it's getting late…"

Stan smiled and shook his head, "Trisha, no worries." He looked down at his feet as he continued, "Necropsy is always open. And besides today is only Tuesday. On Fridays after five we usually get half a dozen submissions because the owners don't want to pay for treatment through the weekend. So this is a piece of cake." He looked up into her eyes and added with a dopey grin, "…horse cake."

Truth be told, Dr. Stan Oblitzski was glad to accept this case for reasons he didn't, and probably couldn't, articulate. First, he was a guy that lived for the science of pathology. For him, each case was a medical mystery that he needed to solve. And second, he was delighted to work with Trisha.

This wasn't because Trisha Maxwell smelled great (though she did remind him of the daisies and wild roses that grew along the borders of the school's pastures), it wasn't due to the magnetic pull of her wholesome beauty (Stan felt that sunsets over autumn leaves paled in comparison), and it wasn't because of a boyish crush (since she was a student, even an innocent crush felt inappropriate to him). It was mainly because Trisha Maxwell represented a tangible link to a foreign land. The land where kind women actually cared about nerdy guys. Every time she waved hello, he was visible. All she had to do was ask, "How are you?" and Stan's passport was validated — he existed in the other world.

Stan and Trisha buckled four leather-wrapped, chain hobbles onto the draft horse's fetlocks and clipped them into the electric hoist. He punched a button on the tethered control and said, "Going up: Second Floor, home furnishings; Third Floor, housewares."

Trisha smiled, "Third Floor please."

"Ah, good choice. Today — and today only — we're having a 20%-off cutlery sale. Gently used hatchets, mallets and band saws included."

As the hoist motor hummed and the chain clinked, the four din-ner-plate-sized hooves gathered together and were elevated. The animal's dependent torso curved into a deep, bold "**U**." Its head and neck sagged on one end and the thick, cream-colored tail hung defeated at the other. As the equal and opposing vectors of gravity and the hoist played tug of war, the increasing abdominal pressure forced out several fecal balls. Steam rose from where they plopped in a pile on the cooler floor. Stan remarked, "Nice and fresh. When did he die?"

Trisha responded quietly, "We put him down 15 minutes ago."

Stan looked up and read the scale attached to the hoist, "2010 pounds."

Trisha whistled softly, "Jeez, he lost almost 100 pounds in the last three days. He really was spiraling."

By now, Trisha's contingent of first years — Sam, Kerri and Rick Larson — were suited up and standing at the cooler doors. Stan and Trisha moved to the animal's rump and began to push the mass on the overhead trolley out into the necropsy room. Sam and Kerri stepped aside but Rick grabbed the upside down mane and walked backward while he acted as if he were helping. By the time they'd reached the middle of the room, and had picked up a fair head of steam, Rick tried to slow the momentum when he realized that his new plastic booties offered little resistance to the ton of gliding horse meat. Stan chuckled to himself when he saw Rick whip his head around to see that he was about to be squashed between the Clydes-dale freighter and a wall of pointy dissection instruments.

Stan and Trisha grabbed onto the tail, planted their feet and skied behind the animal until Stan pressed the "down" arrow on the hoist con-trol and the animal's nose made contact with the floor. The friction caused them to spin around and drag like the basket under a hot-air balloon. Stan, well-practiced at this maneuver, had timed the landing perfectly. His patient slowed to a stop directly over a hydraulic necropsy table that was recessed into the floor.

In the 90-degree spin, Rick lost both his grip and his footing. His feet flailed wildly just like his first time on hockey skates and he ended up doubled over, a mirror image of the Clydesdale, with his hands planted on the floor for balance. Sam grinned behind his mask while Kerri snorted a laugh, drawing a sneer from Rick.

Stan announced, "Going down: First Floor, knickers, briefs and other unmentionables," and then turned to Trisha. "Speaking of briefs, how about a case history?"

"This is a twenty-two year old, Clydesdale gelding named Bud. He presented to the internal medicine service, uh…" she checked the calendar on her watch, "today's the 11th, so six days ago. Initially, he was depressed, moderately ataxic and then went completely anorexic."

Violet Green looked up from her work on a scarlet ibis and asked, "What were your primary differentials?"

"A spinal tap and his vaccination records helped us to rule out EPM," She clarified for the first years, "Equine Protozoal Myeloencephalitis, also Eastern and Western Equine Encephalitis. Rabies is still possible, though less likely." She paused then concluded, "It was awful to watch him go downhill so fast. The owners really loved this guy and couldn't stand to see him suffer any longer." She paused again. "He was a good horse."

Stan said with uncharacteristic sensitivity, "He's still a good horse." Perhaps it was the normalizing effect of Trisha Maxwell's proximity.

Trisha concluded, "The owners would like the hooves returned for burial on their farm." Stan nodded his head solemnly, "Understood. We'd better get cracking if we want to submit samples to the clinpath lab today. Unlike necropsy, they actually do close." He curled his fingers to make two fists and then positioned them just above his hips. His elbows poked out symmetrically and in alignment with his ears. He squinted as he quickly appraised Trisha's first years, "What's your name?"

Having evolved back into an upright, hominoid posture, Rick jutted out his right hand, "Rick Larson."

Stan wasn't exactly sure what to do, so he directed his instructions to Trisha, "Since this is a neuro horse — and you know what that means — how about Rick works with me to remove the head, extract the brain and then the spinal cord. And you three focus on the abdominal and thoracic cavities." He paused while they all nodded in agreement. "Fabulous. First person to find a cool lesion gets 2 points extra credit."

Dr. Stan Oblitzski was a master at taking animals apart. His internship and residency in anatomical pathology combined with the years he spent working the family butcher shop meant that even alone, he could completely disarticulate and examine a horse — even a neuro horse that required taking it down to sections as small as 2-3 vertebrae thick — in under two hours. Working with students actually slowed the process.

Stan raised the hydraulic table two feet off the floor, just enough for the animal's head to hang over the edge. He pulled a slender filet knife from his tool belt holster and said, "Rick, can you steady his head?"

With unwarranted bravado, Rick Larson responded, "Absolutely, done it a hundred times." He reached down with one hand, placed his thumb in the open mouth and a finger in each nostril. It was almost as if he were holding a bowling ball. Stan shrugged his shoulders and made a quick circumferential incision around the neck at the base of the skull. With an additional flick of the razor-sharp blade between the first two vertebrae, the axis and atlas, the massive, once noble head was severed from its body. Rick held on for about a millisecond of the cranial descent, just long enough so that when he released his hand, it recoiled and he slapped himself square in the mouth. He let out an, "Oof!" which was followed by, "Damn…" as equine snot, tinged with blood, dripped down his face shield.

Stan said, "That's why we make you guys wear those things."

Sam and Kerri couldn't help themselves. This time they burst out laughing and even Trisha giggled. Sam said evenly, "Couldn't have happened to a nice-ah fella. Have ya done that a hundred times too?" Their laughter spilled over, infecting the group working up the birds. Even JJ seemed to catch the drift.

Rick, who should have grown accustomed to being laughed at by now, turned on them, "How was I supposed know that would happen? I wasn't warned…"

Kerri responded, "Remember Rick," and she pantomimed with her hand, "tick a lock!"

He stammered, "This is NOT Anatomy Lab."

Dr. Stan Oblitzski, not normally a student of human behavior, realized that Rick was probably wound a little too tight for his own good, so he stepped in, "Okay, okay. Right you are, Rick. I should have warned you. I will give you a heads-up about this next part — it's dangerous." He paused to see that the student was listening fully. "Have you ever used a Stryker saw?" Rick slowly shook his head. "Well then, let me show you how."

Stan looked to Trisha and then Violet, "Hey, can I borrow your students for a quick tutorial on the Stryker?" They both said yes and Trisha smiled broadly under her surgical mask. She remembered this rite of passage fondly.

Stan bent to pick up the horse's head and at the same time scooped a handful of cherry-red, gelatinous blood clots into his left hip pocket. Then, with Rick's help, they mounted the head in the jaws of a massive vise and quickly skinned away the tissues overlying the cranial vault. "Now," Stan held up the instrument, "this is a Stryker saw, its one and only use in this room is to cut through compact bone, and the cranium is composed of multiple layers of dense, hard bone — obviously to provide protection for the brain." He flicked on the switch and the tool came to life. It produced a piercing, grinding, metallic buzz that sounded as if someone had just dumped a drawer full of silverware into a whizzing blender. The instrument's circular head, with its tiny piranha teeth, blurred with vibration.

"We need to make three complete cuts. Here…" he drew a finger across the bridge of the nose just behind the eyes, and then laterally down each side, "and back to connect with the foramen magnum where the spinal cord exits. After that, the skull cap will more or less lift off." To rivet the student's attention and ramp-up the tension, Stan added, with as much awe as he could muster, "This thing," he wiggled the saw in the air, "will march through a skull like a hot knife through butter. So be careful with it." Stan was incapable of lying, everything he said was of course true, but this game was all about intonation, timing and physical execution. He demonstrated by making the first, perfectly straight cut behind the eyes. The buzz of the Stryker deepened as it plowed a thin furrow, spitting up a slurry of gleaming bone flecks, pink serosanguinous fluid and stringy dura mater in the process. Stan then positioned one of Rick's hands on the vise and requested, "Will you stabilize this for me?" And, with a slight of hand that would have impressed Houdini, he retrieved the clots from his pocket and concealed them within his left palm.

"It's important to focus on this part. Don't let the blade dive too deep and destroy the neuroglia." As the rabidly vibrating tool marched caudally towards the foramen magnum, Stan made his move. He blurted out, "Ooops!" just before he let the saw derail and run across his left hand while squeezing the clots between his fingers. The sweeping arc ended as the Stryker made vibrating contact with Rick's left hand. The combination of meticulous buildup, the grinding buzz of the presumably menacing saw, and stunning visual effects caused Rick to instantly, reflexively, and quite dramatically whip back his hand so fast that he slapped himself in the face — again! He yelped like a stricken dog, "I'm cut!"

Stan held up the back of his left hand to the shocked students with two fingers folded in the palm. Remnants of the clots dribbled down as he slowly uncurled the digits with a smile. It was a classic. A perfectly executed pathological joke. Rick checked his hand through his smeared face shield. He counted aloud, "Three, Four, Five…" Stan patted him gently on the back, "Thanks for being a good sport."

After a noticeable pause, Rick replied sullenly, "You're welcome."

The Stryker saw was, in reality, the pussy cat of electrical saws. All growl and no bite. The micro vibrating blade was only effective on rock-hard surfaces, soft stuff like skin and muscle just moved in unison with the tiny excursions of the blade — that's why they're also used as cast cutters.

After a few moments, Stan and the students were distracted from the important business of laughing by a tapping that came from the lab's observation window. The adjacent room allowed the clinicians — the live animal doctors — to see the final outcome of their cases without getting contaminated. The guy inside wore a short white lab coat over jade surgical scrubs and Stan recognized him as a medicine intern. The intern activated the intercom, "Sorry to bother you Doctor Oblitzski, but do you have any results on..." he flipped through papers in a medical record tin-back, "Billy Stolfus?"

Stan's brow wrinkled, "Hmm, Billy... Billy Stolfus?"

"It was an Angora goat submitted this morning."

"Oh yeah, he had a left displaced abomasum, just like you guys suspected."

The intern was visibly relieved, "Okay, great, can I take the body? It was a cosmetic prep."

Stan frowned, turned towards the big yellow dumpster on the loading dock and then back to the intern, "I think one of us screwed up."

The intern's brows moved closer together and alarm hijacked his face. He frantically flipped through the paper record. "It says right here on the form, Cosmetic Necropsy for Private..." And then he realized his mistake, "CRAP! I didn't check the box... *Holy living mother of God!* Mrs. Stolfus is a nightmare." He started to hyperventilate, "She's gonna castrate me..."

Stan raised his still bloody left hand, "Calm down, I think we can recover the parts."

After suiting up in a flash, the intern was at Stan Oblitzski's side holding the hoist control in one hand. Stan strapped on the customized climbing harness he'd made for just this purpose and clipped a large "D" ring in the back to the hook on the hoist. He instructed the intern, "Take me up, motor me over the center and then put me inside." As he was raised, Stan's body slowly pivoted to a horizontal position facing the floor and not long after he disappeared below the rim of the dumpster he yelled, "Stop!"

The intern, still with a stricken look on his face, heard some sloshing followed by, "Very cool!" and, "Got it. Take me up." Stan breached the plane of the rim with two prizes in his hands and a quizzical look on his face, "How about these?"

The intern went shocky as the color drained from his face, "Those are DEER LEGS! Holy crap, I am so dead."

Stan replied with a smile, "Aw, come on, parts is parts… No?" He dropped the deer with a splash, flipped upside down and with his legs pointing straight up he wrapped them snugly around the greasy chain for the next plunge. After a second or two he shouted, "Take me up!"

Stan emerged from the dumpster with a triumphant smile and holding "Billy" by the horns, "Who's your buddy, huh?"

The intern almost fainted with relief.

CHAPTER FIFTEEN

Life on the Edge

Cardiac physiology lecture, Room 13 in the Rosenthal Building, Philadelphia

E ach entity labeled "The Veterinary Class of..." is composed of individuals who tend to cluster in groups. When taken together, these groups make up the whole, much as developing cells in an embryo seek cohorts to form the organs that ultimately comprise a distinct being. And like an individual organism — human, dog, cat or even a fish — a vet school class develops its own unique personality. Over the decades, much idle speculation has surrounded the cyclical nature of class quality. Good year, bad year, odd year. Olympians, dorks, invertebrates. The class year before this one earned the moniker, "The Foreign Bodies" because they just seemed out of place. Their predecessors were "The Whiners," while the current fourth year class had "The Right Stuff." Understandably, theories of class evolution emerged. The presumed, recurrent pattern of cyclicity leaned towards the supposition of an overarching Grand Plan. But a newly emergent, conflicting — almost heretical — theory held that a vigorous, more adaptive student cluster had the potential to sway class embryogenesis. Within *this* nascent class, the four major tissues types had already begun to coalesce: nervous tissue, connective tissue, muscle and epithelium.

The primary lecture hall for first-year veterinary students, Room 13, was actually a subterranean storage bunker that had been renovated, modestly, into a classroom of sorts. It had all the charm of a tomb-robbed mausoleum but met the minimal requirements for teaching: a slender, oak-veneer podium and two blackboards mounted side by side up front;

an AV projection booth for slides in the back; and a light switch so the students could be themselves. Four small, basement-style windows ran along the front wall above the blackboards, their top edges flush with the low-slung, fiberboard ceiling tiles that weighed down on the room's occupants. These windows, which would have looked out on pedestrian feet bustling along Spruce Street, were occluded by dusty institutional blinds. Room 13 was a squat rectangle, much wider than it was deep, and this shape restricted seating to five long rows of 30 chairs each. The design forced the budding veterinary students (and occasionally, like today, the first-year human med students) to unambiguously state their intentions: front row, middle rows, Death Row, or somewhere on the fringe.

Now a solid month into their training, the Veterinary Class of 1992 had settled into a daily seating plan as predictable as chocolates in a Whitman's Sampler. In fact, Sam had sketched out a seating chart, the lid of the box, which sorted the class "candies" into solid chocolates, jelly creams and varieties of mixed nuts. Jack slipped this diagram, anonymously, into a packet of Note Service notes for duplication and distribution. This occurrence, and the resulting ripple of snorted laughter, sneers, and sporadic cries of recrimination for wasting both Note Service funds ($1.70) and paper (85 pieces), signaled "Open Season" for both practical and impractical jokes and may have hinted at the class's burgeoning character.

This afternoon, Dr. Florence Kimball, cardiac specialist and head of the small animal emergency service at VHUP, was center stage in Room 13. With her gushing red hair, sunny green eyes and wrinkle-free complexion, she could consistently spark vibrant life from within the featureless confines of this space. She would use anything, from gruesome props to class participation, to liven up a lecture. In fact, she'd just finished passing around a "sample" from one of her cases — a formalin-filled baby food jar in which bobbed a feline heart ravaged by heartworms. Dr. Kimball carried the prop with her wherever she went — to Wawa for coffee, Friday Night Happy Hour, or even the dry cleaners — so that a commercial for *Eradication of the Heartworm Menace* could be launched on a moment's notice.

After retrieving the jar from a FRoG, she shifted didactics. "Next topic: the cardiac cycle. I know what you're thinking. A stationary bike at the gym…" It wasn't really up to their exacting standards, but the folks on Death Row smiled broadly because any attempt at humor was a welcome transgression during the course of an info-packed lecture. Dr. Kimball glanced at the plain, black and white clock in the back of the classroom,

"We've got about 15 minutes remaining, why don't we break things up a bit with some audience participation."

Flo Kimball had a way of explaining science that made even complex ideas easy to understand and remember. It was the *remember* part that was especially important to her. What good was it to dump volumes of information that just went in one ear and out the other? Sure, it makes the lecturer feel she's done the job. *I showed them. There's tons of stuff you guys need to know, it's difficult, complicated, and most times dull. I did it, now you do it. So on and so forth.* But Dr. Florence Kimball felt different. This caused her to act differently. To teach differently. Simply put, she was enthralled with the process of life — truly, honestly, and unashamedly amazed with life. The physical package life came in did not matter. Whether a sweet puppy, an old cocker spaniel or an overeager vet student, it was all quite incredible to her.

"Every other specialist you'll study under feels that their area, *their organ system*, should be near and dear… to your heart. But mine," she beamed, "by definition, just is." Dr. Kimball closed her notebook on the podium, "Let me tell you a little story. I call it 'Life on the Edge.' The heroine is a trim and fit, well-muscled, four-chambered beauty — the mammalian heart."

"You can live indefinitely if 1/2 of your renal parenchyma dies off. You can surgically remove 2/3 of your liver," she tightened her lips and rethought the sentence, "actually, don't remove your own liver, that's tricky surgery. But, lose most of your liver and you wouldn't even notice it. Go blind, God forbid, and you'll survive while your remaining senses hypertrophy and actually enhance. But," she took in a deep breath, "if your beautiful, warm, ever-pulsing mammalian heart arrests, for any of about a thousand reasons, your brain begins to dissolve in three minutes. Those memories — that glorious Christmas you got the GI Joe with camouflage jumpsuit and matching grenade holster," Jack and Hoss looked at each other and nodded in appreciation, "or the Malibu Barbie with real mini skirt and miniature hair brush, gone."

Jack leaned to his right, muttered to Hoss and shrugged his shoulders, "I was in college; we were just experimenting…"

Flo Kimball paused to see that every eye was focused on her, "And then there's your first kiss…"

Just then, the glass doors at the back of the room adjacent to Death Row opened and Jack looked up to see Anna. She stood in the half-opened doorway leaning over her cane with a scowl on her face and Petunia at her side. She scanned the crowded room for her usual seat down front and, even before Jack could act, Hoss jumped up and offered his seat next to Jack. At first Anna hesitated but when she looked into Hoss' smiling eyes, she acquiesced and nodded her thanks. To make space Hoss took Petunia's lead, sat cross-legged on the floor with his back to the door and Petunia climbed into his lap.

Not only was this seating arrangement unprecedented (with Anna on Death Row), but Jack couldn't remember her ever being late. At first he thought it wise to keep his mouth shut as she levered herself into the seat, and then concern got the best of him. Over the past few days he'd noticed that she walked with a pained gait, and he could have sworn that she slurred when she called Rick a "tolo ass" in lab yesterday. He turned toward the side of her stony face as she stared straight ahead and whispered, "You okay?"

Anna squinted her eyes and without looking at Jack she hissed, "Here's the thing. It's none of your damned business." Though not entirely surprised by the response, Jack pulled his head back, raised his eyebrows and decided to let it go. He turned back and tuned into the lecture.

"Let's examine one functional cardiac cycle, then we'll link it to the sounds you hear in a stethoscope and that ever-present symbol of medicine, the EKG trace. Hold both hands out in front of you like this," Dr. Kimball demonstrated by facing her palms to the class as if she was informing her beagle that there were *No More Treats*. "Now, close the fingers of both hands to make relaxed fists and rest the left directly on top of the right — like one potato, two potato. Your left hand, the one on top, represents the atria, and the right hand is the ventricles. Now, uncurl the fingers of your left hand and clap them shut." The students did as they were told and she heard a muffled clap. "Again. And again. Now repeat this once a second with your left hand." A soft, steady clapping sound filled the room. "Good. Now add in the ventricles, immediately after each atrial contraction." She almost beamed as she looked over her class. "Okay, keep that going for another 60 seconds." The clapping of the mock cardiac chambers was more or less rhythmic and in sync. "That's your heart at rest, but..." She smacked the podium with the palm of her hand and caused the first two rows to startle. "That was a gunshot — not uncommon in Philly. Run! Double time. 120 beats per minute is nothing for your heart. Can you imagine completing 20 cycles per second? A hummingbird does it with ease." The previously synchronous clapping disintegrated. "So, why do we do this exercise?" She bowed deeply, "Because I adore the applause..." and everyone laughed.

During her bow, Dr. Kimball scooped up a tabby that had been sitting on stage at her feet. The cat had been casually licking a paw while seated, gazing contentedly out at the students. Though officially frowned upon, well-mannered pets were often smuggled into class. The species list rarely ventured into the exotic but it wasn't unusual for a ferret or chinchilla to scamper across a desk. Cradling the feline in her left arm and stroking its head with her right, the position placed the animal's purrbox next to the mic clipped to Flo Kimball's lapel. As soft purring blanketed the room she continued, "The mammalian heart is more sophisticated than any engine designed by man. That's *any* engine — stock car, for you country types, nuclear sub, even rocket engines. But just like the internal combustion engine in your car, motion begins with a spark. In this case, the spark is triggered by the Sinoatrial Node — a cluster of special pacemaker neurons located in the wall of the right atrium. When the SA node fires, it sparks the atria to contract and they push blood through one-way valves and into the ventricles." She leaned over and extended the tabby's paw to identify a portion of the diagram on the overhead projector.

"While the atria are contracting, the electrical signal that was initiated by the SA node has been traveling towards the other two cylinders of the heart, the ventricles. But remember your neurophysiology?" She paused and looked around the room at multiple blank faces. "Sure you do. The normal nerve impulse travels at nearly the speed of light. So, when the SA node pacemaker fires, the spark could cause the entire heart to contract at one time. But that does not happen. The heart couldn't work as a pump if it did. What happens is that the nerve impulse gets delayed when it enters the bottleneck of the AV node. This allows the atria to push that last bit of blood into relaxed ventricles. If they were contracted," she cupped her hand then quickly squeezed it into a clenched fist, "blood could not fill them."

It was a true-to-life story, a marvel of nature, and Dr. Kimball's sincere excitement drew the students in. "Now, as I was saying," she fired off, "this impulse gets slowed for about 100 milliseconds. In this time, the atria begin to relax. Just like the spent booster rockets on the space shuttle, they've done their jobs. This relaxation allows the valves between the atria and ventricles to snap shut. As long as they are healthy, these valves stop the backward flow of blood from the ventricles into the atria — you know, like those spiky things in the parking garage at VHUP. Once you drive over them, there's no going back. An interesting and clinically important thing to note here is that when these valves clap shut, they make an audible sound — they make the "lub" part of the "lub-Dub" you hear with your stethoscope. Cool huh? Guess what makes the even louder "Dub" sound?"

A FRoG's hand sprang up and with a little laugh Dr. Kimball said, "No, that's okay, that was more of a rhetorical question. I want to tell this story." She continued, "Now that the ventricles are filled with blood, it's time for them to contract. The impulse leaves the AV node and triggers them to squeeze. When they do, they force the blood through the semilunar valves. The valves open, blood is ejected into the aorta and when the ventricles begin to relax..."

Dr. Kimball paused for just 50 milliseconds too long and in the mounting tension JJ couldn't control himself, he suffered a premature interjection, "And the valves snap shut making the *Dub* sound, the second part of the lub-Dub we hear with our stethoscopes... That's right, huh? It's right isn't it? Right?"

Flo Kimball didn't miss a beat, "No, I'm sorry, it isn't. There is no Dub sound, I made that part up."

"But, but everybody knows that there's a dub. You know, lub-Dub, lub-**Dub**, lub-**DUB**..." JJ wondered if he'd imagined that part — trying on lub-*pause*, lub-*pause*, lub-*pause* for size. The class could almost smell the smoke as his brain churned the problem over a zillion times a second.

Jack leaned toward Sam, "Must be Dub, *must be Dub*..."

Sensing an imminent cranial implosion, Flo Kimball threw water on the flames by saying what JJ desperately needed to hear, "You're right, JJ. That's where the Dub sound comes from. I was just kidding."

JJ paused as his rightness percolated into his brain, dousing the flames of self doubt.

"I'm sorry JJ, I wanted to tell the story myself and you took the punch line, but I am glad you understand the cardiac cycle so thoroughly." She did not intend to hurt anyone's feelings, and knew that a flippant remark from a teacher could crush someone like JJ. She smiled in his direction and noted that he seemed to be recovering.

"Your heart is a marvel. Fantastically dynamic and deeply complex." She went on to describe the heart as a living, respiring, feeling, engine. "Oh yeah, it feels alright. It feels you, your body, your emotions. It 'knows' what you see, hear and touch, and responds accordingly."

She paused as she placed the still-purring cat on the podium, "Now, raise one hand in the air and make a peace sign. Put those fingers together and use them to palpate the angle of your jaw just below and in front of your ear." She paused to give them time to find the spot, "Okay, got it?

Great. Now, drop these fingers down below your jaw line into the trough between your trachea and sternocephalicus. Feel anything?" Some mumbling bubbled up from the middle rows, "Your neck... Yeah good, anything else?" After a moment, heads began nodding slowly. "Yeah, you're feeling your carotid pulse. That intense pulse wave, the most palpable in the human body, is arising directly from your aortic arch. As you know, the aortic arch carries the largest volume of blood at the highest velocity and pressure — it has just been powerfully ejected from the left ventricle. Remember, any significant interruption to this flow and you're stuck with brain damage."

Sam leaned to his right and whispered to Jack, "Or in you-ah case, *more* brain damage."

Jack replied with a smile, "Come on, this is professional school. You gotta elevate your game."

Dr. Kimball continued, "Now, let's be completely silent for a few moments. Palpate your pulse, don't count your rate or anything, just feel it, listen to it. Don't stop until I tell you."

John Fitzgerald Doyle was seated, as always, on Death Row with Sam Stone immediately on his left and Kerri Feinburg beyond Sam. Normally Hoss would be on his right. As a general rule, Jack and Sam didn't take notes. They relied entirely on Note Service to record the details while they took in the big picture. Jack usually just leaned back, stretched out his legs with one toe hooked over the other, relaxed, and listened. And now, in his usual recline, he palpated his neck with his right hand and occasionally picked up what he thought was a pulse, but then lost it. Moving his fingertips under his jaw, down to his thoracic inlet and back up, he began to wonder if he was actually alive. Anna Heywood, seated on his right, was watching him out of the corner of her eye — actually, she'd been doing it since she sat down. After a few moments with no satisfaction, Jack sat up and turned to her with a look of puzzlement on his face. He pulled his hand away from his neck and turned the palm up to silently indicate, *I can't find it.*

Jack was caught off guard by what happened next. While Anna could feel her own strong and steady pulse with her right hand, she reached out and gently placed her left index finger on Jack's neck. He sat stock still because this was the first time since their awkward kiss at the Testicle Festival that she'd even acknowledged his existence, let alone touched him.

Anna waited as minutes seemed to pass and then she felt it. *Boom* — pause, pause, pause, *Boom* — an even longer pause and then finally a third powerful surge raised the tip of her finger. *Boom.* Her eyebrows rose slowly and as she turned to look into Jack's brilliantly clear eyes she thought, *his heart rate is 40 beats a minute.* It was true that Jack Doyle did not appear to have an ounce of fat on his sturdy frame, but this finding suggested he might also have the heart of an Olympian. A hush permeated the room as the students 'listened' to their hearts and Anna let herself get lost. Lost in Jack's strong, slow rhythm. Lost in the warmth of his skin. A feeling of closeness came over her. She lost track of everything else in the darkened space until the throbbing under her digit, the one on Jack's skin, began to quicken. She looked into Jack's eyes and then directly down the row behind him where Kerri was grinning ear-to-ear.

At that very instant, Dr. Kimball exclaimed, "Stop! So, what does your heart feel?" Anna recoiled from Jack as her own pulse galloped. The gel into which she'd been transformed instantly solidified. She squinted at Jack through a voluntary entropion, coughed to clear her throat and mumbled, "I think that's quite enough," and quickly faced forward.

Jack sat there blinking, in silence, staring again at the hardened side of Anna's face. Though he'd never experienced it before, he knew exactly what his heart felt.

Cardiac Physiology, NOTE SERVICE
10/12/88 (1:00–2:00pm)
Dr. Florence Kimball

TR: Kerri Feinburg
DD: Jack Doyle
Page 5 of 5

TR NOTE:

Dr. Kimball gave a thorough, engaging and (and, how shall I say, arousing) lecture.   I reproduced the two diagrams she had on the blackboard. For other illustrations please refer to her handout or the text.

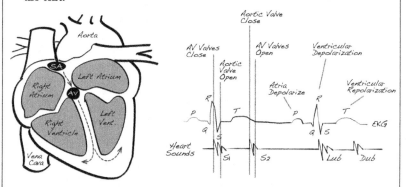

Excitatory Conductive
system: SA & AV nodes,
Purkinje system.

Cardiac cycle: EKG & Ht Sounds,
valvular activities

An Animal Life — Unreal

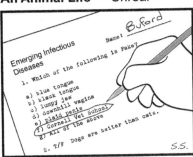

Hoss was off to a roaring start!

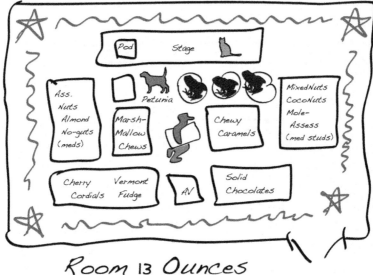

An Animal Life — Charades

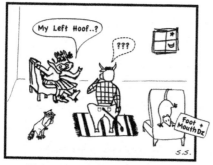

This was Bessie and Gary's first and last date...

CHAPTER SIXTEEN

20/20 Vision

1:50 PM — WEDNESDAY, OCTOBER 12, 1988

Intermission between lectures, Room 13 in the Rosenthal Building, Philadelphia

A flip of the light switch triggered the flickering of overhead fluorescents which yielded to a steady blanket of white. The class blinked as Jack collected himself and then sprinted to the podium for a presidential broadcast. "Two quick announcements, guys." Although he heard notebooks slapping shut, his classmates held their positions. Usually, the "lights up" sequence had the same effect as the Christmas tree at a drag race, people shot to the bathroom or the food trucks on Spruce Street or out to the quad for a quick game of hacky sack.

"Two announcements," he repeated. The first was a decoy. "The Hill's pet food delivery will be delayed by one day. You can pick up your orders at Friday Night Happy Hour."

He glanced at Sam and Hoss. "Now, you've all seen the camera crews around. I'd like to state that the rumors are true." He paused — this got their attention. "The managing editor at '20/20' is indeed a friend of the Dean, and yes, they will be choosing students, either vet students," then he motioned with an open palm, "or human med students, for a video documentary about our four years of schooling." The sheep murmured and baaed with subdued excitement. "And, to generate some interest, they're offering a small yearly stipend for the chosen few."

JJ's hand shot up. He didn't wait to be recognized, "How will they choose?"

Jack realized the irony but, in this instance, he was hoping for this exact interruption. "Good question, JJ. The producer asked me to distribute applications for the audition." He thought about shrugging his shoulders and then just intimated indifference, "Does *anybody* want to participate?" Never before, and certainly never thereafter, was this level of unified interest and agreement displayed by a veterinary class. Jack was astonished. It looked to him as if everyone in the room — except Anna, of course — had their hands raised. And, better yet, most of the human med students elevated both arms as if on a roller coaster free fall. "Wow, okay, I guess I'll need to make more copies and will distribute them via your mailboxes." He smiled toward Sam and Hoss, and then looked in the direction of the human med students, "So, Mr. Cadaver is it? You actually think the TV world is ready for your ugly mug in their living rooms?"

Mr. Cadaver, the first-year med student Class President, usually sat in the mixed nuts section off to one side of Room 13. He stood to face the entire class and answered, "Not only am I ready for a prime-time television audience, I'll bet you the full tab for a Friday Night Happy Hour that the med students will be chosen over you animals!"

A rumbling sarcastic *Ooooooooo* washed across Room 13 and ignited a round of trash talk. *I'll choose your mama again*, etc. Jack raised a hand to quiet his rowdy classmates, leaned into the mic and responded flatly but with a wink to the Death Row Crew, "You're on."

As the applause faded, Jack addressed the last row of the class, "Sam, did you have something you wanted to present?" On cue, Sam Stone collected his favorite mug, a bag of props and a stack of notes, stood up and began to make his way to the stage.

Hoss, who was back in his regular seat on Death Row, grunted a laugh and with a wide grin turned to Kerri, "He practiced on me. It's pretty funny *AND* I have a speaking part!" Hoss wiggled his eyebrows up and down in excitement.

The room lights dimmed and Sam Stone was instantly revealed flipping through notes by the beam of makeshift spot (Jack beamed a flashlight on him). Since the written word tripped him up, Sam had sketched a cartoon storyboard of his jokes for the show. After a final glance, he rested the notes and his mug on the podium, cleared his throat to drop the Mainer drawl and then blurted out in his best Steve Martin, "Thank you. *Thank yoooou…*" even though the class had not yet clapped. "I know what you're thinking, '*I hope this is good*'. And I'm thinking, '*I hope they like it*.' So, why don't we just get this out of the way." He held up one of his props, a small cardboard sign stapled to a wooden slat. It read, "APPLAUSE!" so they humored him.

He responded, "*Thank yoooou...*" and launched into his monologue, "It's great to be here tonight folks. Boy, I have had a rough evening so far."

Hoss bellowed Ed McMahon style, "HOW—ROUGH—WAS—IT?"

Sam replied, "I'm glad you asked," and then faked a nervous shiver. "I'm still a little shaken. I am SUCH an impatient driver. I had another case of road rage on my way here. Last week," he paused, "last week it caused me to hit a cow."

Hoss interjected, "No, not a cow..." He looked over at Kerri and nodded with a self-satisfied grin.

"Yeah, and as you can imagine, it was pretty bad." He shook his head slowly. "This damn cow, she was just moseying along, driving with her blinker on for like 40 friggin' miles. Cows are THE worst drivers." A whoop and brief clap of agreement went up from Death Row. "I'm right aren't I? And, I could see she wasn't paying attention, she was doing her fur in the rearview mirror.

"Well, she's driving a pink Cadillac, you know, one of those Mary Kay deals. It's got a Mary Kay Cow'smetics bumper sticker with the sub-title: 'Makeup tested on animals, by animals, for animals.'" Sam shook his head slightly and made a frown, "I guess that makes everything alright huh? Cows, they think they're so superior, with their little *plays on words*. I coulda' thought of that one.

"So, like I said, I'm driving along and my road rage kicks in. I'm right on her tail and she gives me the hoof! Well, I start laughing. Not like, 'Oh, that's so funny.' More like, 'Ha-ha-ha you silly cow, you don't even have fingers so that doesn't mean anything.' And then I see her mouth the words, '*Eat me!*' in the rearview mirror.

"Well, that did it. I punched the accelerator and I was *right on her tail* when one of my wheels got tangled up in the tip... It's bushy. Whamo, she lost control, her little hooves slipped off the wheel." Sam smirked, "Probably the manure." He stopped to shake his head, "Again, I don't care how speciest this sounds: cows should NOT be driving.

"Anyway, we collide, both of our airbags inflate, but we pull safely off the road. I jump out and march on over because I'm still hungry, I mean *angry*." He paused for the laughter. "I'm feeling like Rocky heading into the freezer." Sam shadow boxed a few times and murmured, "Gimme a piece of dis cow, I'm gonna slaughter dis cow..."

A couple of *Ooos* came from the class so he raised a hand in acknowl-edgement, "I know, I know, she's a girl. But I was upset. Well, I get over there and there's milk *everywhere* and she's crying up a storm. There's French fries and McDonalds' wrappers and special sauce all over the leather upholstery. So I try to calm her down. I say, 'Look, I'm sorry. It was *all* my fault. *Blah, blah, blah.*' So she finally stops crying and looks up at me with those big brown eyes, and then I notice that this girl is S T A C K E D." Sam cupped his hands like he was palming two enormous melons in front of his chest and then, as if realizing his mistake, he said, "Well more like this…" and relocated the gesture further south. "What an udder! I was thinking they *cannot* be real." He shrugged, "But what the hell do I care if they're soy based. They were impressive. So she introduces herself, 'Hi, I'm Daisy Delmonico, my friends call me Double D.' And get this, then she says, 'Let's just cut the bull, what are you doing Friday night?'" Sam moved his eyebrows up and down a couple of times. "That is one thing I like about cows, they're very forward."

"So we went out." He paused, then added with a bashful grin, "It was great…" The class clapped for the sly implication. "But, I don't think we have a future. Actually, we come from pretty diverse backgrounds. First there's the religious differences: she's Hindu and I'm a Green Bay fan. And then finding a restaurant we can agree on is near impossible." He threw his hands up in mock surprise, "Turns out, she's pretty much a vegetarian… And wouldn't you know it, I'm a strict carnivore. But I think it was that *element of danger* that attracted her to me in the first place. Anyway, we compromised and went to Sizzler for the all-you-can-eat shrimp and salad bar." Sam laughed, "The Sizzler lost some money that night, let-me-tell-you. She was just up there grazing, you know, with those four stomachs and all.

"Of course, since she's a Mary Kay distributor, she was all made up. When she came back to the table to chew her cud, she went on and on about her ideas for bovine beauty products. Everything's a *cow* theme with her. She wants to develop her own line of Mooscara, scented fly sprays, and diamond-studded nose rings for bulls. For a domesticated animal, she's pretty wild. She's got a cousin that's a wildebeest and I'd be afraid to go out with her… As it was with DD, I found out later that night," Sam made two slow motion, exaggerated winks with his right eye, "She has a tattoo on the *inside* of her upper lip. It says, 'I'm what's for dinner.' *Holy*…" Sam coughed a couple of times and then cleared his throat.

"But I guess people just aren't used to intra-species dating. I actually overheard a guy saying to the waitress, 'I'll have what he's having, but hold the flies.' People are so damned judgmental. Oh sure, it's fine for dogs and cats to live together, so long as they keep it behind closed doors. Just don't parade it out in public.

"But anyway, the date was fun and we already have pet names for each other." He paused to let the concept sink in, "She's my big old 'Dairy Queen' and I'm her little 'Burger King.'" Sam coughed again but this time into the microphone. "My friends have started calling me, 'Hugh Heifer.'" He raised his eyebrows, "I kinda' like it. But, I can't imagine that we'll actually get married." Sam coughed yet again and this time he said, "Excuse me, dry throat…" He picked up his blue, vet school mug from the top of the podium and took two deep glugs which left a thick white foam over his upper lip. "As my father used to say, 'Why buy the cow?'" Holding up the mug, he said, "This was Free!"

Sam bowed deeply, "*Thank yooooou*, you were great." This time he didn't need the sign, the applause was uproarious.

CHAPTER SEVENTEEN

HypnoGolf

Intermission between lectures, Room 13 in the Rosenthal Building, Philadelphia

Afternoons for first-year, first-semester veterinary students are challenging. The challenges are not due entirely to the long mornings spent laboring in Comparative Anatomy Lab. Nor directly because of the litany presented over hours of lectures — that contributes. More often, it's the mode of information delivery that makes paying attention a struggle. With an energetic, animated professor like Dr. Kimball, time flew and students learned. But most first-year lecturers would have made better hypnotists or anesthesiologists or both — HypnoAnesthesiologists?

Jack couldn't help making fun of one professor: *"Listen very carefully,* the life cycle of the hedgehog pinworm takes three point two weeks to complete, *you are becoming sleeeepy,* the L1 larvae hatch out of the ova in four days if relative humidity and ambient temperature are adequate, *very sleeeepy,* L1 larvae mature into L2 larvae, *your eyelids feel heavy,* L3 larvae mature into L4 larvae, *focus on the sound of my voice,* L4 larvae mature into... *When you reawake, you will remember nothing..."* He snapped his fingers. At least the last part was true. They remembered nothing. The crew on Death Row, however, turned lemons into lemonade. They made a game of it.

They called their game HypnoGolf. Or sometimes DMT, which stood for "Dead Man Talking." HypnoGolf was a more accurate title for a number of reasons. First, there was the hypnotic effect of the lecture. But other similarities were found in the mental gymnastics required by the actual golfer. For instance, in real golf, the choice of club for a particular shot depended on variables such as distance to the hole, direction of the wind, and the location of hazards like ponds or sand traps. This reasoning was applicable to HypnoGolf but the goal differed. In HypnoGolf, the player needed to predict when a specific student would fall dead asleep. Closest to the "hole," without going over, would win.

Certain members of the class were particularly susceptible to anesthetic ramblings and two or three would take the Hypno' plunge each day. But none were more reliable or attracted more gaming attention than José Rizal, the diminutive Filipino circus performer who had been Jack's jockey in deadhorse steeplechase. Despite his best efforts to remain attentive, José was borderline narcoleptic. He could fall asleep at a strip club and, in fact, once did.

José's drowsy sequence usually progressed as follows:

1) After the 10-minute break, José would waltz back to his seat munching a brownie, chips, a cheesesteak or whatever was available from the vending machines in the lounge or the food trucks outside.

2) Install himself in his usual seat in the middle of the middle row. This distance was just within the range that his unusually thick, perpetually smudged, glasses could focus a blackboard diagram. His glasses, really just two magnifying lenses, had to be bungeed in place during the lecture. If not, as he lurched forward during an inevitable narcoleptic nod, they would be hurled to the floor.

3) The third thing José would do was to partially reorganize the entropy that was his desk — it was permanently littered with open notebooks, stacks of reference texts, assorted highlighters, colored pens and pencils, and a pile of indexed Note Service notes. He'd often commandeer a desk that flanked him. In his mind, he sat on the bridge of the Starship Enterprise. He'd mutter, "Screen on Mr. Sulu," preceding every slide presentation. Or, "Scotty, take us to warp factor nine," when he got bored. But unlike the Enterprise with photon torpedoes and phasers, José's only defense against the irresistible force of the midday siesta was stockpiled within the refuse of Coke cans, Jolt cola bottles and Wawa mega-coffee-blast containers collecting at his feet. Each was half filled (he was an optimist) with

a stale, flat fluid. The routine was that he'd take a swig of caffeine and then move on to step number four.

4) Step four occurred when José actually began listening to the lecture, picked up his pen and began taking notes. This was time zero for all those playing HypnoGolf. If you had not placed your bets by Step 4 you were required to wait for the next hole.

Jack played frequently, and, in fact, he was also the sport's bookie. He held the money and predicted times. It was a dollar a hole. There was one good thing about José (Sam would joke, "The *only* good thing about José…"), he was consistent. He would stop scribbling but keep his grip firmly on his writing implement. His head would start to bob — a torpid, forward motion followed by a rapid jerk backwards. As the amplitude of the head bobs increased, and the frequency decreased, you knew he was moving closer to the end. The final event was the pen drop. That was when the HypnoGolfers stopped the clock and tallied the score.

There was one other thing that could, paradoxically, make a mind-numbing lecture more interesting. José sometimes woke up. In fact, José could wake up and fall asleep multiple times within a 50-minute period. Each time breaking the cycle by stooping to retrieve his pen or pencil, mutter a few words to the guy sitting next to him only to return to his infinite struggle to avoid counting sheep — a particular challenge when the topic was ovine medicine.

CHAPTER EIGHTEEN

Heil Vandergrift

2:00 PM — WEDNESDAY, OCTOBER 12, 1988

*Neurophysiology lecture, Room 13 of the Rosenthal Building,
Philadelphia*

T he room lights flashed Off/On, Off/On — pause — Off/On. This was Dr. Vandergrift's adaptation of Morse code. He used it to signal the beginning of his lecture.

Although he was a renowned researcher in Amyotrophic Lateral Sclerosis, placing Dr. Even A. Vandergrift in the lecture lineup immediately after Florence Kimball was cruel but not unusual punishment. Primary research scientists served-up the standard, first-year educational fare — an often bland, albeit nutritious pabulum of essential information. But Dr. Even A. Vandergrift was in a league of his own. He was the quintessential Dead Man Talking. Although he was probably a good guy, probably kind, probably sensitive, and even probably smiled — there was no way to know for sure. He never seemed mean or treacherous or obnoxious or to breathe. He had a slight build and lacked sufficient melanin to be called pale. His unusually long lab coat cloaked his entire form with only his sallow head, hands and (presumably sallow) loafer-clad feet poking out. While Flo Kimball was sweet and real and alive, and Dan Linnehan was over-powering and larger-than-life, Even Vandergrift appeared — if he was noticed at all — *smaller*-than-life. He combed his thinning crop of oily, straight black hair flat across his forehead, and a black mustache had recently sprouted above his lip. He may have secretly imagined that the 'stash made him 10.3 times more virile, which it did (but 10.3 x 0.0 is still zero). Regrettably, he was unable to observe its appearance in a dimmed lecture hall. Presumably, it looked normal enough in the morning mirror — yes, it was thick in the middle, and yes, it thinned abruptly as it goose-stepped out from under the shade of his nose. But otherwise, it was a regular guy's mustache. He was shooting for growth approaching Tom Selleck's, but sadly, from a distance and under weak illumination, most students referred to him by his middle name, *Adolph*.

The Death Row Crew was fashionably late as they settled back into their seats a few moments after the lights finally went off. Jack stretched, clasped his hands behind his head and then looked to Sam Stone, "Answer me this. I know that Anna doesn't have a bubbly personality, but why the hell is she pursuing a PhD with ole Doctor Vandergrift here?" Jack raised his eyebrows and pointed with his thumb toward the front of the classroom, "He could bore the shell off a tortoise." Sam just shrugged his shoulders and gave a quizzical look, so Jack changed topics, "A game of DMT?"

Sam nodded yes then responded, "This was made for HypnoGolf."

Jack looked to Hoss who was on his right. Hoss nodded yes slowly. Hoss did pretty much everything slowly.

Jack enquired further down Death Row, "Kerri?"

Kerri nodded vigorously and chimed in, "Somebody's goin' down and I want in on the action." This was going to be fun.

They decided, after almost no deliberation, to focus on the most reliable subject: José. He was already in the middle of Step 3, tidying up his scattering of pens, pencils and highlighters, so they had to think quickly and evaluate the shot. Some, like Sam, played a more or less intuitive game, quickly scribbling down a number on a sheet of paper, folding it over and inserting a bill. But others, like Jack, used a formula which required more time. Just like a real golfer who adapts to wind speed and direction, along with the lie of the ball and pin position, Jack took several variables into consideration prior to choosing his shot. And this time, he had some insider info from Helga, the operator of the Greek food truck parked on the vet school's doorstep. For only a dollar tip, Jack learned that José had missed lunch at the usual time around noon and had just downed a turkey gyro, two brownies and snack-sized bag of Fritos. From where he sat, Jack could see that the meal was followed by just one can of Pepsi. A full bottle of club soda sat menacingly on José's desktop — a water hazard. If he drank a significant amount of fluid, there was an increased risk he'd need to pee, thus delaying siesta onset.

Jack scratched his head as he considered the audio/visual situation. How many times would Dr. Vandergrift switch from light to darkness and back again? He watched as the professor loaded a full slide carousel onto the projector and then switched on the overhead projector. Room 13's blackboards were still filled with the cardio info Dr. Kimball had presented during the last lecture, and since Dr. Vandergrift usually performed a complete, preemptive erasure if he needed to use the boards, all available information forecasted a lengthy and uninterrupted stretch of relative darkness.

José finished Step 3, his desk was in order, so he took a hit of Jolt cola and proceeded toward Step 4.

Jack usually took other factors into consideration such as the number of FRoGs in proximity to the subject (they might ask a lot of questions and keep José awake), or the number and type of pets cruising the room, but he was out of time. He dashed off his educated guess: 4 minutes and 23 seconds.

Hoss handed in his wager and noticed Jack's shot. "4:23? He don't usually pass out before 5 minutes and it's 2 o'clock not 1..."

Jack smiled. Clearly Hoss was unaware of José's late lunch with a main course of turkey. Turkey contained copious quantities of tryptophan, an essential amino acid that, when consumed prior to sedate situations, like a neuro lecture, aids sleep induction.

All the other shots were considerably longer: Sam — 10:01; Kerri — 10:00; and Hoss — 11:45. Sam's shot sat up nicely in the fairway. He was blocking Kerri, who was effectively out of play. Sam remembered that José's pen commonly hit the floor somewhere between 10 and 12 minutes and got lucky that no one had guessed 10:02, or thereabouts. Jack was the most conservative of the bunch. In effect, he laid up.

Today's Vandergrift lecture continued with neurophysiology. It was supposed to complement what the class was learning in anatomy. Comparative anatomy is about form and structure: *this is the biceps brachii*. Physiology is about function: *this is how the biceps brachii contracts*. In addition to muscle, bone, blood vessels, and the guts — lung, liver, kidney, intestines — the students were also locating nerves.

"*...as you will remember, we were discussing nerve impulse transmission or more appropriately impulse propagation in the peripheral nerve, a peripheral nerve such as the superficial peroneal nerve which innervates the lateral digital extensor is a bundle of both afferent and efferent axons, the axon is the thread-like part of the nerve cell, each axon is encased in a fatty myelin sheath that acts like the insulation on an electrical wire, impulses in the afferent axons are sensory, they tell the brain and spinal cord what is going on in a specific organ and then the efferent axons can send impulses to control the actions of said organ...*"

Jack began to grin. The grin spread bilaterally. As it widened, his cheeks made little pointed creases like arrow heads.

Kerri Feinburg moaned, "God damn..." She saw the writing on the wall (the wall was where the overhead projector was focused). Dr. Vandergrift was just *reading* his notes to the class. Jack scribbled "Quiet Please" on a piece of scrap paper and, just like the Masters, fanned it over Death Row.

"Humph," Sam grunted with a quiet laugh.

Jack squished his lips to one side and whispered to Sam, "What a incredible Cinderella story. This unknown comes from outta nowhere to lead the pack at Augusta..." They quoted lines from *Caddyshack* far too often.

Jack sensed victory but one event started to worry him. José, though initially taking notes, precipitously slowed his pace and then stopped. True, there was no reason to write down what was being said. It was being recorded by the Note Service, it was verbatim from the professor's handout, and, to top it all off, it was deadly dull. But was José going cataleptic already? Dr. Vandergrift had been lecturing only 1 minute and 19 seconds. They could be witnessing a new class record for the 100 yard doze.

Jack scanned the course before him. There was nothing an honorable man could do except *will* something to intercede. The FRoGs were riveted to every utterance, scribbling away intently. Unfortunately they did not look confused or concerned that they were going to miss something for the test (this is one of a FRoG's greatest fears: to miss something that was said). No raised hand threatened the monotonous cadence that was numbly bathing the class's sensory organs. If you want to turn off a sensation, just keep the same stimulus coming and at the same rate. Our sensory nerve endings, in ears and noses for example, are designed to detect changes readily. But expose them to the same "stimulation" (or lack thereof, as in this case) and they acclimate and shut down. Even the sweet smell of a red, red rose can fade into white noise given enough time.

To Jack Doyle, the successive black-and-white diagrams being shown on the screen appeared less and less like graphs, and more like ink blots. He thought, couldn't you at least use a colored highlighter or something to break it up a bit? Though no one ever said it out loud, the exclusive use of an overhead projector was about the least a teacher could do. At the top end, a presentation that included color slides, audio and video clips showed the students that the lecturer cared as much about the audience as he cared about the subject. The University of Philadelphia, School of Veterinary Medicine had a few of these respected and cherished teachers — and, one guy was even, God forbid, humorous. You listened closely to these professors because you couldn't help yourself, it was interesting, it was fun. But today, at 2:05 and 27 seconds, the students wilted as their attention drained from their brains, down their legs and pooled lifelessly on the cold linoleum.

One issue that might have instigated at least a flicker of emotion was the header on each overhead transparency: the date next to the course title "Neurophysiology" proclaimed "Fall 1981." Dr. Even "Adolph" Vandergrift had been using these exact same notes for the past 7 years. This fact should have stimulated at least a subtle murmur of malcontent, but it did not.

"...the nerve impulse is propagated all along the length of the neuronal axon, the axon as you know is encased in myelin, however this myelin coating is not complete, it has holes that allow for the flux of sodium and calcium ions, this flux of ions is the impulse, itself the signal being transmitted, the electrical-like impulse is transmitted down the axon, once started it will continue provided there is no disruption in the path..."

Dr. Vandergrift paused for effect, which was like a flash of lightning in a steady, gray downpour. The class was almost startled, awaiting the potential thunder to follow. Those who were not too close to the black hole of sleep actually tugged their heads up and focused on the screen. As it turned out, his pause was indeed intentional. It was intended to effect the pull of nearby atmosphere reluctantly into his frail, paper-thin lungs. On the plus side, it could now be stated with absolute certainty that Dr. Vandergrift did in fact breathe. But, unfortunately for Jack — and everyone else in Room 13 — Even Vandergrift just resumed his previous drone.

At 3 minutes and 12 seconds, José's head stopped bobbing. Although most everyone in the classroom was sedated, things were just getting interesting for the folks on Death Row. José's pencil, previously held in a nearly vertical position, slackened. Its purposeful motion had been replaced by an impressive imitation of that leaning tower in Pisa. Jack watched the eraser tip so intently he could almost hear the tiny Italian screams.

Kerri Feinburg began a low but barely audible mantra "drop it—drop it—drop it..." It was in their best interest for José to drop the pencil before 4:23. The pool would just carry over to the next hole.

Eight eyes were now silently focused on the gummy tip of the yellow stick as it began its downward acceleration. Jack dutifully raised his wristwatch, preparing to mark the time when the pencil fell. Then suddenly, the Thunder Broke. An enormous CRASH emanated from the shaded windows above the black boards. The entire class, including José, jumped. He bolted upright, blurted out "Mommy!" and, with the reflexive contraction of his hand, flicked his pencil two rows ahead.

The few thin shards of white light that had worked their way between the closed Venetian blinds were now tinged with red. Dr. Vandergrift was so startled that he darted to his right, instinctually away from the sound. But forgetting that the stage was elevated, he fell, crashing into a pile with two or three FRoGs. He gathered himself and stood facing the front of the room, entranced by the red shafts of light.

Hoss exclaimed what nearly everyone was thinking, *"What the hell was that?"*

Only Dr. Vandergrift had a clue. He was afraid that he knew exactly what was going on out there, but then rejected the notion. *It can't be, hopefully just a bird flew into the window and broke its neck.* He thought, *I'm safe here* as he stepped back up on the stage and inched towards the window. He progressed tangentially, not directly towards the window, but more to the side where the control strings hung. He fumbled with the cords — there's three of them and no living human has ever pulled the correct one on the first try. Dr. Even A. Vandergrift briefly examined the threads and ironically thought, *couldn't these be color coded or something* when he made his choice and hurriedly pulled. He chose wrong, as we all do. The metallic horizontal strips rotated quickly around their axes giving the class a horrific, shimmering glimpse — a flash of a surreal image before they slapped shut again in reverse order.

Jack muttered, "Did I just see what I thought I saw?"

The class sat dumbfounded, even though Dr. Vandergrift, immediately recognizing the things he saw, knew he had to confirm his mental snapshot. He blindly chose the next cord and pulled. Another gory, bloody flash. This time a few students gasped, because this time they had an idea of what to expect. Dr. Vandergrift immediately pulled the third and final cord and the blind accordioned upwards. The students were locked onto the sight for the same reason your head involuntarily rotates towards a horrible traffic accident, as if you're controlled by puppet strings.

The window framed a startling, lifeless image filled with dismembered cat and mouse parts and streaks of blood-red fluid. A banner proclaimed "Animal Liberty Militia: Vandergrift is a Murderer! The death penalty for Murderers!" It took a second or two to sink in, but the cause of the crash was now evident. Someone had thrown a container of red paint against the glass. The red liquid arched away from the central point of impact and oddly gave the window a stained-glass effect. This was perhaps not so out of place since the assailants now began to chant with a religious fervor, "Red-Rum-Red-Rum-RED-RUM…"

Everyone was stunned, to say the least, and not a word was uttered for about the next 20 seconds. Dr. Vandergrift was incredulous. *Those are animal parts from my experiments,* he thought, *but how?* Without turning away from the window, he leaned towards the mic on the podium and feebly announced, "…this concludes my lecture for today, thank you for your attention." The string connected to the blinds slipped through his flaccid digits and the shade came smashing down.

CHAPTER NINETEEN

Nothing Ventured

Equine orthopedic surgery suite at the Center for Large Animal Medicine in Kennett Square

D r. Daniel Linnehan reached up and untied the bow behind his head. He let the surgical mask fall away from his face as he said, "Trisha, let's take a look at those rads."

Trisha Maxwell slid three different views of the surgical site onto a view box. The X-ray films made that reassuring *thwap* sound as they connected with the spring-loaded holder along the top of the viewer, automatically triggering the fluorescent back lighting. The first film was a pre-op lateral with four white chunks where the single, cylindrical cannon bone was supposed to be. The other two views were shot at 90 degree angles for intraoperative confirmation of hardware placement. A web of stout screws and metal plates crisscrossed the bone. For a few moments there was silence as Dr. Linnehan inspected his work. Redeemed was exactly the kind of case he specialized in, a high-value train wreck. This three-year-old thoroughbred, that netted nearly $2 million in stakes this year alone, blew out his right front cannon bone in the final turn at Belmont. Concluding his evaluation, Drill Sergeant Dan turned to Trisha and said, "Tell me what you see."

Trisha's thick lashes blinked calmly over her dazzling, wide-set eyes. She had not yet removed her mask, "The shards of bone are perfectly aligned," she paused, "Most importantly, the distal articular surface looks smooth, as if it had never been fractured."

"Agreed," was all Dr. Linnehan said at first and then he looked to her first-year advisees. About an hour ago, they'd gowned-up so they could observe the conclusion of the six-hour procedure. "What's your name?" He was talking to Rick.

"Me?"

Dr. Linnehan nodded once slowly without blinking.

"Rick Larson," Rick stiffened and then added, "Sir."

"Mr. Larson, what's the next critical hurdle for this animal?"

"Uh, well…" Rick began. Kerri Feinburg and Sam Stone sashayed a half step to one side in an attempt to avoid the collateral damage they'd learned to expect. "Well, I couldn't really say. I'm not going to practice equine medicine. I plan to pursue an MBA at Wharton and I'm more interested in the business side of small animal work."

Dr. Linnehan stared at Rick. His eyeballs moved to Trisha and his brow developed two thin, vertical lines. She elevated her eyebrows in response to the unspoken query.

"Mr. Larson, are you or are you not enrolled in the University of Philadelphia, School of Veterinary Medicine?"

"I am, but…" Rick paused, which was both good and bad for him. Good because it probably saved him from digging an even deeper hole. Bad because of the opening it left.

Drill Sergeant Dan interrupted, "But? There are no buts here." Kerri looked to Sam. They both smiled under their masks. The instant tension could have been cut with a scalpel. The only sound was the rhythmic *cusssh*-click of the ventilator and the steady pulse of the EKG. Dr. Linnehan, with an economy of motion, slowly pivoted the point of his jaw one inch to the right. This brought Kerri Feinburg into his sights, "What's the next critical *step* for this patient?" Although he emphasized the word step, even a feline-obsessed, Brooklyn-born, Jewish-American Princess could deduce what he was looking for.

"Recovery?"

"Exactly. Thank you. We've got to get him safely back on his feet so we'll wake him up in water."

Dr. Linnehan pivoted his head back to Rick, "Mr. Larson, since money seems to be your primary concern, please prepare a detailed report describing the break point economics for surgery on this animal. When do economic forces outweigh the humane alternative? Deliver it to my mailbox by tomorrow at zero six hundred sharp." Dr. Linnehan pointed to the surgical-suite viewing window behind the students and said, "See that guy?" The first years turned to look. "He's this animal's trainer. And in two seconds I'm going to give him a *thumbs up* to let him know that we're going for recovery. This information will change his life in two significant ways. First of all, he loves this animal — hand raised it from a foal. Secondly, his family's future is tied to this horse's genes. Even though the animal won't race again, the potential for stud fees could finance the whole farm where he works, thus ensuring his job. His two little girls will likely go to college." He paused, "As long as this," he tapped the black and white chimera of hardware and compact bone on the X-ray viewer, "As long as this heals." Dr. Linnehan raised the thumb of his outstretched arm and relief flooded the trainer's face. The guy mouthed the words, *thank you*. He knew that this could have gone either way. Dr. Dan Linnehan was known in the racing industry as an orthopedic genius, and a hard ass who wouldn't even consider compromising animal welfare for economic investment. He wouldn't operate on, let alone recover a horse — no matter how valuable — if he believed it would suffer unnecessarily. Knowing this fact would have helped Rick shorten his report.

Redeemed lay peacefully in left lateral recumbency on the foot-thick, royal blue foam pad that cushioned the hydraulic surgery table. Dr. Linnehan instructed the anesthesiologist to dial back the isoflurane and then said, "Okay, let's go to 50% room air and be ready with some pro-pofol if things get out of hand." He, Trisha and two surgery techs hooked the patient's white nylon body sling onto the surgical hoist and in one concerted motion, like the practiced surgical ballet it was, he applied gentle upward tension to the sling as the table surface rotated perpendicular to the floor. The patient hung like a rag doll on remote control. A pair of large bore air tubes bridged the gap between the still-sleeping patient and the ventilator while a 20 foot long extension set allowed intravenous access for emergency meds or rapid sedation.

Dr. Linnehan motioned to a surgery tech, "Open the doors," and she peeled back two, 30-foot-tall, sky blue doors to reveal a tranquil inner chamber bathed in subdued lighting and soft country music. Millions of tiny bubbles jetted toward the center of the circular recovery pool in which an enormous black rubber raft floated. Dr. Linnehan handed Trisha the guide tether attached to the halter and then led Sam Stone to the tail rope. "Don't apply any tension until I tell you." He then surveyed everyone in attendance and asked, "Are we ready?"

The anesthesiologist nodded and replied, "O-2 sat is 95% and I'm getting a palpebral reflex." He disconnected the ventilator, leaving the endotracheal tube in place and when he saw a deep, voluntary, thoracic excursion he reported, "Houston, we are good to go."

Lieutenant Dan Linnehan, NASA payload commander, was no stranger to maneuvering large objects that were hovering in three dimensions. During his last shuttle mission, he managed to pluck a wobbling communications satellite out of its decaying orbit on the very first try. NASA engineers worried that the gyrating mass might fatally torque Columbia's mechanical arm, but Lieutenant Linnehan deftly matched its rotational force with light pulses from the shuttle's auxiliary thrusters. Once he'd obtained synchronous alignment, he simply reached out and grabbed the 15 ton craft and stowed it in the payload bay for return to Earth. He accomplished this first-ever feat in half the time the duty schedule allowed, all the while hurtling through space at a mere 17,600 miles per hour. By comparison, docking an 1,800 pound thoroughbred with the recovery raft was a breeze.

Dr. Linnehan drove the yellow crane hoist along the monorail until Redeemed was precisely centered over the deep, blue pool. He motioned to Trisha and Sam with his right hand, "Rotate him 10 degrees counterclockwise. We want his feet in perfect alignment with the socks." They did as directed, slowly shifting position around the pool until the hooves were suspended directly above the four neoprene pockets that protruded into the water from the raft bottom. Dr. Linnehan held up his right hand, "Stop. Perfect. Hold that position," and then shifted his thumb to the down button on the hoist control and Redeemed began to descend. The casted right front leg slid freely into the pocket but when the animal's powerful chest made contact with the float, the thoroughbred suddenly raised his head with his eyes wide open and snorted in alarm though the endotracheal tube. Waking up while dangling in the air over an ominous black raft and a pool of water is an unusual experience for a racehorse. Considering that most thoroughbreds have the stability of nitroglycerine on the Cyclone at Coney Island, it came as no surprise to Dan Linnehan when Redeemed exploded out of his sleep as if someone had just fired the starter's pistol. The animal thrashed, scared out of its mind, but the spongy neoprene craft and warm water cushioned the blows.

"Forty cc's of propofol please," was all he said and 10 seconds later, Redeemed was bobbing peacefully in the raft. "Well done."

Trisha turned to Kerri, "Can you image if we attempted that on dry land?"

The anesthetist reached in and removed the breathing tube just before the patient roused again. This time however, there was no thrashing, no alarm. Sensing the water around him, the horse began to paddle slowly. Just then Dr. Linnehan felt his pager vibrate, it was the front desk.

◄ ● ►

Dan Linnehan turned the corner into the outpatient exam bay and knew immediately why he'd been paged. A greasy, nearly-human object with tobacco-stained spittle collected in the corners of its mouth was anchored to a listless mare by a tattered lead shank. The only things that differentiated this horse trader from Jabba the Hutt were time and location. This was not a long time ago, in a galaxy far, far away — unfortunately for all involved, this was the fall of 1988 at the Center for Large Animal Medicine.

The mound muttered with mild surprise, "Linnehan..." and then leered at a fourth-year student, "So, you called in the cavalry didn't you, hon? I had better not get charged extra." The trader sneezed without covering his nose and then wiped away the snot with the back of his hand. The maneuver left a glistening smear across his cheek. He jerked his melon head towards the horse and added, "This thing's not worth it."

Dan Linnehan drew in a deep breath to steel his self-control, "Always interesting to see you..." He turned to the fourth year, "So, what's the situation?"

The senior flipped a tinback open, "Nothing Ventured is an eight-year-old, standardbred mare. Her temp is 104, pulse 50 and resps run about 15 breaths per minute. According to the owner, over the past seven to ten days she's been dull, partially off feed, and frequently breaks stride."

Jabba the Hutt interrupted by sharply jerking the mare's halter, "Piece of crap cost me seven hundred bucks and hasn't won back a nickel." He punctuated the declaration by flicking the horse's sagging lower lip with the back of his snot-covered hand, "I just want to know if she's lame or sick or — knowing *my* luck — probably both."

Dr. Linnehan folded his arms across his chest, "How about we give her a little jog?"

Jabba squinted as he evaluated the proposal, "Okay, but nothin' fancy. This one don't need no rocket science, Doctor Astronaut."

They exited the outpatient exam barn into the brilliant blue autumn air. While everyone was buoyed by the extra space, Nothing Ventured seemed not to notice.

The senior student on the case took the mare's lead from her owner and scratched the horse between the ears as she whispered, "Come on girl, let's see what you can do." She proceeded, as was protocol, to trot the horse back and forth in front of the group that now included Trisha and her three first years, Sam, Kerri and Rick Larson. With a prompt from Dr. Linnehan, the senior slowed into a fast walk and upon doing so they could all hear the difference in the animal's gait. One hoof clicked less solidly and another dragged across the pavement on the forward stroke.

Dr. Linnehan waved and the girl brought the mare to a stop in front of them. Drill Sergeant Dan gently patted Nothing Ventured on the rump and ran his hand down one hind leg and then the other. The animal's owner pulled out a twitch, basically a wooden axe handle with a loop of cord where the metal blade would have been. He grabbed the mare's whole upper lip, looped the rope over it and cranked down on the twitch, twisting the handle until the cord strangulated the tissue, and the animal, into a submissive lump. Dan Linnehan scowled and said, *"That's not necessary,"* waited until Jabba reluctantly removed the twitch, and then proceeded to check all four feet with hoof testers. After about five minutes, he stood up straight and said, "Well, she's not lame, there's something else going on. I'd suggest we run some blood work and keep her for the night. I'd also like to get a neuro consult…"

The mound of nearly-human flesh scoffed, "Whoa! Sorry to rain on your moneymaking parade Doc, but how much would that run?"

Dan Linnehan folded his arms across his chest again and performed a mental calculation, "Well, we're probably looking at three hundred dollars to start."

Jabba the Hutt spit a stringy wad of tobacco that landed just in front of Dan Linnehan's feet, "Nope. No fucking way that's gonna happen. This thing's not worth fifty bucks to me." He stopped to mull the statement over and just after he licked a strand of brown spit from his lips he said, "Actually, she's probably worth $75 as the secret ingredient in Alpo." He shook his head in disgust, "Damned thing would probably run faster if she knew the dogs were gonna get her."

"So you're telling me she hasn't been on Bute or Banamine in the last 21 days?" For the first time in a long time, this old horse trader was caught off guard. Dan Linnehan knew that if anyone was likely to prop up an ailing animal with every legal and illegal concoction available, it was this guy. "You know she can't be rendered if there's drugs in her system. So, why don't you just leave her here. We'll euthanize her and take care of the rest." He paused and then added what he knew was true, "It'll save you the bullet."

Dan Linnehan could easily imagine the final hours for this sad animal if she went "home" with the trainer. After a rough, careless trailer ride, she'd be off-loaded into an empty box stall with no food and water and held until Jabba found time in his busy schedule to lead her to the farm's trash pit. There, he'd place the rusty barrel of a 22 pistol between those dull eyes and say something like, "Stupid waste of money," and pull the trigger. Then, *if the mare was lucky*, the bullet would pass directly into her brain and it would all be over. But, more likely, the guy would screw this up just like everything else he did. The hastily aimed shot would cause the glancing bullet to partially fracture the cranium and Nothing Ventured would roll into the garbage pit half alive. Then he'd pump two or three more rounds into her chest while she flailed. Eventually, she'd bleed out.

The trainer eyed Dr. Linnehan with contempt, "How much?"

"For you, *my friend*, free of charge. You can just walk away."

Jabba squinted through the permanent sneer on his blubbery face. He rubbed his chin while he tried to figure how he was being taken.

"I don't want to see you fixin' her up and racing against me. That's unethical."

"Sir, I know exactly what's ethical," and after pausing for emphasis, he added, "and I know what's legal."

The horse trader nodded his head slowly and reached up to unhook his lead. His fingers hung on for a moment as he considered if he should also take the filthy halter. But, realizing he was getting a pretty sweet deal, he changed his mind. And then, as Dr. Linnehan had offered, without a word the guy turned and walked away.

All fourth-year students on rotation at the Center for Large Animal Medicine were required to carry their own lead shank and now Trisha Maxwell clicked the snap of her blue nylon strap into the standardbred's halter. Two concurrent transformations took place the instant the slimy horse trader disappeared from sight. Nothing Ventured slumped and leaned into Trisha. There was no longer any need for her to be on guard. And amazingly, at that exact instant, Trisha Maxwell reverted into a 12-year-old girl. She almost pleaded, "Doctor Linnehan, I want to adopt this animal. With my student discount we can at least try to work her up. If all goes well, I can take her home. He'll never know she's alive and I wouldn't race her, I promise."

Dan Linnehan pursed his lips, unfolded his arms from across his expansive chest and looked the fourth year square in the eye. "Ms. Maxwell, we are bound by our oath, *and the law*, to honor our agreement with that man — no matter how odious it may be. This animal was his property to do with as he pleased." He paused, swallowed hard, looked to the first years and then back at Trisha, "Sometimes our only option is the lesser of two evils."

Dr. Linnehan then asked softly, "Trisha, can you sign out a euthanasia kit from the pharmacy, charge it to my research account #R59 and meet us behind necropsy?"

Trisha bowed her head and nodded slowly. After a few moments she responded, "I understand."

Speaking now to Kerri and Sam, he said, "You two go get a bucket with cool, clean water and another with some oats from the feed barn. And mix in some molasses too." Kerri almost whispered, "*We will.*"

Finally, Dr. Linnehan turned to Rick Larson and asked, "Please run over to pathology and let Doctor Oblitzski know that we'll have a submission for him. I'd like a CSF tap and a full neurological workup."

Kerri and Sam performed their tasks and quickly reconvened with their professor and Trisha. They met under a sugar maple, ablaze in fall glory, just outside the necropsy facility. Nothing Ventured seemed to be aging by the minute, her head hung low and her hind end swayed. She stumbled, and, for some reason, seemed unable to lock her stay apparatus; her left and right hips dipped alternately. Although she showed no interest in the handful of clover Dan Linnehan pulled for her, she did munch a mouthful of sweetened oats and took a long drink of water.

Dr. Daniel Linnehan then stood next to the animal's shoulder, facing the semicircle of students, "It's important to remember to take great care when euthanizing a large animal. It can be the most dangerous procedure you'll ever do. Trisha, can you assist me?"

She said, "Yes, of course," and set the equine euthanasia tote on the grass. She located a packet containing a large bore catheter, taking unnecessary care to make sure she didn't contaminate the tip, and, after pulling it from the sterile pouch, attached a syringe. She shook her head and muttered, "Force of habit." In this situation, maintaining sterility of the needle was well beyond a moot point.

Dr. Linnehan smoothed the horse's jugular furrow with his left hand and then gently held off the vein. It took a few moments for the vessel to fill but he guided Trisha as she slid the catheter in place and drew back on the plunger. A billow of red welled up and mixed with the heparin-saline solution in the syringe barrel. "Good job," he said quietly as he taped off the catheter hub. He attached the four foot long extension set and said, "I'll take it from here."

On one end of this IV set was a living, breathing being, on the other, 30 ml of sky-blue, liquid death. Painless, permanent, disgusting. Dr. Linnehan checked on his students, "I need everyone to step back and stay alert. Sometimes there's an excitement phase and things can get tricky."

Dan turned back to the sagging mare. He cupped and then tickled her lower lip as he looked into the cheerless eyes. Dan Linnehan thought, *this is it, your last moment on Earth.* He spoke softly, "I'm sorry girl," and depressed the plunger as fast as he could. Within five seconds her lids drooped and three seconds later it happened. All four legs buckled. Nothing Ventured went down like one of those old, worn out buildings — imploding in a heap were she stood. No flailing, no rolling. Just straight down with a ground shaking thud. It was as if all the natural force of her life was released in an instant. Dan held his position, next to the animal's head. He would never let a student stand so close, but his responsibility to the animal would not let him abandon her.

The sadness was final, it enveloped the little group. How could they feel so much for an animal that they had just met? They had no ties, no history. How was it possible for them to care so much when her owner didn't care at all?

They stood and quietly watched as Dr. Linnehan leaned over and placed his stethoscope on the mare's inert chest. There was no Lub. No Dub. Just the ultimate silence.

And then there was Rick.

Rick had walked up behind the group unnoticed and thoughtlessly, carelessly, did what he did best — he shattered the stillness. "Hey you guys ready for the forklift or what?" Initially, no one acknowledged him but then Trisha turned and, as the saying goes, *if looks could kill,* her eyes would have telegraphed a double-barrel, 60 ml bolus of blue juice into Rick Larson.

He looked back at her in confusion and said, "What?"

Dan Linnehan realized that now was not the time for another Larson tutorial so he just replied, "Yes, tell them we're ready."

CHAPTER TWENTY

Mr. Oliver

5:15 PM — FRIDAY, OCTOBER 14, 1988

The clinical dermatology lab at VHUP in Philadelphia

"Sit, Ubu, sit! Good dog." Mike London smiled at Hoss and said, "I always wanted to do that." Ubu was a mixed breed with the intense, eager-to-please disposition of a pure border collie. The dog sat stock still, rigidly anticipating Mike's next request. He stroked the animal's balding ears, "See the pattern of hair loss? A sparseness that appears to be minimally pruritic. There's scaling and mild inflammation. Considering the age, breed and the clinical signs, it's almost pathognomonic."

Mike continued, "How many dogs would let you do this?" He produced a sterile scalpel blade from a foil packet and commanded, "Hold, Ubu," as he pinched up a fold and scraped the margin of the affected skin just behind the animal's left ear. "Remember, a skin scrape probably won't be diagnostic unless you get down to the capillaries. Unfortunately, you've got to draw a little blood." He deposited the red-tinged debris, a biopsy of sorts, by dragging the blade across a clear slide. Hoss patted the compliant animal on the head and said, "Good boy."

Mike slid into place at the multi-headed, teaching microscope, positioned Ubu's sample under the 4x objective and adjusted the light. He motioned for them to each take a station, "Let's all take a look at this. Jack, can you describe what we're seeing in the field of view?"

Jack Doyle adjusted the width of the eye pieces and responded, "I guess we see lots of hair shafts. They look like tree trunks at this magnification." He paused as they examined the rest, "There's some skin debris and I assume those red clumps are RBC's."

Mike flipped a switch that illuminated a tiny green arrow. He used the joystick to position the cursor, "What's that, at the end of the pointer?"

"It looks like a silver cigar with, I dunno, four pairs of nubs at one end."

"Yup, that's the culprit, *Demodex canis*. It's a mite that's passed from Mom to pup early in life, but only flares up when the dog's stressed and immunocompromised." He clicked the scope off, leaned back and clasped his hands behind his head. "You gotta love dermatology, a satisfying diagnosis is only a skin scrape away. Derm's the country club of specialties: if surgeons drive for show then dermatologists putt for dough." He expanded his arms, "And, when's the last time you heard of a skin emergency?"

Jack looked to Anna, then to Hoss and replied, "Never?"

Mike replied, "Exactly," just before his beeper sounded. "Hmm, maybe this is the first." Mike swiveled in his chair and retrieved the slimline receiver from the wall. He punched in a "9" followed by the outside number.

A female voice responded after the first ring, "HUP ICU."

"This is Mike London, I was just paged to this number."

Mike heard some shuffling of papers and then the voice replied, "Mrs. Irene Oliver has you listed as her emergency contact. Actually, you're her only contact. She's in our ICU."

Mike sat up straight and so did Ubu, who was now positioned at his side, "What's going on? Is she okay?"

"She was admitted yesterday with an unspecified meningitis. She keeps talking about a 'Clancy'? And saying something in French. She didn't want us to bother you but I'm afraid she's going to lose consciousness."

"Okay, I know what she wants, I'll take care of Clancy." He hung up the phone and for the first time since they'd met their advisor, Mike London looked shaken. He stood up, worried his hand through his hair and said, "Remember Mrs. Oliver from the ES?" They nodded yes. "She's ill. I need to go check on Clancy and then head down to the hospital. Can one of you tell Doctor Shanley that we confirmed Demodex on Ubu? He'll talk with the owners and set up the treatment plans."

Anna grabbed her cane and rose from the microscope, "I'm going with you."

Mike started to shake his head no but before he could respond, Jack added, "Me, too."

Hoss stepped up, "It's okay, I can take care of this," he stroked what was left of Ubu's coat, "you folks go ahead."

◄ • ►

As Mike pulled the dirty key from under the doormat, pill bugs scurried among the damp, decaying maple leaves. At the turn of the dead-bolt and creaking of the hinges, Clancy shot out between the gap and skid-ded to a stop in the tiny, fenced in yard. He squatted immediately and with a lolling tongue looked back over his shoulder with an expression of relief.

They entered the street-level apartment of the dilapidated brick building on the corner of 42nd and Spruce, and Clancy led them to the kitchen where he plopped down in front of two empty bowls. Jack said, "He's starving," as he opened the fridge to look for an open can of dog food. He reported, "There's nothing in here, not a morsel."

Mike flipped open the battered, bare cupboards until he came across a stash of kibble and cans. He ratcheted off a lid and spooned out a lump of moist meat. They watched with satisfaction as Clancy gulped down the food and lapped up a half bowl of fresh water. "Let's just give him that for now. I'm afraid he might vomit if we over-do it."

Anna broke away from the guys in the kitchen and stood in the only other room in the apartment. It served as both living and bedroom. She pursed her lips and wrinkled her nose as she drew in the musty air. Moldy travel posters were pinned on three walls, partially covering the cracked Egyptian motif wallpaper streaked with ancient water stains. Jack walked in behind her and whistled softly under his breath, "Phew, would you look at those…" He pointed to the fourth wall, it was almost entirely obscured by framed police service certificates. "That," he moved in for a closer look, "that's the Medal of Valor." This medallion represented the Holy Grail for the Doyle family. "A cop is only awarded the Medal for 'exceptional cour-age, extraordinary decisiveness and presence of mind while attempting to save or protect a life.'" Jack paused in awe as he looked to an adjacent case, "And here are two more."

Hanging next to the tarnished metals was a framed picture of Mr. and Mrs. Oliver on their wedding day. She was the quintessential, petite blushing bride on the arm of a dashing man in his dress blues. Jack counted the medals adorning the groom's left breast, "Seven, eight, nine…" He looked back to Anna wide-eyed, "This guy was the real Superman." Then, as Anna headed back to the kitchen, a framed newspaper story caught Jack's eye. In a rush, the headline's black lettering vaulted from the faded, yellowing page and knocked the wind out of him: 'Decorated Officer Gives Life to Save Drowning Child.' Jack froze. For a brief painful moment, his childhood, the loss of his baby sister, and all those animals his father gave him to rescue came flooding back. Jack reached for his only defense from the deep. He distracted himself. He redirected his gaze and let the joy of the Olivers' wedding photo fill his eyes. He coughed, cleared his throat and turned away from the wall of honor, thankful that no one had noticed.

⊲ • ⊳

After feeding Clancy a small bowl of kibble and fitting his harness, Mike, Anna and Jack made their way down Spruce in the fading October light. Anna kept up with no noticeable problem. It seemed to Jack that whatever her disability, it waxed and waned in severity. Without hesitation, they rushed through the emergency entrance to HUP and into an open elevator with Clancy and Petunia in tow. When the doors slid open on the fifth floor, they were facing the ICU nurses' station.

"We're here to see Irene Oliver."

A nurse spoke up, "Hang on doctor," Mike was still in scrubs and his white lab coat, "Who are you?"

"I'm Mike London from the vet school. I was paged for Mrs. Oliver."

"Okay, but you can't bring those dogs into the ICU." Mike looked down at the two sets of smiling eyes and wagging tails and with mild surprise he thought, *we've got dogs in our ICU all the time.*

Jack took both leads, "I'll wait here with the dogs."

The nurse led Mike and Anna to a glassed-in room adjacent to the station. Mike knew that the proximity of the room did not bode well; this was where the most critical patients were placed. Jack watched as Mike leaned over Mrs. Oliver, said something and then pointed to where he stood with Clancy.

Mrs. Oliver whispered faintly to Mike and Anna, "I was so afraid. Afraid something would happen to me and no one would find him."

Mike replied, "Don't worry, everything's fine. Clancy can stay with us until you are well enough to go home. Mrs. Oliver, did the doctors tell you what they found?"

She turned her head slowly from side to side and flinched, "I don't know, maybe." He lifted the chart from a rack at the foot of her bed, flipped through the thick stack of pages and looked up at Anna, "They've done CAT scans, an MRI and a spinal tap, but there's no diagnosis." He turned and made his way to the door, "I'm going to see if I can find her primary clinician."

Anna moved up to fill the gap when Mike left the room and, just as she'd done when they first met, she cupped Mrs. Oliver's hand in both of hers. The elderly woman turned her head slowly to face Anna and said with a weak smile, "See, like I said, lots of compassion." She paused to take in and exhale two labored breaths, "I'm worried I may never leave here. Can I ask an enormous favor? Can you make sure Clancy is taken care of?"

Anna almost stammered, "Mrs. Oliver, please don't talk like that. You're going to get better."

"Dear, I am blessed. I have had a full life. Although I've never left Philadelphia, this is where I met the man of my dreams. This is where I toured the world."

Anna smiled and paused, "I saw the posters from your trips."

"Oh no dear, that was all Mr. Oliver's doing. We never got to actually travel but he took me to Paris, to Rome and London."

Anna cocked her head and crinkled her brow, "What do you mean?"

Anna felt the woman's pulse quicken between her hands and heard the increasing beep of her EKG. Mrs. Oliver's unseeing but still-animated eyes widened. "My life began the moment we met. He was my own personal hero. It was May 5th, 1930. I was a teacher at the Franklin Academy and on a lunch break when a thief snatched my purse. It was right out here on Spruce Street." She smiled with the thought. "That poor young man yanked the purse off my arm, tore down the block and ran headlong into my Henry. Well, he wasn't my Henry yet." She paused to inhale again but this time she didn't wince. "He was so tall, so solid and broad. After handcuffing the man and returning my property I asked him, 'How can I ever repay you?'" She paused as her excitement built, "And, do you know what he did?"

Anna whispered, "No, *what?*"

"He took my hand and said, 'Come with me to Paris.'"

Her eyes grew even wider as the memory swelled in her heart. "Three days later we met on the top step at the Museum of Art." Mrs. Oliver placed her left hand on her cheek in surprise as if it were happening just that instant. Pools welled in her eyes, "He put a beret on my head, handed me two red roses and said, 'Bienvenue à Paris,' and whisked me inside."

"Behind the red velvet ropes in my own private exhibition of the French impressionists, we glided from Monet to Renoir to Van Gogh. I swear we were dancing. First he'd say, 'Les impressionnistes sont très extraordinaires,' and then he'd translate. I found out later that he'd been tutored by the Academy's romance languages instructor around the clock for nearly two days. And that day, looking into his eyes, I can honestly say that the world revolved around us. Not another person existed. My heart soared and it carried us from the museum to Fairmont Park where we picnicked on wine and cheese." She slowly nodded her head, "He thought of everything — like those posters. I closed my eyes as he read until sunset. I could see the Eiffel Tower, the Seine with les bateaux-mouche, Notre Dame…"

"And you went to Rome the same way?"

Her eyelids fluttered, "And Vienna, and London. We married three months later."

Mrs. Oliver swallowed with some difficultly and closed her eyes. "And then he was gone…" Her voice trailed off, "A little boy fell through the ice on the Schuylkill just before Christmas." She opened her unseeing eyes again, looked towards Anna and said, "Sweetheart, if you find a man who can transport you to Paris just by taking your hand, don't ever let go."

Anna blinked once slowly and then looked towards the waiting area where Jack sat scratching Petunia's ears. She nodded silently and the downward motion caused a tear to spill onto their clasped hands.

Mrs. Oliver smiled, "Oh… you've already found him."

CHAPTER TWENTY ONE

X-Ray Vision

The Seven Seas backup area at The Peaceable Kingdom

D
r. Violet Green still couldn't quite believe it. She stood frozen in the vast space, mesmerized as three male dolphins vaulted into synchronous double summersaults. The sleek animals plunged deep into the sparkling water that served as both their playground and a conservation display arena. Every day that she walked through the massive backstage doors of the Peaceable Kingdom (which was pretty much every day) she was amazed at her inexplicable good fortune. Sure, she was trained during her internship by some of the best zoo vets in residence at this country's first zoo, the Philadelphia Zoo. And, yes, she did have an impressive educational pedigree. But as a recent graduate, she couldn't quite get her head around the fact that she had the opportunity to help design and then run this place, one of the premier veterinary facilities at any zoological park in the world. For whatever reason, whenever she spoke, the architects had listened. Her recommendations for the Seven Seas animal care suite were intricate and exacting, but still, no expense was spared. The main display pool where the three males currently frolicked was connected to a series of holding, treatment and examination pools. A water-filled channel even extended directly into the marine mammal surgery so dolphins and the other small whales could swim in and then be strained up from the water by a false-bottom hydraulic lift — all at the touch of a button.

A duo of perky trainers, a girl and a guy, flanked Violet Green. They kneeled at the maternity pool's edge in full-body, black neoprene suits, each of them with a gleaming bucket at their side. She remembered back to a simpler time in her life when her primary responsibilities at SeaWorld were toting buckets, tooting whistles and working out.

The girl on her right blew twice on her whistle and directed, "Open." The dolphin stationed obediently with its mouth held wide, her pink tongue wriggling back and forth. Another shrill toot and the trainer delivered an icy herring into the waiting animal's mouth, "Good girl, Akai. Doctor Green, she's ready." The trainer got no response so she nudged the vet's leg gently, "Doctor Green…"

"Oh, sorry," Violet Green shook her head, "I'm still amazed at how lucky we are to have this facility for our animals."

The golden ponytail bobbed in enthusiastic agreement, the brass whistle still clamped between her lips. She dipped her left hand into the water which was where Akai dutifully rested her lower jaw. The trainer requested again, "Open." This time Dr. Green swept the beam of her flat-black Maglite illuminating the gleaming arcades of conical teeth. After another "Good girl," a fish-sickle and a command, Dr. Green pointed her newest gizmo, an infrared monitor, into the yawning oral cavity. She tilted the experimental instrument's screen so the trainer could see, "Everything looks cool blue, the inflammation is gone." She reached down and her white-hot finger showed brightly on the screen as she palpated the tooth of concern. Akai held station without so much as a flinch. "We caught that cavity just in time. You guys did a great job." Violet concluded, "How about we get a blow sample and then let's setup for blood."

The perky ponytail bobbed in comprehension, she knew the routine, "10-4, Doc."

Akai's calf, a three-month-old male, mimicked his mom. He hung vertically in the water on her right. His very own private trainer rewarded him, trying to link every good behavior with a whistle toot and a tiny fish that the animal proceeded to toss repeatedly into the air. After he tired of this game, the infant swam in tight circles with the semi-frozen treat perfectly balanced on the tip of his snout. His perky trainer guy remarked with obvious affection, "Doofus, you do everything but eat them. I guess you still prefer your mom's warm milk to cold, slimy mackerel."

The female trainer spoke up, "Keep that up, he's gonna think his name really is Doofus. Remember that the 3rd graders at Independence Grammar School officially named him, Percival the Sea Prince. That's Perci to you, lowly trainer boy."

"His name is Doofus until proven otherwise," the male trainer joked.

Then, in response to a series of hand gestures, Akai logged quietly, parallel to the pool's edge. The female trainer stroked the mother dolphin's slippery back, ending with a finger positioned just behind the blowhole. Dr. Green uncapped a sterile petri dish, extended her arm and nodded. The trainer tapped twice and Akai inoculated the blood-red media with a jet of air that caused Dr. Green's outstretched arm to rebound upward. Perci lined up like his mom, but instead of holding still, he squirmed and chirped with delight every time the trainer "tickled" his back. He blew a small waterspout which was bridged with a toot and another fish. "I suppose he'll figure it out eventually. Right Doofus?" The guy playfully splashed water on the calf's melon which caused Perci the Sea Prince to spin and click with glee, and finally spit water back at him.

"Okay, let's just get the blood and we'll be done with the physicals." The trainer tapped the water's surface with her flat palm three times. Akai responded almost instantly by rolling on her back and laying her broad, flat tail fluke in the girl's hands. The trainer steered the animal like a floor buffer, sweeping her slowly from side to side across the surface. She tooted once more, released her grip and Akai popped up with her mouth open to receive her reward. "Okay, we did our dry run, she's all ready for the stick."

In an instant, Akai lay patiently on her back in the water, holding her breath. Violet could barely make out the faint vascular furrows that radiated outward towards the tip of her tail fluke. She swabbed a site that looked promising and slid the 21 gauge needle into the skin. She applied gentle back pressure on the 3 cc syringe and in an instant received a red flash. "You're the best, Doctor Green, you never miss."

"Oh, I've missed plenty. Just yesterday I had to call it on a humming bird. He was turning into a pin cushion." Violet gently retracted the needle and covered the spot with an alcohol swab.

Dr. Green stood and ejected aliquots of the blood into a series of colored tubes that were wedged in the foam block of a plastic instrument tote. It was labeled, "Routine Cetacean Physicals."

She had just trickled the last crimson drop into a purple-topped tube when her radio squawked to life, "Base to Doctor Green. Base to Doctor Green."

Violet Green capped the tube and reached to her hip for her walkie talkie, "Go ahead Base, this is Violet."

"Violet, there's a Doctor Oblitzski here to see you."

"Great, can you have a docent escort him to the marine mammal surgery?"

"10-4. Base out."

Ten minutes later, Stan the Path Man was waving excitedly on the other side of the surgery doors. Dr. Green motioned that he should come in and before the swinging double doors could close behind him he was already exclaiming, "Wow, Violet, this place is the bomb! It's sooo incredibly cool." He craned his neck and his mouth hung open as his gaze was drawn up into the immense, airy space. Sunlight slanted in through 50-foot tall panes causing rippling sparkles on the water's surface. He muttered, "Like diamonds. Violet, it's a cathedral. A cathedral to life…"

Violet responded softly, "Yeah, I know what you mean." And then noticing the two big boxes, one under each of his arms, she said, "Let me help you." She removed one without Stan noticing; he was still scanning the suite. "You've got large and small animal ventilators, ultrasound and even fluoroscopy. Holy cow! Ab-so-tootly amazing."

Because Violet knew she was standing before a fellow veterinary nerd and true friend, she could be herself, "And you gotta see this, Stan." She drew her hand lovingly over a mobile contraption packed with pumps, heaters, chillers and water reservoirs — it could have come straight out of Dr. Seuss. "It's a mobile fish anesthesia machine; can you believe it?"

Stan the Path Man grinned and was just about to say, *golly gee wilikers*, when Percival the Sea Prince swam up from behind. He poked his perpetually smiling beak out of the water and began chirping away. Stan's face lit up, "Hey there little fella," Perci responded with a squirt of water that splashed on Stan's feet. "Violet, he's adorable. But," Stan shifted into pathologist mode which meant that tact and normal human decorum had vanished, "He's looking a little gray."

"Stan, that's his natural coloration and you know it. He's perfectly healthy."

"I'm just saying," he held up a hand in mock protest, "you never bring any dolphins over to necropsy."

"And my goal is to keep it that way. Besides, we've been giving you way too much business lately."

Violet Green hefted the cardboard box up onto the surgery table and Stan followed her lead, he asked, "We can work here?"

"Yeah, there's plenty of room and lots of great light." She stepped on a floor switch that ignited a massive, overhead array of surgery lights. "I have an office, but I do my best thinking in here."

Stan unpacked the collated stacks of paper. There were manila folders bulging with gross path reports, histo path reports, animal medical records, and line graphs. He extracted a pile of gelled films that resembled X-rays and a microscope slide box that rattled. The little glass plates vibrated in their neat slots as he flipped open the lid. Each glass section held ultra-thin slivers of animal tissue stained in brilliant pink and blue. Finally, he produced a AAA travel map.

Stan said, "How about I cut to the chase?"

Violet nodded, agreeing to the idea.

Stan fumbled with a folder and flipped through a dozen graphs, some computer generated, others hand drawn. He chose a dot matrix plot that stretched out, like a banner, over fifteen sheets held together by the perforated ribbons on both sides. "This," he paused as he drew his right index finger along a line that paralleled the X-axis, "This dark blue line represents the monthly mortality rate at the vet school over the last 12 years. All of these cases have a final diagnosis, a known cause." He then produced a transparency scroll, like the kind used on an overhead projector. He fitted the transparency to the paper graph and took a deep breath, "And these are the undiagnosed mortalities for the same period." He paused, and then pointed to precipitous peak near the end of the graph, "This is August and September, a 350% increase above baseline. Just as you suspected, Violet, nearly every animal presented with neuro signs."

"Did you get a chance to look at the blood work? We drew on the cetaceans last because they seemed unaffected."

"Yeah," Stan slid a series of twelve black and white electrophoretic gels onto the Peaceable Kingdom's massive X-ray view box. He pointed to a fuzzy gray line, "See this thick band?" He went down the line of images pointing, "Here, here and here…" Violet nodded. "It corresponds with IgM production, and compared with your banked plasma samples from normal animals, it's a *whopper* of a response." He let his hands fall to his sides limply, "Violet, this is an epizootic like I've never seen."

"Epizootic? What's going on here, Guv'?" Violet and Stan jolted. They'd both been so intently staring into the light box they didn't notice William Digby's stealthy approach. "It can't be as bad as all that now?"

Stan swallowed, his pointy Adam's apple fluttering. In the shadow of the strapping brawn of William, he was immediately transported back to junior high gym class, "Well, I think it's a novel virus."

William slapped Stan heavily on the back. The gesture seemed designed to have more than a physical impact, "Aw come on now mate, that sounds like something Michael Crichton would invent. In my experience, animals die. Ultimately, that's what they all do."

Stan swallowed again but then regained his composure. They were now firmly in his working realm: death. "Yup, they all die, but not like this." He grabbed the AAA map and unfolded it across the pile of data on the surgery table. It encompassed the eastern half of Pennsylvania, most of New Jersey, and all of Delaware and Maryland. He reached up and aimed two of the brilliant surgical lights so they'd shine a bright circle centered on southeastern Pennsylvania. "The blue dots, and FYI, there are 54 of them, are unexplained equine deaths — including your two zebra and that Przewalski." Stan's hand trembled slightly as he circled the Peaceable Kingdom's location in Chadds Ford. "The 324 orange dots," he spread his fingertips broadly across the region, "are avian mortalities. The majority are corvids, that's crows, magpies and ravens."

For some reason, William bristled, "I know what corvids are, I'm not a drongo, mate."

"Well, then you know that they're the smartest of birds and we've never seen mortality numbers like this in the wild." Stan repeated, "Never," and then Stan the Path Man paused because his next point was a big one. He swirled his finger in a tight circle that included Philly, "Want to guess what the *red* dots represent?"

William rubbed his chin and replied with a smirk, "I dunno mate, how about wallabies, wombats and goannas... you know, important beasties like that." He clapped Stan on the back again and this time Stan actually felt bullied.

Stan squared his shoulders, straightened his back and looked William dead in the eye, "It is an important species alright. Those red dots are humans."

The three stood in silence while the concept of a zoonotic outbreak sunk in. Violet Green's mind raced as she thought, *Is this real? Could an infectious agent spread so widely and affect so many different species — even man?*

William Digby, feeling that this thing was getting a touch out of hand, reached for the walkie talkie mic clipped to his belt. He curled his left arm, purposefully and unnecessarily bulging his biceps as he raised the transmitter to his mouth which was now in the shape of a hard line, "What's your take on all this nonsense, Davaris?"

Violet cocked her head and scrunched up her eyebrows. The speaker on William's two-way radio came to life, "Oh, I don't know, William. It seems that Doctor Green has been safeguarding the health of our collection. She's just doing the job we hired her for. Besides, the data appears quite compelling."

Violet Marie Green ripped the communicator from her own belt and crushed the transmitter under her thumb, "Mr. Davaris, have you been listening in?"

A gravelly disembodied voice replied, "Why yes Doctor Green, and watching too — I like to keep an eye on my investments."

William winked at Violet. Then, as if he were scolding her, he wagged his index finger before pointing to a spot high in the white metal rafters. Violet and Stan tipped their heads back to see a security camera on a motorized tilt and pan armature. It was mounted next to a bunch of yellowing fly strips studded with hundreds of bugs. Violet watched as the body of the device rotated slowly until the lens pointed directly into her eyes; a red LED flashed as its mechanical iris tightened down to a point.

Although Violet Marie Green was, to say the least, taken aback, she quickly refocused and again raised the walkie talkie to her lips. Speaking in a firm, clear voice she said, "If we do have an outbreak and the Peaceable Kingdom is involved, I will have to report it to the CDC."

At this, William took a step towards the two veterinarians but stopped when Davaris broke in, "Now William, I do believe that the good doctor will most certainly do the right thing by her employer and, of course, the animals under her care."

Stan, who'd been mute since the eerie unveiling of "Big Brother's" watchful gaze, grabbed the transparency overlay from the surgery table marched over to the X-ray light box and slid it into position under the clips. He craned his neck back to see the camera pivot in his direction and then he said, "This," he pointed to the red peak, "This is real — this is an outbreak."

William stepped up and dwarfing Stan as he muscled his way into the space. "You're overlooking one important thing mate," and with a single digit he stabbed the exact spot where the blood-red mortality curve plunged back to zero. "Whatever it was… Poof!" He snapped his thick powerful fingers an inch from Stan's nose, "If it *was* an outbreak, it's over. Problem solved." He tore down the plastic strip, dropped it onto the floor and smiled, "I'll leave you Nancy Drews to get to your next mystery."

Then, in the moment that followed, as if nothing had happened, William proceeded as only someone with an ego the size of the Southern Hemisphere could. He turned and placed a hand on Violet Green's waist, "Vi, are we still on for tonight?"

At first she blinked. She was confused, "No William, we are not."

CHAPTER TWENTY TWO

A Note from Buck

*Just before morning oncology rounds in the VHUP small
animal wards in Philadelphia*

Mike London handed back the wrinkled piece of paper and
watched as Trisha carefully folded and returned it to the creased, coffee-
stained envelope. After several moments of silence had elapsed between
them (not counting the background of soft, early morning woofs and
meows of the newly admitted patients), Trisha asked with raised eyebrows
and a hopeful smile, "What's your diagnosis, oh True Love guru? What
does this mean?"

Mike responded as clinically as he could fake, "Well, tops on my
differential list? Hmmm, what you have here is an appreciative client."
He nodded thoughtfully and pretended to conclude, "That's the aim isn't
it? Aside from providing effective veterinary care, we all want an animal's
owner to recognize our value as a clinician." Mike London steadied his
poker face and paused just long enough to induce the first stage of friendly
torment in his classmate and close friend. But when Mike saw Trisha's
brow begin to furrow, he administered the reversal agent, "Nah, I'm just
kidding, I think this means you've got yourself an admirer."

Trisha lowered her eyes, blushed and fingered the shiny ribbon that
had accompanied the note all the way from Florida. Though mailed in
mid-October, the letter had taken its sweet time in finding her. First it
went, as addressed, to the Center for Large Animal Medicine in Kennett
Square. But since the student mailboxes are on the main campus in Philly,
it sat for five days in the basement mailroom waiting for the weekly inter-

office run to the city by the maintenance staff. Once in Philadelphia, since it was addressed to "Doc Maxwell," the letter got misdirected to the faculty on-call room in VHUP where it languished for over a week on a side table next to the perpetually brewing coffee pot. Finally, late the night before, at about 3 AM, Flo Kimball had noticed the name, and recognizing the problem, had inserted the envelope next to the entry for vinblastine in the dog-eared drug formulary she always kept in her lab coat pocket. She did this because she'd just aspirated a lump and presumptively diagnosed a mast cell tumor on a stump-tailed Maine coon named Bob who had been admitted to the ES. Since Dr. Kimball had already set up Bob's 6:00 AM transfer to oncology, that's when she would hand off the note, tucked inside the animal's medical record, to the senior student on the service — Trisha Maxwell.

The circuitous journey the envelope had taken left an impression on both the letter inside and on Trisha. Over the time that the note had been in transit from down South, through stuffy mailrooms and various modes of conveyance, the weight of less significant communications had pressed on the enclosed gift, embossing a pleasing form in the page. What affected Trisha most was the fact that during the time the note had been in passage, she had been doing all she could to keep up with Buck's travels. In her "free time," she had scoured whatever equine publications she could find. But it wasn't until she found the most recent Cutting Horse Association's newsletter, that she finally saw mention of Buck and Suzie placing third at an event in Kentucky. When Trisha first opened the note, she ran her finger along the rim of the molded shape in the paper and whispered to herself, *we were thinking of each other at the same time.*

Trisha slowly raised her head and looked back at Mike with an unmistakable bloom in her sparkling eyes and said, "I'm going to keep this," she said holding up the blue first-place ribbon, "someplace special."

Truth be told, Trisha Maxwell had not stopped thinking about that sweet cowboy since the moment they had met.

October 12

Hey Doc,

I just wanted to say how grateful I am for your help. As you figured, Suzie had a bruised splint bone (I'm so thankful it wasn't broken). After three weeks of stall rest and light breezes, she's as right as rain again.

Last week we took <u>First</u> in the trials here in Gainesville (FL). Please accept this ribbon as token of our thanks— we couldn't have done it without you!!

Yours truly,

Buck Riley (and Suzie)

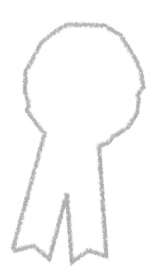

CHAPTER TWENTY THREE

Body of Knowledge

Special lecture series, Intro to Small Animal Nutrition (final presentation of the week), Room 13 in Philadelphia

The laughter and applause trickled off as Sam exited the stage in Room 13. Like an old-time vaudeville act, he framed his exaggerated, smiling face with shaking hands as he shuffled past Jack who was on his way to the podium.

"I'd like to introduce and welcome our final speaker for the day, Doctor Avery Banks." Jack clicked the controller linked to the projector. It activated Dr. Banks' presentation and the title slide appeared. A picture of a perfectly-groomed Bichon Frise, posed for show judge evaluation, was top center. The title read, 'Nutritional Support for the Champion Show Dog, Nutritional Support for Your Practice.' Avery Banks, MS, DVM, PhD The AVIS Corporation.

Jack held up the bio he'd been given and read, "'Doctor Banks is a lecturer and head of veterinary product development for the AVIS Corporation, the parent company that supplies supplements to every major pet food company. Doctor Banks received her MS in sports physiology from Brown University, and completed a combined DVM/PhD degree program at Purdue. She is a board-certified specialist in both small animal nutrition and internal medicine.' Wow." He looked from the paper, down to Dr. Banks. She was seated in the front row next to Anna and the contrast could hardly have been greater. While Anna somehow managed to project terse angles in every direction, Avery Banks was one never-ending, sinuous curve. A radiant sheen seemed to halo from her flirtatious blonde hair. After about three seconds of complete silence and a staged cough from Death Row, Jack realized he was staring. "Um, without further ado..." Jack left the podium and for the first time, did not return to Death Row. He slid into an open seat in the front row.

Avery Banks raised herself regally and mounted the stage. She nodded with a warm smile to Jack, "Thank you, Mr. Doyle," and then opened up to face the rest of the class, "And thank you, first years, for having me."

Back in Death Row, Sam leaned his head towards Hoss and remarked under his breath, "We get to have her?"

Hoss replied quietly, "I don't think she means *that*."

Sam grinned, "I bet Jack does."

Jack's eyes were riveted to Avery Banks as she beamed her luminous, corporate smile. It was perfectly matched and balanced by an ample string of pearls which dipped suggestively into the valley of her cleavage. On another more ordinary woman, the strand might have bowed gracefully in an understated "U," but with Avery Banks, the long string of natural jewels formed a deep V with sides that actually curved inward. This delicious shape was supported by what Jack would have called the superstructure of her magnificent breasts.

Avery Banks strode across the stage exuding power and confidence. The alternating, supple bounce of smooth gluteal curves were transmitted through the second-skin of her black dress. They sent shock waves through Jack's dilated pupils that skipped his brain entirely, but instead, were transmitted down his spine at the speed of light. She held the mic tight to her lips and asked almost breathlessly, "You guys want to see something?"

Jack nodded blindly.

She advanced the 35 mm slide with a click of her finger and the projection came to life. Unlike traditional academic lecturers, Dr. Avery Banks, the professional face of the AVIS Corporation, toured with a battery of presentation equipment. In the back of Room 13 stood a stack of projectors that flashed, faded, and advanced through a series of vivid images. At first, the title slide dissolved into blowing desert sands, shaping and shifting until finally a Sphinx arose.

"This was the ancient ideal of form." Avery Banks stepped back and slowly arced her hand to unveil the next slide like an auto-show model, "But today, this is perfection." The image of the Sphinx morphed with three rapid transitions into the Westminster AKC Best-in-Show, Butch the Australian Shepherd.

She raised her right hand level with her brilliant smile and snapped her fingers twice before lofting a cylindrical object into the air. A black, brown and white blur rocketed down the aisle, leapt into the air and snatched the projectile at its apex. The Australian Shepherd landed on all fours in a perfect show dog pose and then slunk to the side of his mistress. With a wry smirk, and never taking her eyes off the audience, Avery Banks leaned forward and held out an upraised palm in which Butch deposited the can with a brilliant AVIS label, upside down. The class responded with laughter which was immediately followed by applause.

Kerri turned to Sam, "Aw, that was so cute."

Avery Banks barked, "Butch!" The dog stretched up and mouthed the can, turned his head, and replaced it in her palm — this time, right side up. This trick was followed by another — even more clapping from the entranced first years. Everyone participated, everyone of course, except Anna.

Avery Banks bowed deeply, "Thank you. You'll find a doggie bag of goodies from AVIS under your chairs. Pens, pads, highlighters for studying, and I hope you'll enjoy our version of Veterinary Small Animal Nutrition. We sponsor the text and you'll find reprints of all our most recent work in the appendix."

"Today, I'd like to share some startling results from our latest studies. They underscore the critical role nutrition plays in coaxing peak performance from show dogs, show cats *and*," she flashed her tantalizing smile, "the way nutritional schemes can coax peak performance from your practice." She corrected herself, "Your *future* practices."

"As you can see with champion performers like Butch, it's all about conformation — it's all about shape."

Sam Stone whispered again to Hoss, "I'd say Doctor Hot Body is eminently qualified to wax poetic on this topic."

Hoss flattened his lips and nodded, "She does seem pretty smart."

Avery Banks continued, "Nutrition, physical training, and breeding are the top contributors to body shape. Now, I'm going to flash you two sequential images."

The words *flash you*, caused Jack's eyebrows to raise in unreasonable expectation.

"Consider these two boxers." She showed a single slide with two dogs side-by-side for an instant, then switched to a blank. "Which animal was more appealing, which one will be bred more?" She sauntered across the stage, slowed and then turned to look directly at Jack. "Let's meter your choice by applause. Bitch number one?" The picture reappeared. There was a smattering of applause that quickly faded as the clappers sensed they'd chosen wrong. "Or bitch number two?" Nearly everyone clapped. "You're right! The second animal, the Duchess of Burgundy, was Best-in-Breed and the other, I forget its name, was only a runner up." Dr. Banks repeated the shell game two more times with similar outcomes. "So, what was different? What separates a winner from all those losers?"

JJ's arm shot up, "Uh, shape. Conformation." JJ couldn't disguise the puppy love, you could almost see tiny red hearts floating up from where he sat.

"Perfect." Avery Banks thought, *it's almost as if you read the script.*

"Now, I'll show you what your mind recognized subconsciously." She triggered the transition into the next slide. A dotted red line traced the curve on the buttocks of the winner, and a straighter yellow line of the nameless other. "See?" Most of the sheep nodded. "It all comes down to a simple curve. Our eyes are just naturally drawn to pleasing shapes. And a pleasing appearance is what it's all about." She added, "Our eyes have been honed to discern fitness, almost at a glance. Numerous studies have shown that appearance confers a competitive advantage for all organisms. Now let's move on to the exciting results from our most recent studies."

Amazingly, a laser light show ensued. Red, white, and blue stars streaked and pulsed across the ceiling tiles in sync with Thomas Dolby's *She Blinded Me with Science*. Avery Banks plunged ahead and displayed another pair of animals, "As scientists, you know that the only way you can make meaningful comparisons is to control as many variables as possible. So, at AVIS, we only run trials on full sibling pups. They're genetically similar, they've had identical physical training programs and the same total caloric intake. Everything's the same except..." Avery Banks paused for her big finale which usually worked just fine but in this instance was a tactical error.

Anna could no longer contain herself. She blurted out, "Gimme a break!" No one could tell in the dimmed room lighting but her face neared lobster red. Avery Banks was startled; this was definitely not in the script. She looked down on the angular girl in the front row and punched a button to halt the disco ball. Anna went on, "Everything is the same except... The group on the left was fed the new AVIS supplement, let's call it *SuperCurve*. And the group on the right was not." Avery Banks was visibly thrown and Anna didn't wait for her respond. "And if vets sell your new prescription blend," she dipped her voice an octave like a radio announcer, "*Now fortified with SuperCurve*, the potential for profit is immense."

Dr. Banks stood behind the podium and stared at Anna. She reached for her usual tools, flashing that brilliant smile and brushing the silky hair off her right ear. But these charms, the ones that had served her so well over the years, were flaunted in vain. "Do you have a question or...?"

"Yes, I do have a question. What ingredients are in your new diet?"

Avery Banks displayed a mock frown as she tilted her head, "Oh, I'm so sorry miss. The formulation is proprietary at this point in time."

Jack saw his chance to potentially white knight his way into a date so he jumped headlong into it. He stood and interjected, "Anna, until a company actually releases a product they do not have to share such information. It could tip off the competition."

Anna was undeterred, "The can displayed at this moment on our podium boasts salmon fillets as a natural source Omega-3 fatty acids for coat enhancement."

"Yes, yes it does, and we are *very* proud..."

Anna cut her off, "Great, you're proud. But can you tell me where the salmon filets come from?"

"The salmon are grown on fish farms off the coast of Chile which causes no impact on wild salmonid populations."

"No impact," Anna almost hissed, "What are these farm-raised fish fed?"

"My dear, salmon are strict carnivores, *if that's your point*. They need to eat meat. They're fed a high-protein diet manufactured from," she stammered almost imperceptibly, "locally caught smelt, anchovies and herring. A rich, nutritionally-complete and 100% natural food source."

"And how many pounds of wild-caught fish are needed to produce your dog food?"

Dr. Banks didn't flinch but Jack noticed that her succulent lower lip twitched just before she replied, "I'm sure I couldn't tell you exactly."

"I can. According to an independent study funded by ALM, it takes a *minimum* of 18 pounds of wild caught fish, including bycatch, to produce just one pound of your pet food."

Avery Banks squinted and nodded subtly, "So, that's what this is about." Her eyelids fluttered, conveying an expression of tired recognition, "Is this a commercial for the Animal Liberty Militia, or do you actually have a point?"

"Commercial! Pot—Kettle—Black, Miss Banks."

The SuperCurve on the stage finally lost her composure, "That's Doctor Banks to you."

Anna didn't balk, "So, considering your market share worldwide, that adds up to three million metric tons a year taken from wild fish populations that are already in crisis. Three million tons for dog and cat treats!"

"Says you…"

Anna almost laughed, which would have been a first. "Brilliant retort, *doctor*. In order to respond on your level I'd be forced to counter with, 'Oh yeah?'" The two women glared at each other, Petunia, sensing the tension, sat up and leaned into Anna's leg. "The American Fisheries Society has deemed those exact wild fish populations as severely threatened. It's not just me."

Jack bolted from his seat. He shot up on stage and attempted to intervene, "Okay, well, it looks like our time is running short…"

Avery Banks pushed him aside as she came around from behind the podium. She towered over the handicap seating area at her feet, "This is business. This is economically driven." After each sentence she stabbed her finger into the top of the podium and it made a hollow sound. "The consumer wants healthy, nutritious food for their beloved pets. We're providing a wonderful alternative to ground up cow hooves, horse tendons and pig's feet." She cocked her head rapidly to the right and then leveled it to take her final shot, "Miss, as a veterinarian — if you become one — you will be responsible for the health of your patient and that extends to nutritional support."

"As a veterinarian, my responsibilities will go much deeper than that. We're responsible for the health of *all* animals and ultimately the environment in which we live." Anna shook her head slowly back and forth as she gathered herself for her final attack, "It makes no sense to destroy wild animal populations just to get the 'right curve' on an inbred show dog!"

Jack held out his arms like a referee at a boxing match, "Okay, really, our time is up. Thank you." Sam clanged an empty Coke can with his pen, it sounded like a bell. Jack drew a deep breath and expelled it slowly, "I'd like to invite you all to the Halloween Happy Hour at Alpha Mu. This year it's sponsored by the AVIS Corporation, with free beer, wine and uh," he paused, "treats…"

CHAPTER TWENTY FOUR

Animal House

The Alpha Mu fraternity house on Pine Street in Philadelphia

Alpha Mu was the only fraternity on the vet school campus and it was the *original* Animal House. The building, a sprawling 1890s Greek revival originally built for Andrew Carnegie, was neither maintained nor neglected by the club. Its innumerable residents simply cohabited, almost symbiotically, within the massive, honeycombed structure. The white clapboard building did its part by providing shelter, while its inhabitants, representing numerous phyla, gave it life. A pulsing, vibrant, unpredictable animal life.

Every party at Alpha Mu was a species nonspecific melting pot where all sizes, shapes and breeds romped and intermingled. Borzois chased greyhounds, which in turn pursued whippets, which ran in wide arcs around the muddy, fecal-laden back yard. Such a sighthound dash was usually triggered every few minutes by a streaking rodent or occasionally a real live hare. A pack of resident house cats, the kind that knew how to handle any dog, ruled the roost. Some strutted, unconcerned across the kitchen linoleum, others leapt from chair backs and countertops into waiting arms, and all took naps anywhere they damn-well-pleased. Mix-breed moms with kittens, cross-eyed Siamese, and regular old tabbies seemed to check their membership in the Predator's Guild at the door, allowing the lower vertebrates to table their fears. Animals such as Slinky the ferret, a fraternity brother's pet rat, and an avian flock including two peach-faced love birds and José's cockatiel named Flipper, all traveled from room to room entirely unmolested. The only pet under continuous surveillance was Rick Larson's ball python. Rick was required to keep it in its cage, slung around his neck, or on a leash at all times. Amazingly, he'd fashioned a snug fitting, blue canvas, rhinestone studded collar that was reasonably secure behind that triangular, tongue-flicking head. The collar also served to retard the impromptu swallowing of large-diameter pets.

Tonight, Hoss and Kerri Feinburg stood in the atrium on either side of the house's main entrance. As pledges they served a half-hour shift informally meeting and greeting the guests. Everything at Alpha Mu was informal. Kerri wore a full-body, solid pink leotard and palmed a bunch of softball-sized, pink balloons in each hand. Whenever anyone inquired, and they always did, she'd snap to attention bringing both legs together and extend her arms laterally from her shoulders. Her downward curving palms and wiggling fingers embracing each dangling pink cluster. Nine out of ten times she'd have to say, "Come on, you know this. I'm a feline female reproductive tract." This brought rapid nods of recognition and smiles combined with an instant appreciation for her fuzzy brown slippers which were held in anatomical apposition, the toe tips splayed ever so slightly. "Call me, Pussy Galore!"

Hoss on the other hand had taken a detour from animal science and chose a figure from history. In a shiny black stove pipe hat, fluffy Amish beard and with a kite slung over his shoulder, he positively insisted he was Benjamin Franklin. Although he walked around lamenting, "Poor Richard, oh, poor Richard," he was stymied as party goers kept addressing him as 'Mr. Lincoln.' He touched base repeatedly with Sam who assured him with a chuckle that, indeed, his Franklin was spot on.

Hoss and Kerri weren't the only welcoming committee. A small 20/20 film crew documented events while a self-appointed commission of third years stood in a group just inside the foyer, judging costumes. They were uniformly clad in dark coveralls and pairs of big, black, air-filled plastic bags taped over their feet. Each sported a bold capital letter chalked to his chest and if they stood in the right order, they spelled out their purpose: they were the "P-E-N-I-S G-A-L-L-E-R-Y." In this capacity, they shouted any assessment that came to mind as their costumed school mates passed into the house.

A girl, wrapped in yellow vet wrap from her ankles to her armpits, came hopping though the doorway. A frizzle of white, springy spikes poked out from her wig and she waved her arms wildly asking, "Does my ass look big in this?" She spun around on the catwalk as the Penis Gallery pronounced their solicited views and guesses, "Pencil? Vibrator? Shower massager — okay, same thing…"

She repeated, "My ass," hopping up and down as she spun around, "Look, I don't have an ass… I'm a sea anemone you morons!"

Next came a guy dressed in a lumpy white potato sack. He walked in and unceremoniously lodged himself next to a girl in a kidney costume. He stood there with a drink in his hand yelling into the stream of people passing by, "Fight! Flight! Anybody want some steroids?" After about 15 minutes of this, even the Penis Gallery had had enough. They were forced to perform the first-ever adrenalectomy at an Alpha Mu party and he was transplanted to the back yard with the other barking animals.

Mike London and Trisha Maxwell were the lone fourth-year representation at the party. They lounged in plain old scrubs on a dilapidated couch in the fraternity's front parlor. The duo extended their tired legs onto a big, square coffee table in front of a roaring blaze. Mike took a swig of beer, then turned to Trisha and said, "Remember second year when you came as a tapeworm?"

She nodded with a smile, "I was in all white with that diving bell helmet thingy on my head. The ports looked just like a scolex. I think I used white throw pillows as proglottids."

"And," Mike interjected with reverence, "you walked around half the evening holding a tray of liverwurst stuffed with mini marshmallows asking, 'Hydatid cyst? Anyone for a hydatid cyst? They're infectiously good, I just made them myself.'"

Trisha laughed and said, "Yuck, I can't believe you got me to do that."

Mike grinned, "That was the same year I was a big sphincter," then, before his friend could say it, added, "I know, I'm a sphincter every year."

The two friends sat there the rest of the evening, laughing and reminiscing while various pledges refilled their drinks and delivered food as the party evolved around them.

◄ ● ►

"Look at them," Anna seethed, "could she be more obvious?"

Dr. Avery Banks MS, DVM, PhD, Diplomate of the American Colleges of Veterinary Nutrition and Internal Medicine, stood majestically facing Jack Doyle. Her long-stemmed legs supported an hourglass torso, slender arms, and China doll hands. The left hand sparkled with a single gaudy diamond and was wrapped delicately around a champagne flute, while the right was planted flat on Jack's chest.

Avery Banks costumed this evening as Cleopatra and had arrived with an entourage. Her royal litter was carried by two Egyptian slaves who now fanned the Queen and her King with garish peacock staffs (Jack's King Tut costume having been graciously supplied by the AVIS Corporation). A golden serpent posed as Cleopatra's crown and, of course, perfectly complimented her glossy, jet black wig. The head of the gilded cobra rose regally from her forehead, poised to strike, while dark eyeliner exaggerated the pointed, feline symmetry of her emerald eyes. Anna could just imagine the one-dimensional dialogue.

Cleopatra: *Is that so, you big strong man you… You're able to leap tall buildings in a single bound? I don't believe it.*

King Tut: *Well of course you don't believe it ma' lady. You are after all, the Queen of de Nile.*

Avery Banks leaned her head back for an overly dramatic laugh, received a grape from a plebe and eyed the crowd just long enough to gauge her effect. A sea of male drones — including JJ and Rick Larson, an intern who kept checking his pager and two dermatology residents — ringed the Fantasy Island like a shoal of patrolling sharks, just waiting and hoping for something to fall into the water.

Anna huddled with Sam on the back porch, next to the keg, "She's absolutely perfect for him. Someone in tune with his inane banter. A shallow pool of corporate cream."

Hoss and Kerri had just ambled up, fresh from their duty at the door. Hoss said, "Anna, I don't think AVIS makes cream or any other dairy products." He turned, dipped his stove pipe and asked, "Do they Kerri?"

Kerri, her nose below the rim of a red plastic cup, was in mid-sip when she snorted. Foam flew onto Sam Stone, a sudsy blotch clinging to his right cheek. She laughed, "No Hoss, they don't."

Sam raised his eyebrows and wiped the beer from his forearm, "Nice, Ms. Feinburg. Very lady-like."

Kerri blinked once and, as if she'd planned the whole thing, replied, "I'll give you lady-like." She leaned close, placed her left hand in the small of his back, and in one long cat lick removed every bubble from his cheek. Then she looked him straight in the eye and, with a circular swirl of her tongue, licked her lips and whispered, "All better?"

Sam's face (and probably other parts of him) went hyperemic. He nodded and swallowed slowly, "Much better, ay-yuh, thank you ma'am."

Just then, Cleopatra raised her hands high above her head and clapped twice. The sharp, flat sound caused the music to fade and captured everyone's attention. She pronounced, "Let them eat cake!"

Anna spit, "Now she thinks she's Marie Antoinette."

On the Queen's command, two minions appeared from the kitchen with a silver platter hoisted onto their shoulders. On the platter rode a three-foot-tall, cylindrical cake with white icing, flaunting the AVIS company logo and, as if floating on a cloud, globs of puffy white icing encircled its base.

By now the party had grown in cellular mass. Like an unruly but benign tumor, it expanded to fill the space of Animal House. Virtually all of the first-year class was in attendance, along with numerous second and third years, plus a complement of interns and residents. The slaves elbowed their way through the crowd towards the food-laden serving table which was positioned next to the Queen. But, just as the cake was passing the royal couple, a pack of canines blitzed the room, darting around and between legs on its way back to the yard. This mammalian surge was followed immediately by an avian air assault. Fluttering wings of a love bird in hot pursuit of José's cockatiel chopped the air as the birds zoomed back and forth over heads, circled the cake and shot up a stairway. The commotion caused the cake bearers to stumble and bump. The towering can of AVIS teetered left then right, but it did not fall. Jack looked to Avery Banks and noticed that a creamy white blob had landed on the head of her golden cobra tiara. Assuming it was an icing dollop he said, "Don't worry my Queen," and gallantly, smoothly, cleanly scooped the glob off the crown with a finger and popped it into his mouth.

It only took a second for Jack Doyle to realize that something was amiss. His face crinkled. His eyes squinted and his lips puckered just before he doubled over to spit.

Although the apparent subtleties between President Lincoln and Benjamin Franklin seemed to escape Hoss, he immediately recognized what had just transpired. He stuck out a chunky paw, pointed his thick index finger at King Tut and exclaimed as loud as he could, "Jack ate bird shit! JACK ATE BIRD SHIT!"

The party erupted into a raucous laughter that expanded in waves, building and crashing around the royal couple for what seemed like ten straight minutes. Thankfully, Cleopatra had summoned everyone's attention *and* the 20/20 film crew was on point so no one would need to ask, "Have you ever seen anyone eat bird shit?" because absolutely everyone did, or soon would.

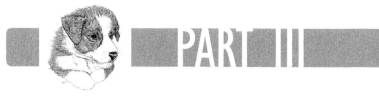

PART II

Veterinary School Interviews (continued)

Two widely-separated rooms in the old veterinary school building at the University of Philadelphia, School of Veterinary Medicine

Interviewer, Room 3: "Philosophically speaking, if you had to be one cell type — animal or vegetable — which would you choose and why?"

Applicant: Buford Hugman was surprised. He chuckled honestly and slapped his knee, "Well ma'am, with all due respect, if that ain't the derndest thing I ever heard." Hoss snugged up his bolo tie, "I'm no philosopher but I reckon you can't choose what you are. You just are. However, if I had to choose, I'd sure as shootin' be a *Euglena*." Hoss beamed a ten-gallon smile, "It can live as an autotroph or a heterotroph like us because it's got both plant AND animal parts — the best of both worlds!"

Interviewer, Room 3: The interviewer smiled and remarked, "I like that answer," bent her head and wrote, "Pollyanna Euglena," followed by a check.

◄ • ►

Interviewer, Room 6: "A Dalmatian breeder, one of your best clients, brings a puppy to your clinic. He doesn't want to sell the otherwise healthy animal because it's apparently deaf. He asks you to euthanize the puppy; what do you do?"

Applicant: Rick Larson angled his head to the right as he considered the question. "I'd have a tech nuke and dispose of the animal." Then Rick squinted and concluded with a nod, "And charge the regular fee. I assume you were wondering if I'd give the guy a freebie since he was a good client." Rick shook his head, "I wouldn't. As they taught us at Stanford, business is business."

Interviewer, Room 6: "Uh," the interviewer paused, "actually, I was wondering if you saw other potential outcomes for this animal." He flipped to the front of Rick's file folder, "Stanford? Your cover letter indicates you attended Harvard."

Applicant: Rick didn't blink, "Oh, yeah, Harvard, that's what I meant. Harvard's a good school, too."

Interviewer, Room 6: After writing a question mark in Rick's file, the interviewer decided to ask a few more.

CHAPTER TWENTY FIVE

The Rhythm Method

NOVEMBER 1988

Mike was, as per usual, correct. His freehand graphic predicting the life trajectory of a typical veterinary student proved true for the Class of '92 with both accuracy and precision — terms which some mistakenly equate. They are quite different. The precision of a rifle, a blood pressure transducer or a student's scholastic performance is related only to the reproducibility of the result. Accuracy, on the other hand, is a measure of "rightness" or "correctness" as compared with a gold standard. The goal in veterinary school, as in most life challenges, is precision *and* accuracy. If two hypothetical students, let's call them Jack and Anna, were testing at 95% more than 95% of the time, well, that would be accurate, precise and expected. But, if a truly hypothetical veterinary student, let's call him Rick, were to produce similar test results at a comparable frequency, we would be forced to wonder.

After a couple months, Jack and the others on Death Row fell within the groove carved by Mike's downward sloping "Test Stress" curve. Jack, Hoss, Sam and Kerri could actually feel the tingle of The Force kicking in. In fact, with 33 major tests under their belts and the new medical ethics course about to begin, the little group, urged on by Jack, decided to up the ante by adding morning calisthenics to their daily routine. They joined the Wildlife Service.

Wildlife, an entirely unfunded and nearly clandestine volunteer service organization, presented the singular opportunity for newbie students to gain actual, hands-on medical experience. A ragtag crew of first-, second-, and third-year caregivers were advised by the only person who had less free time than they, Dr. Violet Marie Green. She'd meet the squirrelly band most mornings for 6:00 AM rounds, follow up by phone midday, and then be on call. Though the case load was heavy — hundreds of orphaned robins, raccoons with road rash, shore and water fowl suffering from high-speed lead injections and pigeons, lots and lots of pigeons — Wildlife was a win-win situation. Animals that would have suffered silently in ditches on the roadside got free medical attention, while budding vets learned medical basics and witnessed response to care.

But the relative ease with which these first years took on additional responsibilities came in the face of a stark reality. When the Veterinary Class of 1992 emerged from the second major wave of testing, three seats in Room 13 were already vacant. One of the absences could have been expected — a frail wisp of a female FRoG who never seemed to adapt. She hadn't gotten close enough to Jack or the others for them to assess her aptitude; in fact, none of them had ever heard her speak. The second casualty was more interesting — a squat little fellow named Claude Francois Dubois. He was a French foreign student, known universally as "Pierre," who had been called unexpectedly, and with dubious cause, back to serve the Foreign Legion. Sam mused out loud, "Why do those Frenchies need Pierre? How many Frenchmen does it take to surrender anyhow?" But the third and — for now — final MIA was a surprise to the Death Row Crew. It was a girl who made up one half of the cute twin pair who had caught Jack's eye on the first day of orientation. Biologically, this didn't make sense. She and her sister were indistinguishable in every way, in every cell. They were two smart, interchangeable peas from the same pod. Actually, the same pea. Presumably, they were both raised in a similar nurturing environment, so what could have caused this egg to split one more postnatal time? Rumor suggested that there was a guy involved. Kerri reflected, "A man? Who would let a man degrade your performance in vet school? There's always another — or hopefully two — around the corner." So, although everyone was aware of the thinning of their ranks, little more was said.

Finally, as Mike's graph predicted, the first years' lives began to be simplified by vet school. In much the same way a magnifier trains the diffuse, wild light of the sun to set paper ablaze — this aggregate of disparate lives, initially wide-ranging and unfocused, was pulled closer by the lens of shared experience. Without even noticing it, a class structure started to emerge, its edges sharpened, emotions clarified. John Fitzgerald Doyle seemed to set the pace for the little Death Row group; he established an easy rhythm which became the form of their function. They fell towards his gravity. Everyone that is, except Anna. Like an electron in nebular orbit around the tightly-packed nucleus, she was ever-present but distant, always on the periphery. And although her association with the likes of Hoss and Kerri was more fluid, she kept a rigid, inflexible distance from Jack.

Regardless of the structure and type of bonds being formed, the little group's life cycle revolved around the tests they took. A precise and reproducible pattern emerged: they studied, took tests and then paused to refuel. Similar to those ubiquitous shampoo instructions (lather—rinse—*repeat*) their lives could be summed: study—test—*drink*. And the next thing they knew, December was upon them.

CHAPTER TWENTY SIX

Wildlife

AM treatments in the Wildlife Ward, in the corner of the old vet school quad, Philadelphia

*J*ack rubbed the sleep from his eyes before pulling a pair of latex gloves from a box. Somehow he'd made it into Wildlife this morning, trudging through the ankle-deep snow along the uneven blocks of Spruce Street and through security at VHUP, without actually waking up. This dawning realization made him wonder: as far as he knew, he'd never dozed off on a stakeout or during those endless hours processing paperwork on legions of Philly perps. Was this new life starting to test his mettle?

Hoss pulled their last tinback of the morning from a towering stack and flipped it open. He grunted softly as he read, "Same treatment for Hootie today — four fuzzies, a multivitamin, 1.2 ml of TMS and 5 mg pred." The two first years swiveled in place to take in a bird with eyes purposefully bigger than its stomach. The cage placard read, "Hootie 15." The formerly great horned owl perched limply on a stout wooden stand in a back corner of a standard 2' x 3' stainless steel kennel. The poor animal's feathers, once puffed and preened to predatory ideal, were matted so flat they revealed its bony, gaunt undercarriage. The two proud feathered "horns" were frayed and poked out at discordant angles while its eyes, those anthropomorphic icons of inquisition and wisdom, lay blank and uneven. In the wild, where masking illness is an imperative, an owl would only be caught dead looking like this. Hoss closed the medical record and retrieved a water-filled beaker from the treatment table. He swirled the floe of furry white mouse-sicles and pulled one out. Rolling the cold, wet little body between his thumb and index finger he pronounced, almost in a whisper and through his half-open lids, "Feels about right. Not too stiff, but stiff enough."

As they say, this time of the morning comes early, and that's entirely accurate for vet students who have been studying late. Most days, the first years shuffled quietly, talking was kept to a minimum with grunts and pointing held as communication. In this manner, these two first years bumped their way around the cramped space gathering medications and supplies, and even though Jack Doyle, the Death Row Crew and Anna had been working the ward for about two weeks, this morning Jack surveyed the space as if for the first time.

Wildlife, aka the "Pigeon Ward," was quite literally an underground operation, not entirely clandestine, not entirely illegal, but on topographical par with the school's subterranean boiler. Pumps hissed. Semi-insulated, asbestos-wrapped pipes clanked. The first years were bathed in sweaty yellow incandescent light as they worked in the dank basement space situated just off the quad near Room A1. Access was effected from the courtyard through a single 2/3 height portal countersunk four feet into the ground. The door's position and size required entrants to first sit on the edge of the concrete well, hop down into the pit and then take a hunchback stance to squeeze through the opening. Once inside however, the students could unfurl themselves to experience the opulent grandeur, as long as they weren't over 5'10". In contrast to the spacious, sparkling VHUP small animal wards with rows of gleaming cages, or the light-filled, airy medical barns in Kennett Square, the Wildlife Ward was almost third-worldly. It was a 12' x 20' catacomb crammed full of animal cages, tired surgical instruments, scrounged pet food, technically-expired medications and, of course, wild animals.

On his first day, Jack had wondered aloud how the service had been started. Initially, his third-year handler feigned ignorance because wildlife wasn't an officially sanctioned vet school club. In an awkward, Big Bird fashion, she flapped her arms and wiggled her head saying, "Who the hell knows?" but then — after peering slyly over first one, then the other shoulder — she whispered from the side of her beak that Mike London was the founding father. Service lore had it that when Mike was an under-grad he had been turned away from the school's ES with an ailing brown bat. So, during his first semester, he acquired a perpetual lease ($1/year) on the crypt from a hospital administrator in an Alpha Mu poker game. Apparently Mike, no gambler when it came to animal health, stacked the deck in his favor with an unusually high rate of aces delivered by a scantily clad dealer whom he knew was, herself, stacked in his favor.

With the space secured, Mike and Trisha Maxwell set to outfit the joint. They begged, borrowed and *borrowed without asking* all the bare necessities. A creaky, streaky, tippy exam table held the center ground of the room (plucked from a demolition pile of a renovated research lab). Above it hung three utility lamps, the kind with a metal basket and bare bulb that you'd find under an auto lift. A rusty, lockable mechanic's chest fit under the treatment table, its drawers stuffed with packs of hemostats, scalpels, bandage materials and medications. Mike worked out a deal with the VHUP techs, who would sterilize the wildlife instruments and pass along any expired or *nearly expired* medications they came across — in exchange, he flirted with them, shamelessly. Wildlife Service represented meatball medicine at its finest (a feathered meatball was in fact the unofficial logo), but with no budget, little space and no paid staff, they flew low under the school's administrative radar.

This morning, as was becoming routine, the students had paired up to complete their treatments: Sam Stone and a female second year huddled around the last of the orphaned squirrels. Sam cleaned the animal's cage while his partner cradled the plump fuzzy rodent, already too tame for anybody's purpose, purring affectionately on its back in the crook of one arm. She delivered synthetic milk with her free hand as the orphan lay trance-like, with no fidgeting, holding two paws around the barrel of the syringe lapping up the warmed formula as fast as she could depress the plunger. Kerri and Anna worked together, mutely, to re-bandage a pigeon's fractured wing. Kerri, allergic to feathered fashion, held the bird at arm's length, tilting her head away from the animal as far as possible. The bird's downy-soft gray head, with beady red eyes, was darting from side to side inspecting its now-exposed wound. But it didn't squirm a bit.

Hoss donned a pair of heavy leather welder's gloves and unlatched the owl's kennel door. Hootie 15 initiated the only defense he could muster, he began to rapidly open and shut his beak, clacking at Hoss Mountain. Jack remarked, "If you think about it, it's got to be terrifying to be trapped in a metal container with a bear-sized man grabbing at you."

Hoss replied quietly, "Aww, sweet little Hootie." Only Hoss would call a raptor with needle-tipped talons and a 60-inch wingspan sweet and little. "I ain't gonna hurt ya. We go through this every day and we're just trying to help." He scooped up the bird's perch and wrapped a glove around the animal's back to steady it as Jack removed yesterday's mouse remains — a neat pellet containing the bones and undigestible pelts of the previous meal.

"Okay, time to get the meds on board." Jack used a pair of hemostats to snag a previously frozen, now vitamin-enriched mouse by the scruff of the neck and squeezed his arm into the cage alongside Hoss's. He dangled the offering an inch in front of the clacking, sharp beak. "I know she's not blind but she doesn't seem to see it."

Hoss cooed, "Just keep it there, she'll figure it out," and almost before he'd finished speaking Hootie struck and clamped down — they heard the mouse's tiny skull crack and Jack released his hold. Although slow to start, once they had their patient going, she took whatever was presented. In this way, they got the two vitamin-enriched and two medicated fuzzies down. After closing the cage door, Jack and Hoss held their position for a moment. Hoss removed the thick leather gloves as Jack said, "I know that this isn't a natural situation, but I rehabbed several owls when I was a kid and none sat like that — it's like she's not really in there."

Hoss's eyebrows raised and he proceeded to scratch his head, "Well, she was hit by a car. Maybe there's been too much damage."

Jack paused and then concluded, "I'm gonna talk with Doctor Green when she gets here for rounds. Those last two Cooper's hawks acted the same as Hootie. Something weird is going on."

"Speaking of which," Hoss paused and took in a breath that showed respect, "just look at him." This statement caused Jack to turn to his right as Hoss elevated a towel which shrouded the front of the largest container in the room. Jack whistled under his breath, *pheww*. A mature bald eagle with a hooked, chisel-sharp beak the size of a dagger and muscular talons sat in much the same stance as the great horned owl. But, unlike Hootie, this bird's massive golden eyes locked onto Jack Doyle with an unblinking stare.

Jack read the all caps and boldly-lettered cage card aloud, "**NO STUDENT TX's**". A padlock secured the latch, reinforcing the overall message of certain danger. A cartoon Sam had sketched was taped to the animal's record. It depicted a severed human head (with a grimace, X-ed out eyes, and blood dripping from the ragged neck stump) being devoured by an eagle. A cartoon bubble curved from the husky bird's mouth which parodied a *Looney Tunes* animation, "You're a chicken and I'm a Chicken Hawk!"

Hoss lowered the towel and spoke with hushed reverence, "We're supposed to let Doctor Green handle that one…"

CHAPTER TWENTY SEVEN

Rectification

Special Anatomy Lab in the teaching barns on the Kennett Square campus

T he senses are curious things. Whether premium products from eons of evolution, the benevolent spark of a greater Creator — or both — the ability to see, hear, smell, taste and touch are endowments to survival. Endowments we alternately enhance, dull and successfully ignore. Taken in the raw, the five senses appear honorable enough. However, if seeing is believing, then why do we doubt an eyewitness? Aside from the obvious — people lie and make mistakes — there's another minor inconvenience. Our brains make stuff up. Groups of well-meaning and likeminded neurons can invent "vision" from vacuum, mercifully shutter traumas or purposely fill gaps. For example, close your left eye and, while staring at the "L" on the page below, bring the image slowly towards you. At about 3 times the distance between the two letters, the "R" — *which we know exists* — disappears.

L   R

This vanishing act is to be expected considering the natural necessity for a hole in the retinal field — no rods or cones can lie where the optic nerve exits each globe, and where receptors are lacking no image can form. But, it's what happens when the "R" dissolves that changes our view. Rather than a black hole in the visual field, our mind improvises. The vacancy is filled with an image lifted from nearby — our brain's best guess at what it *thinks* we should see. As it turns out, our vision, the gold standard for data collection, is just perception filtered and tweaked by a blood and guts machine bathed in crackling hormones, wavering glucose levels, and a mind of its own.

The art of physical examination depends on the skillful merger of senses and mind. It demands both wide-open receptivity and, at the same time, practiced discernment. A veterinary student in his or her primordium is a neophytic deep space probe. A 50-trillion-cell neural net attached to a gel-based supercomputer with a signal-to-noise ratio nearing one. However, over the course of schooling and years of practice, a willing pupil can enhance his standard-issue faculties while developing new ones as well. Having both sense *and* sensibility. For instance, somewhere along the continuum between sight and touch, on the mystical plane of imagination, lies a process called visualization. The ability to tune in and tune out. To feel with your hands and see with something deeper. Because no surgeon, radiologist, nor endoscopist — none except the pathologist — truly gains an unfettered interior view, the clinical vet must rely on her mind's eye. However, two factors can influence the value of this diagnostic modality: 1) a developed talent to translate finger-tip sensations into mental 3D images and, 2) arm length. A vet with long slender arms has a decided advantage, especially in a busy large animal practice. It's all about natural routes of access. But long arms can only take you so far. A person who learns to "see" what he feels is head and shoulders above the rest. At the University of Philadelphia, School of Veterinary Medicine, in 1988, students learned digital imaging the old fashioned way — by hand.

◅ ◦ ▻

For Big Moe Sutton, the highlight of each fall semester came when his little, bumbling first years began the progression from clueless hackers to anatomical visionaries. This transformation brought him quiet satisfaction — quiet because he would never have admitted to squishy soft feelings like caring or pride.

Big Moe clapped his hands and boomed, "LITTLE MOES, GATHER 'ROUND." He stood in the middle of the center concrete aisle of the teaching barn with both hands raised above his head. Even though the inside temperature hovered near freezing, he wore his routine dissection garb, a short-sleeved aquamarine scrub shirt with "MOE" embroidered over the pocket, a crusty pair of tan Carhartts and black hobnail work boots with beefy thick heels. No hat, no gloves. His arms and face were pink from the cold but Big Moe didn't yield to the whims of fashion let alone vagaries of the weather. Big Moe wasn't one to yield — period — and steam rose from his mass just like it did from the cattle milling on either side of the aisle. In contrast, the herd of first years was bundled head to toe. They'd been warned to put on layers, so long johns, flannel shirts and goose down vests were sausaged into the virgin navy coveralls purchased from the bookstore two days ago. Jack's and Sam's still had crease lines from the package folds while Kerri's had been dry-cleaned and pressed — little yellow chick embroidery adorned her standing collar. Hoss was the only one who wore his regular duds: an off-white Ponderosa with a biconcave rim, a brown canvas rancher and blue-jean bib overalls.

On this day in December, the student palpation barns were packed with a dozen horses and twice as many cows, sows, sheep and goats. Standardbred geldings with stringhalt, DJD and chronic bog spavin were here because a racehorse that can't breed *or* race is at a delicate crossroads. Retooling is unlikely and positions in the hansom cab and pony-ride industries were limited. On the other hand, a milk cow with two blown quarters really had no options. If your singular occupation was to magically transform grass and water into vitamin-D-fortified whole milk and you go teats up, there are precious few options that don't include a frying pan or broiler. So, even though the teaching herds didn't know it, along with the occasional, well-meaning molestation and free universal health care, came a reprieve.

Big Moe lowered his arms and continued, "Hell Week is on the horizon." He paused, slowly nodding his head, "For gross anatomy, that means your final cumulative practical and written exams are just around the corner. In fact, I start prepping your specimens tonight." He paused to let this sink in. "A word to the wise," he looked to Hoss, his favorite in the class, "now's the time to get anatomy under control."

"Today, you'll palpate many of the organs you've been dissecting." Big Moe looked again to Hoss and made a lassoing motion with one hand. Hoss, having grown up on his family's cattle ranch near Carson City,

Nevada, moved effortlessly among the 1200-pound steaming beasts. He waded through the foot-deep, brown soupy muck, hooked a halter with one finger and led a black and white beauty out onto the center aisle. Big Moe moved to the animal's rump and lined up along its flank.

"Starting with the female bovine and working from the back end" — he pointed, just to make sure — "you need to be able to identify, in order of appearance: the external sphincter, rectum, the floor of the pelvis and pelvic rim." He slowly advanced his arm laterally, simulating the palpation from the outside. "Then," curving his fingertips downward, "ventrally you should find the cervix, uterine body and both horns." He squinted, looking off into the rafters as he envisioned the rest, "Further along and dorsally, most of you," he paused and looked at Kerri Feinburg's tiny frame, "sorry, probably not you, City Moe." The class laughed a steamy chuckle. "But, most of you should be able to reach the caudal pole of the right kidney."

"In the rectal exam, it's only polite to start out slow." He straightened his back and again raised his right hand. "First, hold your palm flat, bring your fingertips together and lay the thumb in the groove it creates. This gives a slender point to your hand. Second, your partner should elevate and control the tail. And third, advance slowly to your knuckles, wait 15-20 seconds and then go a few inches more. Once you're in up to your forearm, you can feel your way forward as necessary." He clapped his hands and boomed, "GLOVE UP, LUBE UP, and try not to get kicked."

Like a delivery vehicle backing to a loading dock, Jack made a monotone *beep—beep—beep* as he and Hoss maneuvered their animal, Buttercup the moo-cow, into her stanchion. The metal gate clanked, securing the animal's head into place. This whole process, at least for first-time rectal examiners, was awkward, even embarrassing. There's something about inserting your arm into the hind end of an animal that crosses a boundary.

Jack fumbled with the rectal sleeve and bantered to buy some time. "Feels like I should buy her dinner, or at least a drink first."

Hoss leveled a hefty paw onto Jack's shoulder, "Don't worry, these girls are plenty used to this. They've been palpated since they were young."

This got Jack to thinking, so he scanned the barn and spotted Sam Stone just two cows over, "Not so funny now is it, Hugh Heifer?"

Sam was busy taking pictures of his classmates in various stages of involution. Kerri screwed up her face as she stood on a step stool with one finger in her cow. He smiled from under his Red Sox ball cap and held up the camera, "These will be great for the yearbook."

Jack turned back to Buttercup and tilted his head as he examined the long plastic gloves, "Right or left?"

Hoss replied, "They're all the same," and handed him the tube of KY he'd been warming in an inside coat pocket. Jack elevated his right arm as he slid on the plastic barrier and Hoss anchored it with duct tape at the level of his arm pit, "There you go, buddy." The rest of the cows had been moved into the stanchions so that Jack and the others were faced with a row of puckered stars, each with a pouting V notch below and a swishing tail above.

Jack's breath streamed away from him like an old-fashioned locomotive as a cutting wind ripped through the metal-framed barn, "Jesus, it's freezing in here." He stamped his boots and finding no other way to stall, leaned on Buttercup, inserting his hand up to the knuckles. He waited a moment and then advanced. The first thing he noticed was the wonderful warmth. Compared to the bitter draft in the frigid barn, it lulled his senses until a slurry of warm, watery manure began to pour out around his wrist. Unfortunately for Jack, the half-occluded orifice caused the gooey mash to be ejected like water from a fire hose. Most of the fragrant goo ran down his chest, splattering on his boots. Hoss, ever the cattleman, mused, "Great, now you can get a clear feel. Good job."

Jack replied, "I didn't have much to do with it, but thanks."

Jack had no trouble finding, or more accurately, feeling the external sphincter muscle because after a few moments of warming bovine bliss, a pressure hit him like a tourniquet. Jack Doyle, Class President and former K-9 cop, drew in a breath, tucked his chin and grimaced, "Holy cow." The animal constricted like an anaconda and then it passed. He advanced his arm further and after what seemed like days, said flatly and in defeat, "I think I feel the pelvic floor, but I can't find the uterus." He looked up to Hoss who'd been stabilizing the cow's rump with his hip and elevating the tail.

Hoss stammered, "Well, you're kinda' on your own in there. There's really no way for me to help you. Except..." He paused and thought, scratching the side of his face with a grubby finger, "If you think of the rectum as a watch," Jack grinned, first at the thought of a rectum clock and then as he issued their standard retort, "Rectum, damn near killed 'em!"

Hoss continued unfazed, "Close your eyes and remember our dissection in the lab. The uterus will be at the bottom, at 6 o'clock." Jack did as his friend instructed. He extended his first and second fingers and smoothed them along the circumference of the distal colon. Eventually and with his eyes closed, he discerned a bulge and smiled, "I think you may be running late, 'cause this one says 6:30..."

After about an hour of redirecting errant palpaters like JJ, who had one hand in the air and the other mistakenly in the repro tract while making the diagnosis of colonic atresia, Big Moe eventually made his way back to the middle walkway leading a blue ribbon bovine. He clapped his hands twice and then cupped them to form a megaphone, "LITTLE MOES, YOU SHOULD BE ABOUT FINISHED." Jack nodded when Big Moe looked his way. "Now that you've visualized the normal anatomy, I've got a challenge. This here is Clover, and she's special." Clover was as beautiful as a cow could be. In spite of the sloppy winter conditions, her coat gleamed. She had a robust profile. A massive pendulous udder, and her eyes sparkled as she casually chewed her cud. The only trace of ordinary bovine was the glob of manure on the tip of her tail. "There's at least two things that make this animal special, and one is this," he pointed to a rubber disc about ten inches in diameter and protruding from her caudal left flank. "She has a bonus port of entry — a permanent fistula." Big Moe reached over with his ungloved hand, grasped the raised edge of the central disc and turned, "Just like a bottle cap, Righty tighty, lefty loosey," and with a half rotation the cap came off. Big Moe reached inside. Clover didn't take notice. After a moment of fishing, Big Moe retrieved a fist full of greenish pulp, brought it to his nose for a long draw and pronounced like a connoisseur, "Ahh, now this is normal rumen contents." Fluid from the gooey mass dribbled down his bare arm as he elevated the steaming lump so that everyone could see. "I want you to find the second thing that makes her special and I'll give you a hint: it could result in a reproductive emergency." Big Moe canvassed the barn and settled on Jack, "PRESIDENT MOE, you're first."

Jack pulled on a fresh rectal sleeve as he watched Clover's tail swish in big arcs as if flies were circling her rump. "CONFIDENT MOE, how about you give him a hand and control this tail." Anna Heywood, another of Big Moe's favorites, hobbled forward. Whatever her condition, the cold surely made it worse. Even though she walked without her cane this morning, her movements were clearly labored. Big Moe helped her re-glove and before he turned back to work with the others he said, "Gimme a holler when you guys have the answer." Adding, with a wink, "If anyone can figure it out, it's you two." Without a word, Anna grasped Clover's tail in her right hand and, gently curling it forward, she took up position along the animal's left flank near the fistula.

Even though she and Jack had attended all the same classes, worked shoulder-to-shoulder in the wee hours of every morning in that cramped Wildlife Ward, and studied in conjoined anatomy groups, they'd hardly shared a word since the *situation* with Avery Banks two weeks earlier. Jack, standing with hands on his hips wondering how he should proceed, said, "Are you ready for me?" Anna looked him straight in the eye, shrugged and nodded once. Since Jack was right-handed, he placed his left on Clover's hip and began. This time, he had a feel for the environment. He identified the successive parts along the "path" without hesitation but then, while almost up to his armpit, he came upon a hard, pointy structure and then another. Jack leaned in, closed his eyes and, as he'd seen Hoss do earlier, he rested his forehead on the cow's rump. Anna faced him and watched as he worked his way along the darkness. Through the bowel wall Jack's fingers splayed and rolled until he counted what he thought were five little protrusions in all. He raised his head while still leaning over the animal's hind end and blinked.

"I've found something special, I just don't know what to do next." Jack stared into Anna's darkly intense eyes. He tried to visualize what was going on behind her mask. As he began to wonder if she might just push him aside and take over, without saying a word she unscrewed the fistula's cap, inserted her slender left arm and reached in towards Jack. Clover's rumen, the fabled first of four gastric chambers, was an enormous vaulted space half-filled with a sweetly fermenting blend. Anna ran her fingers along the wall of the caudal pole. She could imagine the fimbriated lining that felt for all the world like shag carpet, and then bumped into the focus of Jack's confusion. As she laid into Clover's side to count, her face was now inches from Jack's. He raised his head again with his eyes still closed; she could see them darting back and forth under his lids, and then suddenly they stopped. She'd found the specific objects that held his attention and with her palm manipulated the rumenal sac just enough to guide his fingers. Jack's eyes popped open, then a soft grin spread across his face as he realized what she was doing.

Jack whispered in her ear, "She's pregnant... and there are two of them."

But before Anna could respond, Sam Stone, who'd approached unnoticed from the other side, clapped his Death Row mate on the back and quipped, "Jack Doyle, I hear you should be pretty good at diagnosing this sort of thing. Didn't you have a *reproductive emergency* with Doctor Avery Banks the other night?" Anna watched as Jack lowered his eyes again. And when he came up with a big sheepish grin, it was too much for her to bear. In one fluent motion she straightened her back and let Clover's tail fly like a medieval catapult. It swirled and whipped low and high until finally finding its mark — the soggy, manure-laden tip slapped Jack square across the mouth.

Sam and Hoss doubled over with laughter as Anna capped the fistula and silently hobbled away. Jack spit and sputtered, wiping his mouth with the back of his free hand.

"First bird crap, now this," Sam said, holding his side, "Maybe you shoulda been a para-shit-tologist!"

V'92 Note Service - Special Anatomy Lab @C-LAM   TR: Jose (Sam)
12/15/88   (8:00-11:00am)   DD: JJ
BIG MOE   Page 9 of 11

Rectally speaking (per ass), we shouldbe able to palpate the following:

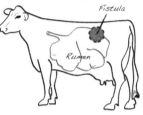

Bovine (female)
- pelvic inlet, pelvic/pubic brim, iliac shafts
- vulva, vestibule, vagina, cervix, uterine
  body, uterine horns, uterine tubes,
  infundibula and ovaries, as well as the broad
  ligament which suspends these structures
- Lt, Kidney: right of rumen, midline area
- Small bowel, cecum ventral right of lt kidney
- Rumen: left of midline and cranial

Equine (both sexes)
- lt side, distal left ventral colon, the pelvic
  flexure, the proximal left dorsal colon, the
  spleen, the left kidney and the left ovary.
- ventral abdomen: bladder, inguinal rings,
  cervix, uterus
- rt side: cecum, small colon
- cranial aspect of the dorsal abdomen: the root
  of the mesentery and the nephrosplenic
  ligament

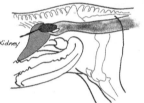

** Big Moe's tip: think the "5F's"
(5F's,just like Jack's report card...)

What you feel could be: Fat, fecal, fluid,
flatus (Hoss...) and/or fetus...

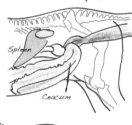

An Animal Life — Samurai Moe

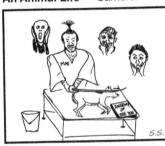

S.S.

Oddly, Moe Belushi wasn't all that popular with his
dissection group...

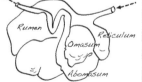

*** Reminder: If you want to audition for
20/20, see Jack for an application ***

CHAPTER TWENTY EIGHT

Can of Worms:
Part I (A Plum Job)

9:25 PM — THURSDAY, DECEMBER 15, 1988

Violet Green's office at the Peaceable Kingdom

*D*r. Stan Oblitzski stumbled over a pile of defeated running shoes as he tiptoed his way into Violet Green's office. Violet was on the phone and raised a finger to let him know she was almost done. He looked down at the mound of beaten Nikes and Reeboks and said to himself, *they look like I feel.* These past few weeks Stan and Violet had been burning the candle at both ends and the middle because even though the incidence of mysterious neuropath submissions had ceased entirely by November, they couldn't just ignore what had happened — whatever it was. Besides, they still had those live-animal cases Jack Doyle discovered in the school's Wildlife Service.

Tonight was Stan's first visit to Violet's new work space in the Tree of Life. Though she'd had a perfectly serviceable office onsite during park construction and launch, Davaris was always expanding and enhancing his empire. He "requested" that Violet design an aesthetically pleasing office complex for the husbandry staff, one that would blend seamlessly with the park's wild facade, so she scribbled off a few quick sketches of a design she never thought would be built. The result? A towering stand of phylogenetic "trees" — massive concrete faux oaks, each one representing a different animal family line from the ground up. The workspace penthouses, camouflaged by fake foliage and branches, were accessible via elevators concealed in the massive trunks and connected to a warren of underground tunnels. When viewed from a distance, as the visitors did on their safari rides, the "animal health forest" appeared natural and scaled to fit the landscape. Functionally, the setting did give the keepers and veterinary staff the high ground to monitor the park's collection. From Violet's tinted and outwardly pitched windows, she could look down into the primary captive breeding pens and medical treatment areas. And what she couldn't see directly was displayed on a bank of monitors with video and infrared feeds from locations all over the zoo.

Stan's mouth hung open as he stood near the entryway and took stock of a room that looked like a fantasy cross between an air traffic control tower, medical library and science lab. It was, in his mind, the most ideal tree fort any kid could imagine. Outside, during the warmer months, the horizon would be filled with herds of roaming hoofstock, rhino, elephant and flocks of fluttering birds. While inside, inside it was a veterinary geek's dreamland.

An industrial-grade lab bench with a chemical resistant sink ran along the trunk side of the 8' x 12' space. A gas valve next to the sink was connected by thick black hose to a Bunsen burner with a 500 ml Pyrex beaker balanced on a stand above. Stan noticed, with a smile, that a half-eaten container of Lipton's Cup-A-Soup sat nearby and Violet's toothbrush rested in the crease of a tube of Crest, its bristled head drip-drying over the sink edge. Nearer his position, Stan eyed a double-headed compound microscope fitted with both SLR camera and video display while next to him, a slowly tumbling blood tube mixer kept the anti-coagulated samples in purple and green topped tubes from settling. Above the bench was an X-ray view box plastered with 20 or more radiographs. They were layered 2-3 deep in spots, the faint purplish-white light showed through the multiple radiodensities of overlapping femurs, humeri and skulls.

The remaining office "space" was crammed nearly floor-to-ceiling with books, file folders, and stacks of medical records. Stan decided to try to sit in the lone visitor's chair, but it was surrounded by columns of medical texts piled almost four-feet high. Blank spots of the Astroturf carpet showed through an expanse of veterinary journals that lay splayed open on the floor. Some face down, holding their place, others paper-clipped open with long sections of text highlighted and festooned with Post-it note reminders. The trail of carpet patches created a dotted line marking a footpath from the door to Violet's desk.

In the olden days (two years ago), when they were both residents, Stan loved to visit Violet's office at the Philly Zoo. It was a mess. But Stan adored the mess because it showed, in no uncertain terms, exactly where

Violet's priorities lay — with the animals under her care. Stan and Violet had been close for years; in fact, she had been looking out for him like a big sister from the moment she'd befriended the squawky and overly ebullient, undersized front-row geek from her seat in the third row of Room 13.

Tonight, despite the lofty mess that surrounded him, Stan saw only one thing that was out of place. One thing that made him sad. The framed picture of Mya propped up on the desk directly in front of his friend. As far as Stan knew, Dr. Violet Marie Green was more attached to that sweet lion cub than any other patient she'd ever cared for — and now Mya was gone, shipped off to some park in Texas.

Violet replaced the handset on the receiver. "Sorry Stan, sorry to keep you waiting. I was just checking on our newest additions," she pointed to a monitor labeled NIC-U, "a new pair of baby addax." A doting mom licked at the two, spotted forms as they wobbled to stand and nurse.

Stan faked bewilderment turning his head slowly back and forth, "Vi, your office, this place… It's insane. Insanely great that is!"

Violet averted her eyes. It appeared to Stan she was embarrassed. "Yeah, well, that's Davaris… We have all the high-tech gear we could ever want, but," she paused, "he won't hire enough staff to care for the animals. I dunno, it seems like all he wants to do is show off the collection of gee-whiz gadgets and endangered species to his CEO cronies." She shook her head, "But you're not here for my *poor little rich girl* complaints."

Stan glanced toward the ceiling and then over his shoulder to the corners of the room as he pushed the door closed, "Vi, can we speak freely in here?" He was alluding to their previous "big brother" experience with the park's owner. Violet nodded yes, "I swept every nook and cranny before I moved my stuff in and, other than the phone line, I feel certain we're alone."

Stan's face mutated into instant glee, "I got us some help with the neuro cases! I found exactly the right person to evaluate the histo and data we compiled — and, he wants to talk to us tonight." Stan the Path Man waggled his head from side to side, barely containing his excitement, "A longtime *friend* of mine has just been named Director of the US Infectious Disease Lab on Plum Island." He reeled off a number, Violet dialed and put the call on speaker.

It rang once, "Hello, USID."

Stan responded with a sly grin, "Could I speak to Doctor Oblitzski please?" Stan wiggled his eyebrows, "Tell him Doctor Oblitzski is on the line!"

"Doctor Oblitzski this *is* Doctor Oblitzski!"

"Pops!"

"Son, how are you?"

"Couldn't be better and guess who's here with me? Violet Green."

"Violet!" The caller didn't pause for a second, "You have to come for Christmas again this year! Vi, do you remember the time you and Stan showed up on our doorstep with tissue samples and gross path reports from your open cases? I trimmed them in, fixed and stained the slides and then we read them together..?" What fun! Now that was a great Christmas Eve, remember that?"

"Yes, Doctor O," Violet smiled, she could have measured how far the apple had fallen with a micrometer, "I do remember, that was last year... And, I had a wonderful time."

After a few minutes of catching up, with Dr. Oblitzski Senior relaying that his new position was indeed a *plum job*, followed by some reminiscing about the vet school and older professors, Dr. O assured Violet that their communications were secure and they got down to business.

"Violet and Stan, I reviewed your slides. In the crows, ibis, flamingo and equine cases I see definite cytopathic effects suggestive of a viral etiology. From this history, timeline and the distribution of cases, it sure as hell looks like an infectious disease." He paused, "Only problem, and it's a biggie, you've got no causative agent — I couldn't find a thing. And of course, if it is an infectious disease process, the mode of transmission is still unknown."

Dr. Violet Marie Green slumped in her chair, "Yeah, and we've isolated affected birds, pairing them with healthy controls, but there's not been any spread. If the living animals are carriers, then they must not be shedding. I can't figure it out."

"Well, this really is a toughie. A fabulous conundrum!" But then, as he paused they could hear Dr. Oblitzski Senior draw in a deep breath and sigh, "My real concern is when this thing resurfaces — and I'm willing to bet my brand new ElectroScan microscope that it will — if we don't nail down the cause, things are gonna get ugly."

The two veterinarians in the tree fort faced each other in silence as this likelihood sank in. Then Stan the Path Man raised his right arm, made a defiant fist and blurted into the speakerphone, "What's the one thing that can save the day?" In synchrony with his father on the other end he exclaimed, "PATH-POWER!" and said good night.

Violet stared at Stan and the hefty gold signet ring embossed with a bold "**P**" on the fist of his still raised arm. "I always wondered about that ring..."

CHAPTER TWENTY NINE

Can of Worms:
Part II (The Oath)

Veterinary medical ethics class in Room 13 of the Rosenthal Building

S am stood just inside the entryway to Room 13 with a flashlight slung over his left shoulder and his right hand out, palm up. "Tickets? Tickets please. The matinee showing of *Star Wars: Return of the Jedi* will begin momentarily. Please, take your seats." Now, almost four months into their first year, the class had become acclimated to Sam's clowning — not that it wasn't humorous, often he'd come out with gold, but for the most part the first years just smiled and played along in the fantasy land that sprouted from his frontal lobes.

"Ticket, miss?"

Anna, encumbered with a heavy parka, a loaded backpack over her shoulder and two dogs in the lead, stopped, cocked her head and responded, "You're a moron." Sam was undeterred. He saw Anna Heywood as one of his most discerning critics and he valued her reaction.

"Ay-yuh, that may be true but I still need a ticket."

Lifting her cane with mock menace she replied, "How's *this* for a ticket?"

Sam nodded, "Ah, you're down front."

In this way, on this day, the class filled the square, squat room and though no one mentioned it, nearly a whole day after their Large Animal Center palpation excursion, the sweet aroma of cow, horse and goat still hung in the air. A contingent of "announcers" lined up next to the podium before nearly every lecture waiting for a turn at the microphone. At this moment there were only three, Jack Doyle, Mike London and Trisha Maxwell and since this class was led by their faculty advisors, Dr. Florence Kimball (whom they'd already grown to love and respect) and Dr. Dan Linnehan (whom they'd instantly grown to fear and respect), the proclamations were kept lovingly, fearfully and respectfully short.

Jack motioned for Mike and Trisha to go first. Trisha clicked the mic on and began, "Class of 1992, we know you're fast approaching your first-semester finals and we remember them fondly…" She looked to Mike as she said, "How many did we have?" and didn't wait for a reply, "About 14 as I remember it. That being said, you guys will need a study break and tomorrow is the Student Chapter of the American Veterinary Association's annual spay, neuter, and vaccination clinic. This year it's sponsored by the AVIS Corp — they pay for the materials, supplies and biologics with all proceeds going to the student scholarship fund."

Mike leaned toward the mic to chime in, "These scholarships support your fourth-year external rotations."

They'd obviously rehearsed because Trisha countered with the next point, "And low-income families receive affordable health care for their pets."

JJ's arm sprang upright. Mike, seeing that he was in the front row, frowned, "JJ, I can't hear you from there."

JJ sputtered, "But, I'm…" and then realizing what he meant, grabbed his notebook, bolted to an open seat in the second row and tried again.

"JJ," Mike said, turning his head no, "how about I answer your questions tomorrow at the clinic? I know you wouldn't miss this opportunity to give back." He opened his attention to the whole class, "We hope you'll all come out and lend a hand. Thanks." Mike handed the mic to Jack who checked with Dr. Linnehan to see if he could proceed. Drill Sergeant Dan was tightlipped but nodded yes, once.

Jack's blue eyes flickered with a covert excitement as he spoke, "Quick reminder, next Friday is the last Happy Hour of the semester. There will be skits, awards and the 20/20 folks will be in attendance." He paused ever so slightly for effect, "As I understand it, they'll be filming and conducting auditions for the show. If you want to be considered, bring your resume and be prepared for a screen test." He added, making it sound like an afterthought, "And please remember to encourage our human med student counterparts to participate — we want to trounce them fair and square." Jack hastily snapped the mic into the stand on the podium, bowed his head to the professors and jogged back to Death Row where he received oversized grins and a disproportionate number of high fives.

As one of their responsibilities, the class's faculty advisors, Drs. Flo Kimball and Dan Linnehan, organized the Veterinary Medical Ethics class for the first years. The topic was no afterthought but the course felt like one. An already crammed four-year curriculum required it be compacted and shoehorned into the last month of the first semester.

Dr. Kimball took the stage and the podium, "I rarely do this but I have a short commercial, too!" She smiled warmly, "I wholeheartedly encourage you to attend the clinic tomorrow. Most of the faculty participate." Flo paused, and then continued, looking at JJ, "It's not only a great way to give back and learn... we gotta push the heartworm prevention!" Flo Kimball reached into her lab coat and produced that jar stuffed with gobs of heartworms. After waving the prop in the air for a moment, she pocketed the jar, ducked her head to separate the context and then continued, "Okay, class, in a moment, you'll break up into groups again and debate your answers to last week's ethical challenge. But, before you do, Doctor Linnehan would like to say a few words prior to your final exam for this course."

Dr. Daniel Linnehan flicked on a battleship gray overhead projector and slapped a transparency sheet on top. He dialed the lens up and down to bring, at first, the concentric rings of the lens into focus and then the words of a pledge:

The Veterinary Oath —
At the time of being admitted as a member of the veterinary medical profession:
I solemnly pledge myself to consecrate my life to the service of humanity; ***
I will give to my teachers the respect and gratitude which is their due;
I will practice my profession with conscience and dignity;
The health of my patient will be my first consideration; ***
I will respect the secrets which are confided in me;
I will maintain by all means in my power, the honor and noble traditions of my profession;
My colleagues will be my brothers and sisters;
I will not permit considerations of religion, nationality, race, party politics or social standing to intervene between my duty and my patient;
I will not use my veterinary medical knowledge contrary to the laws of humanity.
I make these promises solemnly, freely and upon my honor.

He took a red felt marker, circled the two lines with asterisks and then looked up to the class. "If you are an MD, a human physician, who is your boss?" He opened his hands and then answered himself, "It's almost silly. Your responsibility is to the patient alone." He looked to the class with a half smile. It was something they'd never seen on Drill Sargent Dan before, so it really got their attention. "But as veterinarians, we consecrate ourselves to the service of humanity *and*, as you see from the oath, our patients must be our first consideration." His smile disappeared, "So, which is it? Whom do you serve?" And then, quite unexpectedly, he began drawing a cartoon-like figure on the transparency — as the image took shape it appeared to be an animal in mid-stride and as the marker squeaked, a deer with a prodigious set of antlers materialized. He looked up from his drawing and reverted into Terminator mode the way they'd met him in September, "Where does the buck stop?" He scanned the room from left to right with only his eyes, not moving his head. There was no reply. The class knew where they were (on murky ground surrounded by quicksand and the occasional land mine) and who was asking the question (Dr. Ethical Responsibility). "This one's not rhetorical… consider the oath as you tackle today's case and the final exam next week." He replaced the oath with a different transparency.

> Signalment: Three-year-old, male, intact, pit bull terrier.
> Presenting complaint: Severe trauma, bite wounds and deep lacerations to the head and neck, likely blood loss.
> Physical exam (PE): TPR (Temp: 100F, Pulse: 170 thready; Resp: 60 BPM, shallow) CRT: >5 seconds. General body score of 5, fit. The left external pinna has been severed and the left eye has been dislodged from the orbit, dangling, 2 cm of the optic nerve visible. Animal unresponsive.
> History (Hx): Animal presented to the Emergency Service at approximately 2:00 AM. The owner (who must live in west Philly because you've seen him with a gang of youths on your late-night route home from work) states that the animal got out of his apartment and must have been HBC. The owner becomes agitated when you don't buy the story and then confides that he fights the dog to make money to support his family.

After giving the class a few moments to mull the situation over, Drill Sergeant Dan asked, "Sound far-fetched? Tell that to the current

ES intern." He paused and then concluded, "Break into your groups and develop your course of action."

The class segregated themselves into their naturally emerging organ systems. The FRoGs clung together in clusters near the front (on the outside chance that this was just a massive game of musical chairs, they wouldn't dare risk losing proximity to the podium). The middle-earth groups, like the one with José Rizal, formed comfortable associations in rows three and four. While, in the back of Room 13, the Death Row Crew of Jack, Sam, Hoss and Kerri assembled.

But, before the FRoGs could tremor, "We didn't come to a consensus but felt compelled by client confidentiality so we would treat the animal and return it to the hoodlum owner." And before José could respond, "Our group needed more time to make a sound decision, so we'd stabilize the patient with IV fluids, pain meds and turf it to the ICU." And way before Jack could stand up and report, "We'd confiscate and treat the animal immediately, then inform the perp that he was under arrest." Before all that could transpire, the class was interrupted.

Standing where Sam had previously collected tickets was a real-live uniformed cop and a barely-alive professor — Dr. Even Vandergrift. Dr. Linnehan motioned for them to come to the stage.

Sam poked Jack in the ribs, "No offense, and I hate to stereotype, but that cop could be your cousin." Sam was right. The cop had ruddy cheeks, brilliant blue eyes and carried his boxer's build in Jack's sure and confident way. By comparison, it appeared that a stiff breeze could blow Even Vandergrift away. After a few moments of muffled discourse between the professors and new arrivals, Dr. Vandergrift took to the mic. If you didn't know better you might have guessed he was just continuing the topic of his last lecture, with one exception — this time his shaky voice was directed entirely at Anna.

"...and as you know my laboratory attempts to elucidate the mechanisms and etiologies of neuromuscular transmission diseases, we study amyotrophic lateral sclerosis or lou gehrig's disease, muscular sclerosis, and others, we were closing in on a study funded by the national science foundation when, last evening, our facilities were compromised and intruders absconded with our testing animals and computers with data on axonal transmission rates and myelin regeneration, these results were proving to be quite fascinating, likely leading us toward further investigations and even a potential treatment..."

Whether it was a natural instinct or one developed on the streets, the cop could sense that this approach was heading nowhere slowly so he gently tapped Dr. Vandergrift on the shoulder and they conferred. He took over the mic and continued, "What the good doctor is trying to say is that the vet school's ALS lab was broken into last night between the hours of 11:00pm and 1:00am. At this point the masked assailants are presumed to be from the Animal Liberty Militia."

Without raising her hand, Anna blurted from her seat, "Why do you *assume* that?"

The cop paused and looked Anna over before he answered, "Because they left their calling card. They spray painted 'ALM' on nearly every surface." He continued with the description, "The perpetrators released over a hundred mice, fifteen cats and one squirrel monkey into the street." Anticipating a challenge, he turned to look at Anna, "We know they let them go just outside the school because three white mice were found squashed on 38th Street and two cats were recovered when they came to the Emergency Service doors — one had a white mouse in its mouth. The whereabouts of the monkey is unknown." He paused, "There appears to have been insider involvement because they used keys and secure combinations to gain entry." In all the time that the officer was speaking, Dr. Vandergrift never broke his mournful stare at Anna.

The cop continued, "There was one human casualty," he pulled a 3x5 note pad from his chest pocket and flipped it open, "A Mr. Maurice 'Moe' Sutton, 51, gross anatomy instructor, was on campus preparing examination materials when he heard a commotion in the lab. He engaged the intruders, apparently breaking an assailant's leg before being overpowered and rendered unconscious — he's currently at HUP under observation but should be released in a few hours."

Anna exclaimed, "Big Moe! But, the Animal Liberty Militia is supposed to be nonviolent..."

The cop looked Anna in the eye and turned his head slowly, "Yeah, supposedly," and then addressing the larger class he concluded, "If you know anything or have any hunches, please contact me. My baby brother, Officer, uh, I mean Mr. Jack Doyle in the back row has my number."

CHAPTER THIRTY

Mr. Right and Wrong

8:15 PM — FRIDAY, DECEMBER 16, 1988

Murphy's Tavern on the corner of 44th and Spruce

The news of the ALM attack cast a shadow which settled onto the Class of 1992. Its effects even subdued and attenuated the Friday Night Happy Hour. Jack hung out in the lounge outside Room 13 with an assortment of students, interns and residents for a while. He was half engaged in idle speculation about both ALM motives and the class's impending final exams, but he couldn't get Anna out of his mind (he'd watched as she stormed out of the classroom at the end of the period and disappeared). After a couple hours of small talk and beer, he gathered the Death Row Crew and headed over to Murph's where he, Hoss, Sam and Kerri settled into their usual booth in the far back corner of the bar. This booth was where they'd usually end Fridays swaying in song, singing Don McLean's "American Pie," but tonight they shared something different.

Jack sat in the middle, with his friends flanking him on either side of the 3/4 round booth. Even though the place was abuzz, smoke-filled and raucous, the little group hunkered down like a cloistered jury, weary from a grisly trial. At first, Sam and the others stared silently at the empty table in front of them, but then turned their attention to Jack. Their friend and classmate sat slumped with his hands folded in front of him. His face, battered from a youth of sibling rivalry, Philly street fights and then adult "scuffles" with errant law breakers, appeared heavy, weighed down. In his friends' experience, Jack Doyle was a paragon of unflappability but tonight worry had him on the ropes.

Jack finally broke the dismal silence when he stated, after a long sigh and without raising his eyes, "Folks, I don't like this situation."

Sam responded, "Me neithah, we need a pitchah."

Jack shook his head in slow motion, "Nah, I'm talking about the Animal Liberty Militia, the break in — the whole thing stinks. I mean, how did they get keys and access codes? How did they know what was in the lab?" He stopped, still staring at his folded hands on the table top.

Hoss leaned back, hooked his thumbs in the arm holes of his vest and spoke with a perplexed look on his face, "What I don't get is why? Why us? If there's one place that cares about animals, it's the veterinary school — we all got into this because we love animals. Didn't we?" He was moon-eyed and soft as he surveyed the table.

Kerri smiled, "Not me, I'm in it for the men. Well, perhaps there's some overlap, I love men that are animals."

Sam chimed in, "It's the moolah that I'm banking on..." and then chuckled, "See how I did that, sort of a pun?"

Hoss appeared as if he were about to respond too, but he was cut off when a sudsy pitcher and a fist full of mugs were plunked down in the center of the table. Though it was true that Murph's was the official off-campus vet school hangout, occasionally the med students slummed.

"Couldn't help but notice that you little vet-in-nannies looked sad — I'm guessing you're preparing your concession speech for next week. You know, when *we're* chosen for that TV show." Mr. John A. Cadaver, the med student Class President and a couple of his buddies stood in the deficit of the booth with broad self-satisfying grins.

Jack Doyle transformed himself as he leaned back with a smirk and stretched his arms along the back of the curving vinyl booth, one behind Hoss and the other behind Kerri, "So you think you got this thing locked up?"

The guy leaned into the jury box. He placed a flat palm on the tabletop and looked to each of them as if he were telling a secret, "Well, let's put it this way, the 20/20 production crew filmed our biostatistics class this afternoon, and the camera guy told me that we were *ideal* subjects."

Jack's eyes widened in response, "Biostatistics — riveting cinema, I'm sure..."

"Shit," the med student straightened up, "compared to a flea dip, human medical biostats is rocket science." He concluded with a sly smile, "So drink up little vetties because the next Happy Hour will be on you!" And with a wink to Kerri Feinburg, Mr. Cadaver and his friends marched back to the bar.

Sam declared under his breath and through a fixed grin on his handsome face, "Ain't that a pissah! Pretty confident for a buncha' flatlanders, wouldn't you say?" At first Jack looked to Sam and smiled, but this quickly faded as his thoughts rebounded to the reason they'd assembled.

"Look, I'm just gonna say what's on everyone's mind — I think Anna was involved with the break in." He paused for a moment and then proceeded to lay out the evidence. "She's in the vegan club. God knows why, but she's working in Vandergrift's lab on her PhD, this gives her access to keys and codes. And then, remember her little performance during the AVIS lecture when she spouted all that ALM boilerplate?"

The little group sipped and turned the deposition over in their minds. Hoss mulled with a fleshy frown for as long as he could, then he pushed his mug away, rejecting both the beer and the notion. He sat there for two seconds slowly rotating his head topped with that seven-inch crowned, Dan Blocker hat, "No way, no how — Anna is one of us. I don't believe it for a minute. Underneath all that bluff and bluster, she's a good person." Kerri nodded to show her agreement.

Jack countered, "I know how you feel, Hoss, but we all saw her reaction in ethics today, *and* the way Vandergrift was staring at her." He slumped, fixing his gaze on the foam of his undrunk beer, "I know she is one of us, and we care about her. So what am I supposed to do? My brother expects my help." Without altering his view he began to look inward, "My dad was a beat cop on this very street for twenty years. In our family's world, right and wrong are pretty clear: you break the law, you're wrong." Jack paused while he gathered his thoughts, "As my dad would say, good people do bad things all the time."

Hoss sat like a continental impasse. He smushed his lips back and forth as he stewed, but then, holding his ground, he repeated, "I just don't believe it — something else is going on."

CHAPTER THIRTY ONE

Synapse

The Annual Student Chapter of the American Veterinary Association (SCAVA) spay/neuter and vaccination clinic in the old veterinary school quad

I t was a perennial debate: exactly when should SCAVA hold its annual spay/neuter and vaccination clinic? One camp held (and quite logically) that the clement weather of spring or early summer leaned the schedule toward May. December on the other hand, with its snow and sleet seemed about the worst possible choice. But two logistical factors routinely tipped the odds in the 12th month's favor: first, late December was when the juniors finished their small animal surgery block. They'd just spent 10 weeks performing successively more intricate procedures, starting with laceration repairs, moving to laparotomies, and then GI anastomoses. And second, with the holidays just around the corner, almost everyone was in a festive, giving sort of mood. The clinic provided a win^3 (cubed) opportunity — students honed their technique by performing dozens of spays with a faculty member at their shoulder, low-income pet owners received top-notch care for a pittance, and SCAVA raised student scholarship funds. And though the timing occasionally varied, the event location did not.

The old vet school quad, a tucked away space, shielded from the din of the city world, was quite literally designed for this purpose. For nearly a hundred years this site was the heart of the school's outpatient care. In the olden days, everything seemed to happen within these four high walls. In fact, it was here, way back in 1884, that Eadweard Muybridge invented the first moving pictures (movies) of galloping treadmill beasts hauled over from the Philly Zoo. And, just as in the time of horse and buggy, today's communal flora escorted their fauna in from the street for care on the hoof.

Processing was stepwise, systematic and thorough — reflecting the structure and philosophy of a teaching hospital. First there was "Admitting" (performed just inside the massive stone archway), followed by history and physical exam, a consultation with a hospital clinician, and finally off to surgery or vaccination. Room A1 was converted into a waiting room where cocoa and cookies were served. And though it was not publicly broadcast, a supply of donated pet food was on hand for those who needed the help. With Trisha and Mike's early morning efforts to deck the halls — twinkling lights and boughs of holly — the atmosphere in the old courtyard was transformed from a stark, cold parking lot into the veterinary equivalent of a holiday soup kitchen.

◄ • ►

Admitting —

This morning Jack Doyle, Hoss and Anna were on the receiving end. They greeted the patients and their owners, and started the paperwork. Along with a couple fourth years and two, second-year SCAVA reps, they worked at a "U" of folding tables under a vinyl banner that proclaimed "SuperCurve (TM), AVIS Pet Foods, Inc." Front and center and free for the taking were stacks of SuperCurve flyers, AVIS logo mugs brimming with multicolor AVIS pens, and piles of AVIS-branded chew toys. A banner of show dog winners was draped and wrapped around the front while clipboards with paper registration forms and tethered pens were stacked on the side tables. The whole setup flashed a trade show vibe because that's exactly what it was — Avery Banks had her minions transport the booth over from the convention center last night.

Jack and Hoss posed, arms folded, chests out and with cheek-bulging grins next to a photo enlargement mounted on the brick behind the booth. The aging photo, taken at this very spot, depicted an unsmiling all-male veterinary class in black bowlers, bow ties and full-length, brilliant white uniforms — those in white pants and short white jackets looked like Good Humor men while others in high barrel collars were clad in spotless white, ankle-length frocks. Off to the side in the image stood a stout, impish man in drab, grubby clothes. His face, though soiled like his gear, wore a beatific, nearly toothless smile. You could see the laughter in his eyes as he balanced a hefty sledge over one shoulder and held the reins of three massive draft horses. The caption on the brass plaque read, "Horse-shoeing Lab, Class of 1902." The school's blacksmith clearly knew what lay ahead for the dandies in white.

Jack, his arms still folded across his chest, appealed to Sam through a fixed grin, "Snap the damn picture." Sam replied, "Someday, you'll thank me for recording this," and a flash of light blanketed the space.

Anna Heywood, bundled against the cold in a flat green army sur-plus jacket that had been her father's, eyed the forming line that now stretched out through the arch and around the corner. She turned to face Jack and Hoss and complained, "Come on guys, we need to get to work."

Before Jack could respond, and unbeknownst to Anna, a shapely form materialized behind her, "Now, don't push Mr. Doyle too hard, he's got a big night ahead of him." Anna spun on her cane and found herself face-to-face with Avery Banks. Avery continued, "Besides, he looks almost edible in that pose wouldn't you say miss, what's your name again?" Anna got all angular, flat and sharp, but didn't reply. "Oh, that's right, you don't eat meat... you're more of a fish girl." Jack broke from Hoss and pushed between the two women.

Avery asked, "Did you get the tux I sent over?"

Jack nodded, his face flushed. He was embarrassed by his position and, feeling like a kept man, he said sheepishly, "Yeah, I did."

Avery Banks reached over to give his biceps a squeeze and speaking loudly enough so that Anna would most assuredly hear, "Did it fit these big arms and broad shoulders?"

"I better get back to work," he answered awkwardly.

"Fabulous. I'll have the car pick you up at eight. Don't let this thing run too long today."

Anna piped, "If, by this *thing*, you mean our spay and neuter clinic for low-income families?"

Avery Banks replied with a dismissive wave as she floated through the arch and out of the quad, "Yes, I mean the clinic I'm paying for..."

Jack looked to Anna, but before he could say anything, a young wom-an swathed in an array of woolen scarves and looking something like a tech-nicolor mummy grunted to lift a cat carrier up to the booth. Jack reached out to help and was astounded at the heft. It felt like thirty pounds. He glanced through the mesh of the carrier's door to confirm this was in fact a cat, not a Shih Tzu, and was met with an unmistakable feline growl. The kitty's normal-sized head seemed wholly out of proportion to his portly torso. Jack thought, if Orson Welles were reincarnated, this would be him.

As if performing a practiced wintery striptease, the woman began to slowly unwrap.

"This is Spartacus and he needs to be neutered."

Jack thought, *he needs to be neutered of 15 pounds of fat*, but replied, "Sure, we can certainly arrange for that. Is there anything else?"

The woman hesitated, "He needs the special kind of neutering. The kind that makes him a girl."

Somewhat confused, Jack said, "Well, the surgery will remove his testicles, but he'll still be a boy... at least mostly. He may not be quite the gladiator he once was, but I think you'll hardly notice."

"No, Spartacus has a pee-pee problem and he needs it cut off."

Jack blinked.

The woman's countenance took on the seriousness of a Shakespearean actor. She leaned in and continued in a hush, "He has trouble going #1 and I read that he might die if his thingy blocked up again, so I want you to amputate."

Jack was a amazed by her directness and confused by the request. Mike London, who was also manning the booth, overheard the exchange and stepped up to explain that Spartacus must have been the victim of a urethral obstruction, a potentially fatal condition if left untreated. Though medical management was usually the first course of action, it didn't always work and the procedure she was referring to was called a perineal urethrostomy. It involved widening the urinary tract and removing the penis to make obstruction less likely.

Jack turned, wide-eyed, to face the woman, "Well, I'm not sure that's something the surgeons can handle today, but how about we get the ball rolling, as it were..."

◄ ◦ ►

History and Physical Exam —

If nothing else, JJ was at least consistent: if a teacher or authority figure, even a fourth year, told him to do something academically oriented, he did it. This blind fidelity resulted in him working the patient history booth alongside other more altruistic students and practicing vets. Since the annual event drew in professors from both the large and small animal clinics, there were dozens of new faces working side by side with the first years. So it was no surprise to JJ to be paired with an aging, bushy eye-browed vet in a long white lab coat whom he'd never seen before. As a matter of course, he treated the elderly gentleman with the respect that was his due (as per the Oath) but that didn't stop JJ from whining.

"I know Doctor Kimball said we should be here today, but honestly, I think it would be more productive if I were home studying. I've got 12 final examinations next week and my class rank is at stake." The kindly old man patted JJ on the back, "Son, I graduated in 1943 and I can tell you after 45 years of practice, class rank doesn't mean a wit. The essence of being a veterinarian is being well rounded — and what's most important of all are people skills. Study humans not animals." JJ was mildly dazed but before he could stammer out an objection their next patient came through the pipeline. The old vet nodded and JJ watched with interest as an equally ancient woman shuffled toward them. She wore a filthy, floor-length fur coat that looked like it had mange and the bottom edges were stained with sidewalk salt. When she finally got situated in front of them, she pulled down her hood to reveal a greasy mat of hair plastered to one side where no doubt she'd slept and then plunked a heavy purse on the table — a small head poked out of the open top. The tiny, quivering pug half recoiled when the old vet introduced his thick but gentle hand.

"Madam, how are we doing today? What a grand little fellow you have here."

The woman didn't remove her heavy, scratched sunglasses, "He's my Rex, Rex is his name."

JJ was staggered by the burst of alcohol fumes, but soldiered on, "How's Rex been feeling? Any coughing, is he eating well, drinking plenty of water?"

"Oh, yes, he eats like a champ — I know a butcher and I get all the chicken bones Rex can eat."

While the older vet continued asking questions, JJ found that Rex's right eye appeared bluish and opaque, its center cratered and raw. A thick crust of debris had collected in the corner and along the lower lid. Rex worked hard to keep the eye open, but it was clear from his squinting that he was in pain.

The woman noticed JJ looking at the animal's eye, "My poor little Rex has had something wrong with that eye since October. I've tried everything, washing it with soap and water, the stuff I use on the dry parts of my feet and," she winked, "a little scotch every now and then, but it just keeps getting worse."

The aged vet deftly applied a drop of fluorescein dye followed by a saline flush and pronounced that Rex had a corneal ulcer.

The woman scooped up and clutched the little dog. Her speech suddenly became stilted and her composure faltered as she started to cry, the tears cutting a path through her unwashed face, "I don't want him to suffer." She pleaded, "But, please don't put him to sleep!"

JJ didn't know what to say. Taken aback by the unfiltered emotion, he turned to his partner with a look of confusion. The old timer took over, "Oh, ma'am, don't you worry. Nobody's going to put Rex down and you can be sure that the surgical team will be able to treat that bad eye of his."

The woman was visibly relieved. She produced a flask from somewhere deep inside her mammoth wrap, took a swig and extending it to JJ, whispered, "Besides this, Rex is all I have."

◅ • ▻

Consultation —

The consultation area, the last stop before surgery or vaccination, was staffed by several clinicians, including Drs. Flo Kimball and Violet Marie Green. Also present were Trisha Maxwell and two of her first-year advisees, Sam Stone and, never far from him, Kerri Feinburg. Trisha's other advisee, Rick Larson, was nowhere to be seen and his absence was refreshing.

Dr. Green was working with Trisha as she helped an owner lift a dog carrier to the exam table. In it were two Corgis. "Okay, sir, it looks like Angus and Argyle, uh," she paused to crinkle her upper lip, "are just slated for the rabies boosters today. Is that correct?" The disheveled man carried a subtle but permanent smile while his ruddy cheeks gave him a cherubic glow that seemed entirely appropriate for the season.

The man surprised Violet with an almost indecipherable brogue, "Och aye, that's reit yoong lassie."

She paused as her mind processed the translation, "And, I notice it says here that neither dog has been receiving heartworm preventative?"

Dr. Kimball's ears perked up.

"Aye, again. Ah wasnae sure whit it was, tae be honest."

"Well, after we check to make sure they aren't already infected, I'd like to recommend that you begin monthly heartworm medication. If these little guys get the disease, it could shorten their lives considerably. But it's an entirely preventable condition and I can assure you that the cost of prevention is considerably less than what it would be to treat should either dog become infected."

Dr. Kimball sidestepped into the conversation, "Please forgive me for interrupting, sir, but can I show you something?" She reached into a cardboard box under the table, produced a glass pickle jar and plunked it down. Flo Kimball leaned forward and pointed to the right atrium and ventricle. "Can you see those squiggly things that look like spaghetti?" The man was intrigued. "These little spaghettis are what killed the gorgeous dog this heart came from." Then she reached into her purse and retrieved a mini photo album. "These are some of my patients, and this was Brutus," an enormous swatch of Great Dane brindle filled the frame.

"Those wee things killed thes big loon?"

"Yes, the heartworm has an amazing life cycle." The man screwed up his face, there was no hiding his emotion and Flo Kimball knew what was confusing him. "We call it a life cycle. It means where the eggs are laid, how they are born and live their lives. With heartworms, the babies live in the blood. When a mosquito bites an infected dog and then goes on to bite another, it can spread the offspring, or larvae, from one animal to the next. The mosquito is what we call a vector."

"A weck-tur?"

"Yes, a wecktur, I mean a vector. A vector is something that helps transmit a disease."

The man, reached up under his cap, scratched his head and then bent to pick up some snow from the ground. He held it in his outstretched hand to make his point, "Och aye, but thaur arenae onie mosquitos noo ur thaur, yoong lassie?"

"Aye, I mean, yes. You're correct, but they will come back. The mosquitos die off in the fall, return in the spring and then continue to spread the worms." She paused to see if her words had room to sink in.

Violet Marie Green stood and stared at the heartworm tutorial with an intensity that made a laser gunsight look diffuse by comparison — then, it all clicked. The synaptic gap was bridged. She turned to face Trisha, placed both hands on the fourth year's shoulders and whispered in amazement, "A seasonal vector... That's why it fell off in October. *That's why the cases stopped.* I've got to talk to Stan, we have to get our hands on some mosquitoes!"

CHAPTER THIRTY TWO

Love is Everything

8:30 PM — SATURDAY, DECEMBER 17, 1988

*On Spruce Street outside the main entrance to the Hospital
of the University of Philadelphia (HUP)*

*J*ack Doyle performed as instructed. While Anna was helping to discharge the last patient, Jack broke away from the SCAVA clinic so he had time to shower and dress. He was fiddling with his stiff new cufflinks (a present from Avery Banks) when he heard the limo's horn and didn't get them toggled into place until he was standing before the tinted glass of the sleek, shiny behemoth. The driver, who had double-parked with the flashers on in front of Jack's apartment at 4431 Spruce, jumped out when he saw Jack approach. As the door was pulled open, Jack was nearly razed by two staggering blows. The first was a dense, sickening wall of honeysuckle perfume that billowed outward as the door swung through its long arc. And this assault was countered almost immediately by an electrifying upper cut — the slit of Avery's dress. Before Jack stooped to get in, he couldn't help but trace the gap in the shimmering black gown from delicate ankle to sinuous calf. Past silky knee and across milky thigh along the serpentine course of the sartorius to the delicious outer contour of hip. From there, Jack let his eyes dive medially toward the origin and insertion of Avery Banks' power over him. He stood there in the dark, you might call it transfixed, with snow swirling and the chauffeur politely looking the other way until an elegant hand conveying a bubbling flute of champagne appeared in the opening. He took the glass and a sip, then climbed in.

As they motored down Spruce, splashing through icy slush past Murphy's Tavern and mountains of graying snow, Avery Banks laid out their evening. They'd begin by having drinks and hors d'oeuvres with the CEO of AVIS, the dean of the vet school and the head of the National ASPCA. This mixer would be followed by a dinner and awards for local *do gooders* — which she punctuated with a roll of her eyes — some requisite dancing and then hopefully, "dessert." Jack knew what Avery meant by *dessert*. He'd been successfully curbing his sweet tooth while deflecting her offerings for the past few weeks, but tonight he wondered if he'd have the will to pass on the last course. Despite his unrelenting maleness and a wandering visual appetite, John Fitzgerald Doyle was something of a rarity — he was waiting and looking for *The One*.

So tonight, after settling into the car's plush black leather, Jack sipped the bubbly, nodded where expected, and kept his eye turned toward the street. Though snow was piled high against the buildings and in the gutter, Jack found what he was looking for as they neared the entrance of HUP. He could tell, even from a distance, that it was Anna in her rumpled army jacket — the silhouette was unmistakable, especially with the cane and two dogs at her side. As the limo slowed for a red light and rolled even with her, Jack discovered his classmate engaged in a knockdown shouting match with a guy cloaked in a parka. Having been on the receiving end himself many times, this observation alone was not surprising. But, as the vehicle began to pull away, Jack realized something was wrong when he saw fear streak across Anna's usually hardened face. Without hesitation or consultation, Jack barked, "Stop the car!" kicked the door open and sprang from the still moving limousine. He dodged a cab and then another car, horns honking, and hit the sidewalk running about fifty yards downstream while yelling her name. Unintentional though it was, the bellow of "A-N-N-A" came out with the same intonation as "A-D-R-I-A-N" from every Rocky picture ever made. The guy who she was fighting with turned toward the shout and from under his dark hood developed an expanding appreciation for the 180 pounds of tux and tails barreling his way. In his past life, the instant that *Officer* Jack Doyle gave pursuit, his brain began calculating: closure rate to the thug, potential for weapons involvement, escape routes and body mass discrepancies. But tonight, while his flexing quads drove him forward as fast as his flat-soled dress shoes would allow, Jack had only Anna on his mind. Reflexively, he reached to his hip for his service revolver but before its absence could register, he saw the assailant shove Anna down and take flight. In the span of just one of his six-foot strides she disappeared completely from sight. Jack skidded to a stop where he'd seen her vanish and descended a slippery concrete stairwell to where Anna lay with Petunia and Clancy nuzzled into her cheek.

Jack dropped to his knees and anxiously whispered while stroking her hair, "Anna, my God, are you okay?"

As if waking from a nightmare, the kind where escape is mired by waist-deep brine, Anna looked up to see Jack crouched over her and felt his hand on her cheek. Even with the streetlamp behind him, she could see everything she needed in his face. She blinked slowly and a half smile developed as she spoke, "It's you..." Then as a metallic taste came to her mouth, she drew a finger gingerly across her lips and realized she'd bitten her tongue. Anna looked down at the blood and then up at Jack again. Behind him was a halo of light and falling snow, "Where did you come from?"

"I was watching you," he paused because he realized how that sounded, then added, "We were driving by." He scooped her to her feet. Petunia and Clancy licked her hands and burrowed into her legs as they climbed back to street level. Once at the top, Jack held Anna's arm, faced her square on and said softly as he shook his head, "Who the hell was that?" He paused, and when he realized she wasn't going to answer, he continued, "You knew that guy, didn't you — was he with the ALM?"

Anna straightened her jacket, brushed the snow from its creases, and reached up to sweep the hair from her forehead. She could feel Jack's gentle touch giving her strength as he cupped her elbow to steady her weakened body. She looked down at her cane, wondering if perhaps she wouldn't need it anymore, and then began, "Yes, well..." but trailed off because his face was so close she could smell the soapy clean scent of his recent shower. When she finally let herself look directly into Jack's eyes again, it triggered something. She began reaching out to him.

And then, suddenly, a horn blared. The two jolted apart and Jack spun to rediscover the long black limo with a window rolled halfway down. "Are you about done visiting with your little friend? The mixer starts in five minutes. Chop-chop!"

Jack turned back to Anna to find that a stricken look had replaced the softness and connection they'd just shared. She yanked her elbow from his grasp and, without a word, gathered the dog leads and began hobbling towards the entrance of HUP.

Jack waded through the snow mound in the gutter and leaned down to the open car window to tell Avery to go on without him, but by the time he'd caught up with Anna outside the revolving hospital doors, everything had changed. He called her name again and without turning Anna let out a low growl, "Get away from me. Go back to your Lois Lane," and pushed her way inside.

Jack stopped and watched the limo's tail lights fade into traffic. He waited as if cast in bronze for nearly 10 minutes with snow melting into his suit while he considered chasing Anna. Finally, he turned, pulled up his collar and began slogging his way back home.

◄ ● ►

Once Anna had cleared the revolving door and was out of Jack's sight, she limped robotically to a chair in the lobby next to a sickly ficus and collapsed. Both Petunia and Clancy pulled in close as she slumped and her body tremored. Clancy curled at her feet while Petunia rested her head on Anna's thigh, looking up into her eyes. Anna could do little more than pet away the tears as they fell.

Over the past weeks, Anna had convinced the nurses on Mrs. Oliver's floor that Clancy and Petunia were therapy dogs and thus should be allowed on the ward — this wasn't entirely untrue because Clancy was a trained service dog and both animals did have a therapeutic effect. But tonight, as she made her way off the elevator and past the nurse's station with the two canines in the lead, she could see that something had changed. Mrs. Oliver's room, the one directly ahead at the end of the hall, was empty. The head nurse came around the desk, "Miss Heywood, I'm sorry but Mrs. Oliver has had a set back — she's back in the ICU." The nurse looked over her left shoulder and added with a sadness that belied her professional facade, "She's in a coma."

The nurse proceeded to explain that the doctors had ruled out all known causes of encephalitis including bacteria, protozoa, viruses and even autoimmune disease. They were stumped. Then she stated that Mike London was up to speed because he called in regularly, but wondered if Anna could relay this information to her classmate, Jack Doyle — she assumed Anna knew that Jack sat with Mrs. Oliver at lunchtime most days. Anna did not.

Anna blinked a few times and took a deep breath as the realization set in. Maybe her heart *was* right. Her thoughts swirled and then she was jogged back to Mrs. Oliver's reality.

"Mrs. O left an envelope to give you, if something happened. Unfortunately, I think this qualifies." The nurse returned behind the counter and pulled open a drawer. Anna could only nod her head slightly as she acknowledged with a whispered, "Thanks."

Anna stood at the ICU window and, after watching the serenity on Mrs. Oliver's face for nearly an hour, she opened the envelope. There was just one page inside:

Dear Anna,

Whether a four-legged friend or the man of your dreams, Love is Love.

And Love is Everything— I'm going home to mine.

Thank you for taking care of my dear boy, Clancy. I know he can help

you find your way too.

Mrs. Irene Oliver

CHAPTER THIRTY THREE

Mostly, There's Love

8:30 PM — TUESDAY, DECEMBER 20, 1988

Equine soft tissue recovery barn at the Center for Large Animal Medicine in Kennett Square

The waning days of December are, for fourth-year veterinary students, short on daylight and long on stress. December is when most fourth years take the National Board Exam (NBE). Add this dinky, little, career-defining hurdle to the rotational load in clinics and few holiday seasons hold more shining light than the one in the final year of vet school. That is, unless you're Mike London. Mike took to clinics like a FRoG on a front row log. And, as Trisha described for their first-year advisees when they met to share the transcendent power of old tests and vet pictionary, he had already sat for *and passed* the NBE in his third year.

So, though Mike was unfazed by the dizzying jumble and restless demands of senior rotations, for most students, the two- and four-week rotational experiences were aptly named because just as soon as the seniors got acclimated, they were blindly spun and plopped into a brand new world. Since the administration's priority was hospital coverage, students were launched Wimbledon-style from dermatology in the city to field service in the country, from companion animal dentistry to passing gas for race horses, from equine neonatal intensive care to small animal oncology — and then there were the electives. Some fourth years doubled up on their local favorites, two scoops of dairy medicine for instance, while others ventured further afield to learn fish surgery in Woods Hole or pachyderm medicine on the Serengeti. And along with the serial jumble of topic and technique, rotational staffing took a bingo wheel approach to combining the students as well. This whole grand contraption churned out configurations unknown in the wild.

In this way, Mike was recently paired with his class's variant of Simon JJ Harding III (every class had one). For over three, years Mike had erroneously pegged the beanpoled kid with Dumbo ears as the ultimate FRoG. It took a theriogenology rotation where they collected 15 randy stallions, impregnated a herd of Angora goats, shared a stinking, moldy dorm room, and several tepid six-packs of PBR to discover that the kid was actually alright — an uncool retro nerd by nearly every measure but, as it turned out, sweet, kind and funny as hell. Earlier in the day, Mike showed Trisha the only picture currently in his wallet; it featured his newfound friend mounting a phantom mare while striking a front row pose with a beer in elevated hand. The fleeting experience of his last rotation taught Mike a lesson, lumpers may stay sane but splitters can find gold. A goofy gem lay hidden beneath that FRoGy veneer and all he had to do was look.

But even with the curricular tumbler set to full scramble, and the benefits of cross-pollination acknowledged, Mike and Trisha were happy to find themselves working their current rotation together. Large animal soft tissue surgery or "soft tissue" had been unusually busy the past couple of weeks. Although late December was outside the traditional colic season — where equids presented with signs ranging from pawing at their bellies to bruxism to repeated flehmen — the duo was coming off their fifth consecutive night of belly-busting surgery. Colics were gory, messy, high-stakes ventures. When a horse presented to the school's referral center for colic, it usually meant that the local practitioner had exhausted all palliative medical options and the animal was just hours from total collapse.

Tonight, Mike and Trisha had just finished PM rounds with the soft tissue resident in Barn A, a bantamweight kid who looked like he might not survive even the first year of his three-round training program. In between patting bandaged bellies, he complained bitterly and nearly under his breath about the "dick of a senior clinician known to dump work on residents under the guise of *teaching* so he could dedicate more time to chasing nurses." The resident knew better than to commiserate directly with his subordinates, the fourth years, but when you average 3 hours' sleep a night for weeks on end, you tend to get a little surly and disregarding of protocol.

After Mike had squared away the last of the evening treatment plans, he turned to his platonic girl friend and said, "You got the service beeper tonight?"

Trisha placed a palm over the black plastic bulge on her hip and yawned, "I'm on deck."

The two of them stood in the dull yellow glow of the nurse's station at the end of the barn and, even though they'd both been through the same soft-tissue organ grinder, Mike London looked as fresh as the proverbial daisy. Trisha crossed her arms and examined her classmate. She shook her head slowly and said to Mike, "Look at you… Did you sleep at all last night?"

Mike crinkled his eyebrows and pursed his lips, thought for a moment and then replied, "Nope, can't say I did. One belly after another." Then he added with a wistful look and a broad, comfortable smile, "It was awesome."

Trisha continued, "But you're off tonight, so what's your plan?"

This question caused Mike to stop and plant his hands on his hips. It wasn't that he didn't have an answer, it was just that this kind of question had never occurred to him. Trisha watched as Mike's face made the shift from serene to sublime just before he replied, "More of the same, thank you," and then he turned to open the door.

They plodded the snowy ten yards between barns and Mike angled towards the outpatient clinic while his friend continued to poke fun, "More? Mikie, and I can't believe I'm saying this to you, but my dear, I think you need to jump start your social life. Have a beer or even, gasp… go on a date."

Mike grinned as he opened the clinic door, warmth and light spilling out onto the snow all around. He ushered his classmate forward with an, "Apres vous," and the two entered a space that was pleasantly snug, fragrant and softly abuzz.

Mike nodded to himself and then whispered over Trisha's shoulder, "This is my favorite time."

Trisha glanced at a feeble string of blinking lights and garland strung around the Pharmacy window and replied, "Christmas?"

"Naa," he paused, "The night. It's bonus time. During the day, Monday through Friday, that's the work week. On Saturday and Sunday, we have weekend duty. But the nights are play time." He paused to knock the snow off his boots on the rubberized floor, "Cases admitted between now and morning rounds are gravy — I know it sounds crazy, but I just want to see if I can help fix 'em." He turned back to the door they'd just entered and put his hand on the knob, "In fact, I think I'll head over to the NIC-U and then I guess on to post-op."

Trisha remarked with a friendly smile, "You troll for cases the way mere mortals bar hop for chicks."

As his eyes swept the clinic space they'd just entered, Mike's placid smile returned, "Where else would you want to be? I swear it feels like the world is revolving around us. Look…" He used an extended arm to reveal what was there all the time: Dan Linnehan scoping an Arabian mare, a seasoned field service clinician examining a show cow, the yellow ribbon still hanging from the halter. Nurses and students buzzed, and buzzed peacefully around a Staffordshire ewe and her fuzzy, out-of-season lambs. Though fluorescent lighting can be harsh, in this place on this night, it served as an ocular solvent, picking up and melding the teal of surgical scrubs with the chestnut of withers. It dissolved and mixed the blacks — Holstein patches, the Arabian's mane and the shiny blackness of the endoscope. Everything about the scene was supportive, soft and caring. Mike added, "I know it's winter, but this feels like the Dairy Queen back home on a midsummer night. It's all here, everything you need — the drama of life and death, honor, conflict and comedy. It's got everything, but mostly, there's love."

Trisha Maxwell did a double take, then stared mutely back at her friend of nearly four years. He stood in front of her with a battered stethoscope slung around his neck, grizzly stubble along his jawline and a subtle grin. The silence stretched on until Trisha asked, "Love?"

Mike nodded his head and replied softly, "When you're exactly where you're supposed to be, there's nothing left but romance," then he pointed towards the family in a corner exam stall. "Those kids love that ewe and they won't sleep until they know she's okay. Over there, in the steel stocks, that farm manager loves that Arabian. I'll bet that animal represents his entire life's work." Mike didn't stop there, "Look at Doctor Linnehan driving that endoscope; he loves being the best he can be. And, see those two from our class?" Trisha spied two front-row denizens clumsily flirting as they percussed a cow in all the wrong places, "Those are FRoGs in love. You tell me, what were the odds they'd find each other in the real world?"

He sighed and concluded, "Hell, I may not be able to tell the difference between hook- and pinworm ova but I know True Love when I see it." Mike's grin spread and took control of his face, "See you at 5:30 for morning rounds." The door clicked shut behind him.

Before Trisha had even a moment to reflect on the miracle she'd just witnessed, the pager clipped to her waist vibrated to life. She looked down and read the number. It was the admissions desk.

Trisha crossed the buoyant sea of life and love in front of her and made her way into a hallway that led to admissions. After walking silently for a few seconds she took a left and then froze. Trisha whispered under her breath without taking her eyes off the guy about 20 yards away.

"*It's him…*"

As she took in the rugged-built man, faded jeans, spurs and Stetson, the synaptic clicks made her feel flush. Buck stood facing away from her in front of a floor-length window. She couldn't take her eyes off the back of the sturdy frame silhouetted against the cold night sky. Trisha nodded to herself so slowly her head didn't move. She thought, *well I'll be damned, Mikie was right, again.*

The cowboy must have been deep in thought because he didn't hear Trisha Maxwell approach. Afraid she might be dreaming, she stopped a body length from the man and quietly called his name, "Buck?" As the man turned, Trisha could have sworn she saw him catch his breath and then she noticed his arm in a homemade sling.

He said, sounding relieved, "Doc, I'm so glad you're here."

Trisha paused, and with a growing smile replied, "Me, too."

Then something rare happened, something that does not happen every day. Trisha Maxwell and Buck Riley held their positions and just stared into each other's eyes. Two, then three, then four seconds passed and neither said a word. Trisha placed a hand on the counter next to her. She needed to steady her balance because the world had begun to spin. *So, this is what it's like*, she thought, and then, even though she didn't want to, she broke the trance. She took a step forward, reached to the sling and asked, "What happened?" and before Buck could reply she added, "Where's Suzie, is she okay?"

Buck's eyes dropped, "No, something's wrong — something's really wrong with her, and I don't know what to do…"

Trisha said, "Tell me what's going on."

"Well, we've been on the circuit down South for the winter and doing really well — I was saving up," he paused and raised his eyebrows, the memory of his recent purchase made him smile. "But yesterday at a trial outside of Raleigh, Suzie went down." He gingerly lifted his right arm and winced, "That's how this happened." Now Trisha noticed the dirt all down his left side and a laceration with some fresh blood above Buck's eye. Instinctively, she reached for something to dab the cut clean. The only thing she had was Buck's own handkerchief, which she always kept in her back pocket. As she began to raise the white cloth to his forehead it unfolded and a blue ribbon fluttered softly to the floor between them. Trisha blushed and Buck smiled.

"Have you been to a doctor?"

"Nah, I'm fine, Suzie's what's important. A couple of days ago she seemed depressed and then this... It's not like her at all."

"Why didn't you go to NC State? They have a great vet school there." Trisha shook her head in wonder, "You must have driven all night."

"I did drive all night, because I wanted you... you're the best," he paused and then added, "The best for us."

Trisha blushed, "Buck, I'm just a vet student, I don't graduate until spring."

He replied softly, "I know that," then added, "And I knew it before, but a piece of paper isn't what makes you a good vet." He added as his face brightened, "And that's not why we were coming back to you."

Trisha blinked. She felt a catch in her throat. Was he saying what she hoped he was saying? She closed her lids hard again. When they re-opened Buck was still there, his arm was still injured, she could still see into those eyes filled with sincerity. She lowered her gaze and whispered, "I'm glad." After a moment she looked back up, "I want to see her."

Buck pushed open the door and they went into the night together.

"Buck, can you unload and walk Suzie slowly in a circle around me?" As the snow kicked up, Trisha glanced to the tall xenon lights that ringed the back parking area, "I should be able to see well enough here."

The animal backed out of the trailer awkwardly, stepping all over herself. Once they were out, Buck cupped Suzie's nose with both his hands and, ignoring his injury, he cooed, "Okay sweetie-bug, we're just gonna walk slow," and then gently kissed her muzzle. There was no reply. No horsey purr. So Buck began to cautiously lead his best friend around the lot.

The first thing that Trisha noticed was the most subtle. Suzie's head hung slightly, her ears were lax and her eyes, they were somehow empty — she thought, *it's like this horse is not here*. Trisha continued to watch as Suzie moved with a sluggish, weary gait and then she saw it. The slight drop of the animal's left hip, the dragging of the toe. Then, Suzie staggered. This wasn't subtle and it scared Trisha. Her mind vaulted. Sure, there could be a dozen different causes — EPM, EEE, WEE, or hepato-encephalopathy, but it just didn't feel like those. Trisha's heart tightened, her pulse and pressure elevated. This man came all this way to her. He believed in her. He brought his only family to her.

Buck stopped because he saw the alarm in Trisha's face. "What's the matter, what did you see?"

Trisha didn't respond at first and then she said, "Hold her steady, I want to get her temp." Suzie was inert, she didn't even notice when Trisha lifted her tail and inserted the thermometer. It read 105.3 F. As Trisha stood in the exact spot where they'd first met, now in the blustering swirl of December snow, a magical thing happened — her fear vanished. The gravity could have hobbled her, she could have buckled or bailed, but there was something about the presence of this man that freed her. The years of training and experience came together under those icy lights in that lonely parking lot and she knew in her heart what had to be done. "Buck, we have to get Suzie into the ICU. She'll need a full CBC and chemistry panel, a spinal tap, intravenous fluids, probably anti-inflammatory meds and broad-spectrum antibiotics to start." She paused and gazed with concern into Buck's watery eyes, "There could be days of intensive nursing care. We can sign her in under my name for a discount, but this," she took a deep breath, "this could cost thousands," and then she wavered, "and I don't know if we can save her."

Buck didn't hesitate, he glimpsed the truck and trailer in the background, "I can sell my rig and," he reached for his wallet, "I have some savings left." Even in the winter darkness, Trisha could see that Buck's weathered, ruddy face had paled. He was shaken, but replied without doubt, "We have to do the right thing by Suzie."

Trisha blinked once, "Okay, I know just who to call."

CHAPTER THIRTY FOUR

Overwinter

The Equine Intensive Care Unit at the Center for Large Animal Medicine in Kennett Square

*T*risha whisked Buck and Suzie directly to an empty stall in the Equine ICU and called in everyone she trusted. Mike was, of course, first on the scene. He materialized in about 30 seconds with the nursing staff just moments behind. After consulting with Dr. Green on the phone, Trisha raised the horse's jugular, drew blood and ran a quick PCV and glucose at the nurse's station. Seeing a HCT of 60%, Mike worked with Trisha to place a large-bore IV catheter and hung 20 liters of Lactated Ringers while Nurse Linda hurried the purple and red top tubes to the STAT lab for a full panel of tests. Dr. Linnehan showed up five minutes later and was in the process of listening to Suzie's heart and lungs when Drs. Green and Oblitzski arrived.

After the two clinicians and pathologist had evaluated Suzie and heard Trisha's history and physical exam findings, they conferred amongst themselves. The assembled conglomerate was truly a mixed bag of specialties representing the fields of zoological medicine, equine orthopedic surgery and diagnostic pathology — and though no one was the designated lead on the case, Stan Oblitzski spoke first because he could barely contain his enthusiasm.

"It's kind of amazing that we're all here at this very moment because I've just finished a series of gels, immunoassays and EM work proving that Violet is a genius!" He paused, flashed a toothy, geeky grin and then plundered onward with excitement, "She put all the pieces together and the missing link was glued to the fly strips at the Peaceable Kingdom. We were looking for the etiological agent and a seasonal vector and *voila*, those mosquitoes were crammed with viral particles." His eyes got wide as he turned to face Buck, "It is the coolest, most insidious neurotrophic disease I've seen in the *looongest* time. Highly contagious and eminently virulent, it appears to be universally lethal in crows, infects owls, ibis, flamingoes, equids, other exotic species and even humans!" Then, uncharacteristically, Stan slowed his freight train of pathological glee and a series of deepening furrows developed across his forehead, "But, with this new case, it means that the virus has spread south and now," he gulped and Trisha watched as his pointy Adam's apple bobbled up and down, "it can overwinter."

Seeing the confusion and fear in Buck's eyes, Violet Marie Green stepped forward, "Mr. Riley…"

Choking back his worry, the man replied, "Ma'am, just call me Buck."

"Buck, there are several possible causes for Suzie's neurological signs, and we'll run tests to rule them out, but we think she may have a new disease, one that's just been discovered. It's called West Nile Virus — it's never been seen in North America." True to form, Dr. Green didn't say, *A new disease that we discovered.* Her work wasn't about taking credit; it was about the Mission.

In a flash, Mrs. Oliver's mystery condition was clear to Mike. He excused himself and stepped away to call the HUP ICU.

Buck tried to speak but his voice cracked, "A new disease? Will she die?"

With calm and steady compassion, Dr. Green replied, "Buck, it is possible. There are no specific treatments for West Nile but Trisha has taken exactly the right steps — you and Suzie could not be in better hands." Buck beamed at Trisha with an emotion that was unmistakable to everyone, even Stan Oblitzski. The cowboy's eyes locked onto Trisha because he knew that this was exactly where he was supposed to be.

After coordinating with the ICU nurses, double checking the medication plan and listening to Stan rave for a half hour more about the malignant qualifications of the West Nile Virus, Violet Marie Green came to two realizations: 1) it was time to re-sequester Stan the Path Man from the general public, and 2) she needed to lock down the Peaceable Kingdom.

◅ ❖ ▻

Though it might seem as if Suzie was receiving extra special treatment, she was and she wasn't. The truth is, though the University of Philadelphia clinicians are the best of the best, this is the standard of care at vet schools almost everywhere. This is the way things are done, the way it's always been done. Clinicians run themselves ragged, students rarely sleep, and no one wants to give up on a case. In fact, most private practitioners, when empowered by an animal's owner, can rally a staggering array of diagnostic tests, surgical techniques and medical treatments to care for their patients. It's just that most of this professional compassion and quietly-skilled dedication goes on without fanfare behind-the-scenes in clinics, barns, shelters and stables across the land.

However, on this night in late December of 1988, Suzie was somewhat of a special case. She had the good fortune that Buck Riley had fallen for Trisha Maxwell — Trisha was a favorite of the Center's staff. So, after spreading an extra deep layer of clean rice straw, dimming the barn lights and getting the animal to bed down, the nurses looked the other way as Trisha and Buck curled up in a corner of Suzie's stall. The winter storm rose and howled outside as Buck whispered the stories of his travels since they'd met, all in the cozy warmth of horse and sweet clover. And though they talked in each other's arms for hours, they must have dozed off in the early morning hours because Trisha woke to the gentle tickle and sniff of Suzie's soft muzzle. The animal stood over them, eyes clear, ears erect and munching a mouthful of hay. By the AM rounds at 5:30, Suzie could *almost* qualify as BAR — she'd clearly begun to improve.

CHAPTER THIRTY FIVE

Violet's Choice

6:40 AM — WEDNESDAY, DECEMBER 21, 1988

The Peaceable Kingdom's large animal surgical suite behind the dolphinarium

"Yes, that's absolutely correct." Dr. Violet Marie Green closed her eyes momentarily as she nodded with the phone to her ear. She and Stan had had a long night moving susceptible animals into isolation. "That's right, the whole rainforest exhibit is closed to the public." She nodded again, "Mmhmm, the aquarium and the dolphinarium too — all of our warm, indoor spaces where mosquitoes could potentially breed." She turned her head back and forth the way you sometimes do when you're not getting through to someone, "No, I'm sorry. They're closed until further notice." She listened without a word for nearly a minute and then replied, "We'll just have to refund their money. These are animals, not machines, they get sick. Good, please do communicate the situation to Davaris."

Violet clicked the receiver, ran her finger down the list and dialed the next number on the husbandry phone tree. She'd paged William last night twice and again this morning, but with no response, she moved on to the park's front line of curators. As she began to talk with the head of the aviary, the double doors to the surgical suite flew open with a *BANG*, cracking one of the glass viewing panes. Completely ignoring Stan who stood at the surgery table, William Digby stormed to within a foot of Violet's face. He bore into Violet's eyes with an intensity that was upending and before she could fully explain the species predilection of West Nile Virus for the birds under the curator's care, William reached up, yanked the phone from her hand and slammed it down on the receiver.

"Vi, what the hell are you playing at?" He slapped a thick file folder down on a surgical instrument tray, noticing that the shiny scalpel handles reflected his image like series of tiny mirrors. "You pulled the scarlet ibis, toucan and three-toed sloth off exhibit from the rainforest?" He seethed, "And you shut down our dolphin facilities?"

William's anger stunned Violet but before she could respond Stan broke in. He waved both hands above his head as if he were trying to distract a marauding bear from his favorite classmate. "Lookie, over here, this is what we're playing at." William broke his glare. "Violet figured out the transmission vector which led us to the etiological agent!" Stan the Path Man proceeded to tell William that the virus was likely imported into the States either in the body of an ill animal or as a blood meal inside the belly of an Asian tiger mosquito. He pulled open a manila file folder and spread color-enhanced electron photomicrographs, one after another, across the gleaming surgical table. The brilliant operating lights made the little polyhedrons, stacked like cordwood, almost jump off the page. He then went on to explain the most salient part: when you looked at the geographic distribution of the cases — he'd updated the numbers and his map — and triangulated, the Peaceable Kingdom was at the epicenter of the outbreak.

"And," Stan looked William dead in the eye, "*You* hit the nail on the head when you astutely noticed the decline of cases in the fall — it's the hallmark of this kind of transmission. It's almost..." he hesitated only because he loved to use the word and he let the anticipation build in the back of his throat, "pathognomonic! Even though there were still plenty of susceptible birds and mammals around, as it got colder the local mosquito population died off and the number of new cases plummeted." His eyes got wide again and, though he didn't for one second forget he was in the presence of a menacing bully, he stammered on with full-bore excitement, "It would have taken us months to isolate the virus from the dead corvid and equid cases but the insects on your pest strips were like concentrated packets of disease — it was all right there," he pointed up to the yellowing coil next to the security camera above. "SO incredibly cool!"

Stan the Path Man had been floating around in the sequestrum of veterinary pathology for so long that he'd been almost entirely insulated from the perverse forces of the outside world. But in this moment, something happened that brought Dr. Stan Oblitzski tumbling back to Earth from his ever-exuberant orbit. William Digby reached out, slid the photographs together in a pile and crushing them between his meaty paws, snarled, "I've tolerated your little wormy face for long enough, mate."

Violet Marie Green clicked the dial on her radio to select the park's secure, internal channel and hailed for help. She called out to the park's owner, "Doctor Green to Davaris." With no response she clicked the button and tried again, "Mr. Davaris, we have a situation."

The radio hissed to life in her hand, "Ah, Doctor Green, yes, from what I hear, we do indeed have a situation."

William came back around to his original stance; he stood squarely in front of Violet Marie Green and once again ignored Stan. Violet continued her transmission without breaking visual contact with the tower in front of her, "Mr. Davaris, we have a zoonotic on our hands here and it's quite possible that it began at the Peaceable Kingdom with an infected carrier. We need to take all reasonable precautions — quarantine susceptible species, eradicate potential vectors, and officially report our findings to the CDC. William seems to be opposed..."

Davaris cut her off, "Doctor Green, please get William *on the line*, as it were."

William unclipped the walkie talkie from his belt, brought the device to his mouth and gave it a squeeze. Violet could hear the metal housing creak, "Go ahead, Guv, Digby here."

"William, I need to spin the PR from this unfortunate situation. Could you take over where you are and remind Doctor Green of the confidentiality agreement she signed when she became the Chief Veterinary Officer at the world's largest zoological park? All information about our animals is, of course, proprietary. Report back when you have this mess cleaned up." The walkie talkie clicked twice and went silent.

A smirk crawled across William's thick facade, "He says you pledged your allegiance to us. If you report this, you'll be out on your lovely ass, all on your own."

Violet didn't hesitate for an instant, "I don't care if I'm out. I know what independence means. My allegiance is to my profession and my patients — I took that oath when I graduated."

William's smirk turned into a full-blown smile and with it he appeared both ominous and satisfied. "But luv, who's gonna believe a vet that was fired for transferring her own captive-bred animals to a hunting park? *Hmmm?*" He pulled a stack of papers from the folder he'd carried in. They were animal health certificates. "Come on now, don't be a daft sheila. Do you really want to give up your position," he stretched out both massive limbs like a beefy ballerina, "and this incredible opportunity for a hunch?"

"A scientifically confirmed hunch. I ran the statistics with the school's SAS software on the mainframe and with a P-value of < 0.05, well, I'll tell you that means we're more than 95% certain." Stan nodded his head.

"Sorry that, a hunch scientifically confirmed by a *pimply runt*."

Dr. Violet Marie Green had never been a talkative, effusive or demonstrative person. She wasn't one to wax poetic or debate vociferously, even on topics of much import. But, at this instant, she went entirely mute. She rifled through what must have been more than a hundred 'veterinary health certificates,' each with her forged signature. She felt bile, outrage and heartbreak welling up as she remembered the individual animals represented by each sheet — the gemsbok, the scimitar horned oryx, a dama gazelle, that pair of kudu twins...

And then she came to the lion cub, Mya. The very same lion that she'd hand-raised against all odds. She couldn't reconcile the image in her head of this beautiful animal life in cross hairs or mounted on a wall somewhere, but then William did something extraordinary, he shook Violet Marie Green to her core. William Digby, the trophy hunter from Down Under, opened his wallet to reveal the only picture it contained — one of Mya prostrate on the hood of a Range Rover and William posing with his gun.

Violet slowly lifted her head, looked up at the glistening brawn that was William Digby and whispered, "You're a monster. I can't believe I almost let you..."

Since William thought he'd recaptured control, his composure returned in spades. He stood like an Adonis ablaze in the shaft of dawning sunlight that streamed through cathedral windows from above. William Digby thought he knew a lot of things. Like the other species in his charge, he thought he knew women. But, when you're an egotistical swine who's easily distracted by your own reflection you tend to miss things.

William sneered and replied, "Don't flatter yourself luv, if I wanted, I would have just taken you."

As Violet began to subconsciously calculate the distance between the heel of her right palm and the point where she'd drive it into William's nose, from out of nowhere came something to which William Digby should have paid more attention. Dr. Stanley Leonard Oblitzski, an unapologetic veterinary medical nerd and proud Front Row Geek, roared, "YOU SON OF A BITCH!" as his arcing roundhouse terminated by a clinched fist caught the strongman in the jaw. The punch, Stan the Path

Man's very first, was perfectly timed and released. The force corkscrewed the golden column nearly 360 degrees clockwise, dropping the Aussie like a side of rejected beef into a dumpster. Apparently, hauling hundred-pound slabs of meat around the path lab had fortified Stan with something more than knowledge.

Violet Marie Green was, for the second time this day, stunned, but she collected herself and knelt to confirm William's strong pulse. As she felt the rebound of his carotid, she cocked her head and looked up to see her former classmate in a new light. She blinked twice and asked, "Above all, do no harm?"

Stan grinned and rocked his head from side to side, "Yeah, well, oopsie…" and then continued as he shook out his stinging right hand, "But, wasn't it totally cool how his mandible took the impact? I caught him almost exactly on the left mental foramen and then the momentum spiraled down the vertebral column with the centrifugal force causing his arms to spin outward. And now, look at that swelling and hyperemic response!" He began to reach down toward the redness and then noticed the impression left by his heavy signet ring. He depressed the spot marked by the reverse "**P**," it blanched and quickly rebounded. "CRT under 2 seconds, so cool." Stan the Path Man paused and then added with a goofy grin, "Never underestimate Path-Power…"

Stan and Violet scooped up their charts, photos and path reports and exited the suite just as the baby dolphin, Percival the Sea Prince, swam up the med channel behind the crumpled mass of Mount Digby to revive him with a playful squirt.

CHAPTER THIRTY SIX

Jack and Anna

Jack's family home in west Philly and Dr. Vandergrift's
laboratory in the old veterinary school building, Philadelphia

Jack Doyle was confused. And when Jack was confused there was only one place for him to go — the paved courtyard behind his childhood home.

This space was where he spent his youth. This was where he cared for all those animals his parents' friends and neighbors had delivered. Like other Philly row homes, stony wells and shafts penetrated the compressed structures, providing a little light and air to the backsides of the dwellings. With the help of his eternally gruff and stoic father, he'd constructed the dozens of chicken wire cages, wooden hutches and runs that still crammed the tiny bricked quad behind their home.

Jack stood in the frigid space with his hands buried deep in the pockets of his heavy winter coat. This time of day, at this time of year, it was dark — only a single dim spot illuminated the snow piled two-feet deep on the now empty cages. He'd shut down the operation when he released his last patient, a sweet little saw-whet owl, the day he joined the force. Though Jack never really connected the dots, this whole adventure — little Jack Doyle's wildlife ward — was part of his father's plan. A plan to keep his youngest son distracted from feelings of loss and unwarranted responsibility for the drowning of his baby sister.

Tonight Jack was so distracted that he couldn't really see the once bustling animal cages or feel the cold. He just kept turning one problem over and over — Anna Heywood.

In his mind, and probably in reality, Anna was conflict personified. Jack had been drawn to Anna from the moment they met. Some times she seemed to care for him, but then, when push came to shove, she usually did both. Regardless, for some reason, he felt a need to protect her, to save her. And though his father's remedy had worked for years, keeping him distracted, keeping him from thinking and feeling deeply, the treatment had begun to lose effect. Staying in the shallow end of life was indeed safer than going deep, but then Anna Heywood surfaced. His heart drew him to her. And his heart told him she wasn't involved with the break-in at school even though the evidence said otherwise. In the literal shadow of the family home where right and wrong were as clear as the written law his father and brother enforced, Jack Doyle didn't know what to do.

As Jack turned to leave, he heard a flutter from within one of the snow-covered enclosures. It was that little owl. She'd returned and huddled in the corner of her old cage. She was in rough shape, nearly comatose and frail. Jack scooped up the tiny bird, nested it in an inside pocket of his thick warm coat and headed back to the vet school.

◄ • ►

Anna Heywood sat surrounded by mess. It had only been five days since the ALM break-in and Dr. Vandergrift's lab was still in ruin. Since yesterday, when the police removed the crime-scene tape, she had been doing what she could to regain order from the chaos the protestors had created. Though Rick Larson, their nearly useless work/study student, had swept up the shards of shattered computer screens and beakers, paper files were still scattered on the floor. What the group hadn't destroyed, they stole — taking records, computer hard drives and, of course, the animals. Anna shook her head slowly in disbelief as she took in the words "Animal Liberty Militia" scrawled in blood-red spray paint on the wall in front of her. Although she understood the ALM's rage at animal experimentation, because she felt it herself, this wasn't part of the bargain.

Anna was at a place in her life where she'd never been. She was nearly defeated. It had taken all of her declining strength to confront her convictions on animal welfare to work in this lab in the first place. Her decision was both selfish and selfless. Though she couldn't know if her work would ever help find a cure, she felt certain it would come too late for her.

As Anna thought back on the thousands of animal lives sacrificed to generate the years of data now lost, she felt sick. What was the point of it all, what was the point of going on? She knew her prognosis, she understood the sentence of gradual, inexorable decline that her disease imposed. She'd read the texts and medical journals, she knew what lay ahead for her. Isolation and imprisonment within her own body. Absolute loneliness. It was at this moment that Anna thought nothing could ever change the course of her life. Anna was wrong.

CHAPTER THIRTY SEVEN

Letting Go

AM treatments in the Wildlife Ward, in the corner of the old vet school quad, Philadelphia

Most mornings, the treatment rounds in the pigeon ward were quiet, subdued affairs. It was early, people were tired. But today, nearing the end of hell week and on the eve of the final anatomy exam, the mood in the ward was more solemn than a tomb. Repeated cycles of cramming until 3:00 AM, followed by testing, more testing and cramming, rendered the first years nearly incapable of full sentences. This morning, with grunts and pointing, the students worked on autopilot.

Despite Jack's wild animal experience and innate leadership skills, Anna had morphed into the de facto crew leader for their little group. And though today she was even less vocal than usual, she seemed able to get her point across without ambiguity. "JJ, mice." This meant that JJ was assigned to the container of three white laboratory mice returned to the school after the ALM break in. The animals weren't ill, so JJ had only to change their bedding, give them fresh food and water, and check off their record. But before he could accomplish this 10-minute task, Simon JJ Harding III began to squeal, "Stop, *stop*. Awww, come on, please, stop squirming… *Ouwwwww-ouch*! Mickey's got me!" JJ held his hand up, exactly as FRoGs are known to do, but this time a white ball of fur was clamped to his index finger.

Sam raised the bill of his greasy ball cap with the back of his hand to get a better view, "Chill, dude, it's just an iddy-biddy mouse, not a tigah shahk. Put your hand in the cage and let his feet touch the ground, he'll let go."

It was a surprise to everyone that JJ had joined Wildlife — mostly, it was a surprise to JJ. He'd had a long talk with that local practitioner at the SCAVA clinic and, though it was counterintuitive to him, JJ began to wonder if giving back, even just a little, might not be part of a veterinary life. Besides, he thought, how much could it hurt? Now he knew. And though the addition of JJ to the early morning crew was indeed a surprise, no one could have imagined what happened next.

As JJ was returning the clean cage of mice to the rack with a heat lamp, the 2/3 height door to the ward blew open. It swung wide and an icy blast filled the tiny space. Sam groaned, "JJ, you forgot to latch it again." But it wasn't JJ's fault this time. Rick Larson poked his head in.

"Sorry."

"You're late," snapped Anna.

"Yeah, well, traffic was God awful and…"

"Bullshit, you live at Alpha Mu, that's three blocks from here," she cocked her head and then continued, "Just close the damn door and give me a hand with this pigeon. Grab that tube of gentamicin and coat the lesion."

To his credit, Rick kept his mouth closed for at least the next five minutes. He dabbed antibiotic ointment in wounds, scribbled in medical records and puttered around, generally making himself look busy. But when the AM chores were not concluded, as he assumed they would be, by the time of his tardy arrival, he made his first significant mistake of this day. He whined, "Look, I really should be studying, this is ridiculous, how are we going to pass a cumulative anatomy final if we're in here packin' pigeons all day?"

No one looked up except Anna, "Rick, this was the deal, you are allowed to study with us this week — with your mouth shut — if you contribute to AM treatments." She stretched out her right arm which tapered to a point, "That sink full of dirty food bowls has your name on it."

Rick slunk over to the grubby porcelain janitor's sink, stopped up the drain and turned on the water. He pantomimed ticking a lock, so Anna began the final check of the tinbacks to make sure they'd not missed any treatments. With heads bowed the crew mutely plowed toward the end of their chores so no one noticed when Rick Larson wandered away from his work. No one noticed the beginning of his second, even bigger mistake of this day. No one noticed, that is, until he squawked, "We've got one more and we're outta here — a little help?" Anna turned, ready to admonish Rick, and gasped. The sound startled Sam, Kerri and JJ. Jack lifted his gaze from the little saw-whet owl he was treating and froze. He whispered between fixed lips, "Rick, do not move… do—not—move!"

Even though the kennel had been clearly marked in bold letters and skulls and cross bones… even though the cage door had been locked… Rick had ignored it all. Whether in defiance of his menial dishwashing assignment or in haste to finish treatments or just stupidity, Rick decided to "treat" the newest patient in the Wildlife Ward: an adult male great blue heron transferred in from a southern rehabber. Even though the record instructed, again in bold lettering, **"Only when accompanied by a clinician, wear proper gear when handling this patient,"** the long, thick welder's gloves and wraparound shop goggles lay, unused, on top of the bird's cage. Rick stood in the center of the room grasping the football-sized middle of the animal's body while its snake-like neck swayed from side to side directly in front of his face. The only thing that was saving Rick was the total shock of the animal — it had never been handled like this and was distracted by the other humans who ringed the ward.

With clenched teeth, Jack directed, "Hoss, you move s-l-o-w-l-y around to the right to keep his attention diverted. I'll approach from the left and, when he's focused on you, I'll restrain the head with a towel… Rick, if you move, even an inch, he'll spear you."

Hoss did exactly as he was told. With arms extended and palms facing forward like he was moving in to hug his mom, Hoss advanced slowly to within the bird's striking distance and then whispered, "On the count of three…"

But before the countdown could begin, Rick — of course — moved. He shifted his stance which instantly aligned the bird's attention. The animal's dagger-shaped head whipped around and locked onto Rick's beady eyes. With the four-inch-long, needle-sharp beak pointed directly at his classmate's face, Jack blurted, "Three!" and looped a heavy towel over the living spike just as the bird drew back to strike. The cloth settled over the flailing bird and in the struggle that ensued, Rick got a grip on what he assumed was the bird's neck. "Got him! It's all cool, I got him."

In the moments of stillness that followed, the little group breathed a collective sigh and then, with a newfound and entirely unwarranted level of confidence, Rick directed the next step of the process. He commanded, "Jack, stabilize the body," and for some reason, perhaps it was the fatigue, Jack followed the order. This was unfortunate because, without thinking, which was primarily how Rick operated, he peeled back the towel to discover that he'd only had a grip on Hoss's wrist. With the towel lying at their feet, the bird's head was completely liberated and by now he was fighting for his life. In a flash, Rick let go and jumped backward in retreat. As he fell into a line of cages, the massive great blue heron turned on the one left holding the bag. With two lightning strikes, the terrified bird stabbed at Jack's eyes. The report of beak on bone made a sickening sound like the thump of a blade into a melon. As the animal reared back for a third, and perhaps fatal attack, Hoss snared the animal's neck between his thumb and forefinger.

Anna, with an agility never before witnessed by her classmates, swooped in with clean gauze to cover Jack's wounds. She cradled the back of his head with one hand and applied pressure with the other. Still holding the bird's body tightly to his chest, Jack acknowledged to Anna, "Pretty stupid, huh?"

Anna replied warmly, "Yeah, you always have to be a Superman, don't you?" As she held Jack close, a peaceful feeling came over her. But this feeling wasn't long-lived because in the next moment Rick clambered back upright, extracting himself from the pile of creaking, wrecked cages. Anna tore her attention from Jack and, glaring with a force only she could produce, she skewered Rick, "YOU DON'T BELONG HERE!" The power of her words physically bowled Rick over. He tripped backward and landed with a crash back in the mess he'd created.

As Sam, JJ and the others finished treatments and closed up the ward, Hoss and Anna led Jack through the old vet school courtyard and over to the VHUP emergency room. As luck would have it, Dr. Florence Kimball was on duty. While they waited for the ambulance, she quickly cleaned and expertly evaluated Jack's wounds. She announced, with much relief, that both globes were intact.

CHAPTER THIRTY EIGHT

The Kiss

11:20 PM — THURSDAY, DECEMBER 22, 1988

Room A1 in the old veterinary school building, Philadelphia

Since the moment of the heron incident, Anna had only left Jack's side twice. She rode with him in the ambulance and then grilled his doctors (Jack would have two black eyes, but miraculously only the left eyeball had been grazed by the beak's serrated edge). The doctors at HUP assured Anna (and Jack) that he'd be able to replace the full bandage wrap, which completely blocked his vision, with a less bulky version in about 24 hrs. This way, he could take the anatomy final on time.

Anna organized his treatment orders, picked up his meds (azithromycin to cover the most likely avian bacteria and prednisolone to check the swelling), and retrieved their lunch from the food truck in front of the Rosenthal building. She changed his bandages twice and schooled Jack in the basic operation of Clancy. Anna noticed that Clancy's tail swooshed a little higher than just the day before — this new found responsibility seemed to restore the golden retriever's laughing face.

Jack was lucky. Not only because he'd have his sight restored, but because of some kindly accommodation with the biochemistry final planned for that afternoon. Though modern college students are granted a make-up exam for so much as a botched pedicure, in vet school in the late 1980s, if you had a pulse, you took the test as scheduled. Since Jack most definitely had a pulse, a semi-retired and universally beloved biochem professor, Dr. Delluva, sat Jack in her office, read the test questions and wrote out his replies. This was the first time that Anna left Jack's side this day.

◄ • ►

The entire group (Hoss, Kerri, Sam, JJ, Anna and Jack) studied together from late afternoon — after the biochem final and through the quick spaghetti and meatball dinner Hoss whipped up in the Alpha Mu kitchen — and into the early evening. That is, the entire group minus Rick Larson. Rick wasn't actively shunned, he just disappeared and though everyone noticed his absence, no one brought it up.

Another occurrence observed and overlooked by most, was Anna's proximity to Jack. Kerri Feinburg, an accomplished student of human behavior, was an astute observer of male/female interaction and she'd been monitoring Anna's progression throughout the day. She watched as the spiral of Anna's orbit around Jack tightened. It appeared to Kerri that, from the instant Anna cradled Jack's head in the Wildlife Ward, she'd maintained almost continuous physical contact with this guy that she seemed to abhor just the day before. Whether guiding him with Clancy or gently replacing his soiled bandages, the cleft — that previously rigid gap between them — was gone. Kerri didn't pry, she didn't need to. If there was one thing she knew besides fashion, it was attraction. But this realization triggered a cascade of events that led to Anna's second separation from Jack that day.

At about 7:00 PM Anna was extracted from her adherent position at Jack's side. Sam took over nursing and tutorial duties when Kerri coaxed Anna up to her room on the third floor of the frat. Kerri's pretense for the excursion was a "study break," but when she got Anna up the stairs and had her positioned facing away from a mirror, she simply said, "Close your eyes" and surprisingly, Anna did. Kerri brushed out Anna's silky black hair and then applied a thin foundation. Within minutes, the long lashes that had always been there became visible. The brow that was so often furrowed, relaxed. Thick, curvaceous lips emerged with almost no effort, and when she finally spun Anna around, Kerri was tickled to see real-live dimples flank a voluptuous smile. Anna's soft brown eyes radiated a brilliance and, starring back at her friend, it spoke volumes without a word. A transformation, no matter how transient it might be, had occurred in that room. The change, though seemingly superficial, was anything but, and it wasn't for Jack. This was for Anna.

When the two women returned downstairs, Hoss lifted his nose from deep within a pile of books and let out a low whistle in conjunction with a wide-eyed, "Whoa…" Kerri, following behind Anna, stopped him and the others with an upheld palm, this was a delicate moment. Anna smiled demurely and then silently gave Hoss a sweet hug.

The group packed up their books, notes and old tests, and headed back to the school's Anatomy Lab where over the ensuing hours they splintered into smaller and smaller aggregates. Ultimately, Hoss and Sam stayed in the lab, hunting and pecking their way through the animal parts dangling from meat hooks that Big Moe had left out for the purpose. Kerri returned to her room at Alpha Mu while JJ, with an unexpected wink and nod to Sam, befriended two female FRoGs and relocated to Room 13 to run old tests. And, since Jack was visually impaired and wasn't getting a lot out of lab, he and Anna excused themselves, ending up at the table on the cobbles, center stage in Room A1.

◄ • ►

Room A1 was a coveted place to study. It was coveted most by Anna. From that very first day of orientation she felt a presence in this space. A thrilling, supportive hum. Though difficult to put into words, she sensed a continuity and connection going back through the decades. It didn't take a grand imagination to realize that every student who braved these halls, at some point, crossed the exact spot where she and Jack sat this evening. The challenges they all faced were inextricably personal and professional. On these hard stones, men and women opened massive beasts with shining blades, they diagnosed compound fractures and assimilated mountains about worms and flies and biochemical pathways, and they listened to thudding hearts. Whatever the call that originally drew them, their lives going forward would forever be linked by the excitement, fear and reward of healing animal life. Though Anna didn't say it aloud, she felt the pulse of that life most strongly here in this aged amphitheater.

Tonight, Anna Heywood sat directly across from John Fitzgerald Doyle. She'd positioned their chairs with the small table between them (the fear of rejection is as tenacious as they come). The only light in the auditorium streamed down from the massive chandelier with the crystal facets spreading faint star points across every surface. The seats the class had occupied during orientation, rose into the darkened vault while the two dogs, Clancy and Petunia, lay curled up and snoring at their feet. The two worked through the limb muscles of the cow, sow, horse, cat and dog — origin, insertion and action. Arteries, veins and nerves.

As the hours passed, Anna surprised Jack in a couple enjoyable ways. He wasn't surprised that she'd committed every muscle, vessel and nerve to memory (and there were hundreds of them). And he had expected her to know every answer on tests going back ten years or more. What did catch him off guard was when she made him laugh. First, there was her cartoonish description of Rick Larson, skulking around the Philly Zoo randomly releasing the lions, crocs and zebra because he'd been asked to wash dishes at Alpha Mu. Then, in reference to the bandage encircling Jack's head, she delivered a string of retorts such as, "*Ahh, the mummy speaks,*" and, "*This ain't 1776 and you ain't got a fife.*" But, when they got to the reproductive system of the common bitch, Anna nearly laid him out with the line, "How about we leave Doctor SuperCurve out of this?" Her timing could hardly have been better because Jack had just raised a can of Coke to his mouth. The less-than-subtle zinger caused Jack, in mid gulp, to spew bubbling soda from his nose. At any other time this would have been a crude and funny occurrence, but with his current injuries, it was crude, funny *and* painful.

Anna's second surprise for Jack was more of a gift. It was her laugh. Jack couldn't remember hearing it before. It was soft and sweet and intimate. It was, in a word, intoxicating. So, in this way, going system by system, Anna quizzing Jack and laughing at each other's jokes, they made their way forward through the night. From muscular to skeletal, digestive to urinary, respiratory to reproductive to endocrine, they made their way to the system usually taught last — the nervous system.

As per convention, they began on the input side, exploring the afferent components of sensation. Anna described a diagram called the "homunculus brain" for Jack. It came from one of the texts she lugged around. Even though the extra mass was almost crippling, Jack noted she always carried human medical books along with their required vet school materials. He chalked it up to her research in Vandergrift's lab, but still, he always wondered if there wasn't another reason. The famous schematic of the homunculus brain that Anna described portrays the relative amount of sensory cortex devoted to specific regions of the body. Out from the curving gyres bulged oversized images of hands, fingertips, face, lips and genitals. Though Jack couldn't know it, Anna blushed when she described that the lips, tongue and cheek were so well endowed that, per square inch, they made the retina seem almost redundant. This thought tipped the scales and triggered something deep within Jack. He leaned forward so his face was only inches from hers as she read from the text.

Anna looked up to discover that nothing more than silence lay between them and even that evaporated when finally Jack uttered, "You rescued me today." He paused and then continued softly, "Why do you keep so many things hidden?" And though he didn't say it by name, they both knew he was talking about her condition when he whispered, "Is it getting worse? Is there anything I can do to help?"

If Anna weren't already there, this foray into the darkest, most private part of her life would have certainly brought her to the edge of tears. The clash between hope (which she barely let herself feel) and fear (which was ever-present) left her paralyzed. She tried but couldn't respond to the strong, gentle man before her. She just stared in total silence at Jack and his bandaged eyes. She knew deep within her beautiful, four-chambered mammalian heart that this man was the One for her — but how could she tell him that this was impossible?

Maybe it was fatigue, maybe it was justifiable impatience, or maybe it was just inevitability, but Jack Doyle held back no longer. He reached out with his right hand and found the soft curve of Anna's cheek. His touch guided his lips and they met hers. The kiss that ensued was deep and soft and so filled with tenderness that Anna dropped her final guard and let thousands of receptors, the same ones they'd been studying for months, launch wave after wave of desire straight to her heart. She completely forgot that Jack had not asked permission and she forgot how terrified she truly was. The only thought that came to her was: *I want to live.*

In Jack's mind, this kiss — the best one he never imagined — could have gone on forever. Though, or perhaps *because* his eyes were bandaged, Jack could visualize the whole, complicated, subtly gorgeous face and life he held in his hands. He could see the strength he admired, the softness he craved, and also the fear he wanted to quell. Mostly, he could see his life with hers.

But only moments after this tidal wave surge had been sparked, two forces pried Jack and Anna apart.

The first and most formidable came from Jack himself. Because of his misguided sense of "right," "wrong" and Anna's presumed role in the ALM attack, Jack recoiled. Breaking the spell, he blurted, "I can't..." *What would his father say? His brother? How honorable were his actions knowing that laws had been broken and people hurt?*

The second wedge occurred before Anna could respond. The heavy wooden doors of A1 creaked as Mike London entered the hall. Mike shuffled, head down, with his pager held out in front of him. He made his way up to the last row, slumped in one of the rigid wooden seats and stared at the numbers as if that could make them disappear. Even with only the dim light all the way in the back, Anna noticed his scrubs. They had been, no doubt, clean when he put them on, but now were absolutely covered with the remnants of his day — animal hair, blood stains and spills. As Mike began to speak, Jack turned to face the voice but could only hear the sadness in Mike's eyes. "Anna, Jack — I know she was important to you both… Mrs. Oliver is gone."

Bewildered and not knowing what to do, Jack and Anna took turns quietly hugging and petting Clancy (and Petunia, of course). After a lengthy period of total silence they packed up their books and prepared to leave. But just before they ventured out from this sanctuary into the dark December night, Anna stopped and looked to Mike and then settled her gaze on Jack when she said, "She's with her True Love."

CHAPTER THIRTY NINE

Tradition

5:35 PM — FRIDAY, DECEMBER 23, 1988

Room A1 and the quad bounded by the old vet school building, Philadelphia

Tradition is a human necessity — it connects, grounds and secures us.

First-year skits are tradition. A bawdy circus of tradition that began in 1894 with an all-male musical review of "Grimm's Veterinary Tales." Such scholastic rituals serve as tonic, release and bookend. Wrongs can be righted, truths revealed. And if they're done right, they can make you split a gut in the process. Tonight, in the final hours of their first semester, the Class of 1992 crossed a threshold. After months of right brain trials and industry, they entertained their peers with a long-overdue left brain romp. A sanctioned venue for professorial critique in memory of numbing lectures and crushing exams, skits can also be gelastic, bombastic retaliation served cold. The University of Philadelphia, School of Veterinary Medicine's skits night is Saturday Night Live, just with more goats.

Few students, staff or clinicians missed skits. Large animal interns and residents carpooled in from the country and a VHUP relay team handled small animal chores so nobody missed too much. Recent grads within a 30-mile radius, if they could finagle the night off, made the pilgrimage. And the first years turned out in force, of course. Even the most socially stunted FRoG made an appearance.

But winter comes to Philly just like elsewhere in the Northeast. The temperature drops and normal humans head indoors. However, humans of the animal persuasion tend to ignore deterrents like sleet, snow and frostbite, especially when there's a raucous party to be had. As the winter sun on this shortest of days faded below the rim of the quad, a dozen SCAVA reps and a delegation from Alpha Mu descended on Room A1 and the old veterinary school courtyard. Directed by Sam, Kerri and Hoss, the worker bees transformed the venerable lecture hall into an olde-tyme theater. Programs were printed. A deep purple curtain was strung. Candles flickered from the massive chandelier, casting hundreds of dancing stars to mingle with the ancient constellations that adorned the domed "sky" above. Outside, in the quad courtyard, club booths hocking barbecue, mulled wine and beer sprouted and lined the walled space. And with nighttime temps hovering near zero, the second years took the initiative to flood the center, curbed island creating a serviceable skating pond. All that was needed was a bonfire and that would be lit after skits wound down. In fact, with the wrought-iron gates secured, a mixed-mongrel pack romping and the band fired up, a throbbing, soothing, playfully irreverent oasis emerged from within the dark, cold city night.

◄ • ►

Tonight, high up in the nosebleed section of Room A1 sat a cluster of vet students, two fourth years and some of their advisees. Mike London in jade surgical scrubs and a white lab coat had his tired stethoscope draped around his neck and a pair of hemostats clamped to his lapel. His 6 o'clock shadow had metamorphosed into a scruffy, nearly-full beard. He sipped from a plastic cup and surveyed the scene below while his closest friend, Trisha Maxwell, who sat next to him, giggled like a schoolgirl. Mike watched with a deepening grin as the first years scurried last minute, confirmed their marks and ran scripts. His grin turned to pearly satisfaction when Trisha extended her left arm to display a promise and new life. She held out her hand so that, from their vantage point, the tiny but brilliant gem on her ring finger lined up with the twinkling eye of Pegasus on the ceiling above.

Down front, Dr. Florence Kimball and Dr. Daniel Linnehan, the class's faculty mentors, kicked off the event. Flo Kimball, decked out in shimmering reds and greens and with two shiny Christmas balls dangling from her earlobes, triggered the microphone and tapped the grill trying to capture the boisterous crowd's attention. Seeing no effect, Drill Sergeant Dan boomed, sans amplification, "AAAAAH-TENNNN-SHONNN!" (which worked), and then, with an open hand bid his colleague to begin.

"First years, upperclassmen, faculty, staff and dear alumni, welcome to the end — the end of fall semester!" Applause erupted, bubbled and built. A human wave, begun by Sam and Hoss, swayed, crashed and reflected back and forth across the amphitheater until Flo Kimball concluded with a beaming, "You made it!"

Drill Sergeant Dan leaned into the mic though he didn't need it and interjected, "Just three and a half more years to go." This proclamation was followed by slightly less applause.

Flo Kimball's face morphed, "Although, we did lose a few good students," she paused to glance at Anna Heywood seated in the front row, "and one *not so good*, tonight is a celebration."

Jack Doyle, with one eye still bandaged, was precariously perched in a seat way up in A1's Death Row. He turned to his advisor, Mike London, and asked over the cheers, "What's she talking about?"

Mike shrugged and shook his head, "Damned if I know."

Back downstage, costumed in a long flowing robe and fake white beard, Sam Stone bowed deeply after receiving the microphone from Dr. Kimball. He turned to face the packed, standing-room-only crowd and announced in his best Obi-Wan Kenobi, "Ahhh, you will never find a more wretched hive of scum and villainy. My fellow scum and villains, let's get this show on the road!" On cue, the band launched into Star Wars *Cantina* and as Sam signaled, the spotlight dimmed and a slide projector hummed to life.

Sam continued, "For as long as there have been veterinary students and animals with more than one orifice — there has been..." he paused for a drumroll, "The Wrong Hole Award!"

He paused again but this time for the applause.

"Our first award winner came from behind and took a very wrong turn. This year's deserving winner is... Simon JJ Harding the Third!" Sam depressed the clicker and a slide appeared showing JJ up to his elbow in a Holstein repro tract. With a look of consternation and a grimace on his face, a stream of manure streamed out from the *correct* orifice only an inch away. "This is a shot of his fifth attempt, proving that JJ is at least precise if not accurate — get on down here you palpation machine you."

JJ jumped from his seat with his advisee group in a middle row. Agilely hopping down the aisle, he made his way onto the hallowed cobbles and waved both hands to the audience. Sam handed him the mic, "There are so many people, animals, *and holes to thank*, I hope I don't miss any." The crowd roared their appreciation for the ad lib attempt and Sam bestowed JJ with a "right hole" rectum wrist watch. JJ held it aloft to thundering applause, gave a huge smile and exited stage right.

"Since we're on the topic of rectums, let's consider Officer Jack Doyle!" The crowd guffawed at the innuendo. "Jack seems to have a predilection for GI tract products. If it pleases the court," Sam winked, "and I think it will, I'd like to present exhibit A." He advanced to the next slide, it showed Jack in the recent palpation lab with manure splattered across his face. "And Exhibit B." This announcement triggered the projection of video shot at the Alpha Mu Halloween party. The clip began with the aerial fly-by fecal bombing run and ended with a close-up of Jack licking a gooey white glob from his finger and then spitting in disgust. "This year's recipient of the 'Shit-Eating Grin Award' goes to none other than our Class President, Jack Doyle!" The throng applauded wildly as Jack waved in acceptance of the honor from his seat on Death Row.

Sam segued to the next award, "Now, it's happened to all of us, *you know*, saying the wrong thing at the wrong time," he looked around at the nodding heads. "But the recipient of the 1988 'Foot 'n Mouth Award,' has really raised the bar. I swear he might be able to fit his whole leg down his gullet. You all know him, you've all been offended by him at one time or another — will Mr. Rick Larson *COME ON DOWN...*" The mass burst into applause and the spotlight swept the crowd but after a prolonged goad of *Foot—Mouth—Foot—Mouth—Foot—Mouth*, it was clear that the honoree was absent. Sam quipped with raised eyebrows, "Well alrightie then. I'll just keep that one for myself — probably need it before the night's over."

"In all seriousness, folks," he made a quick transition, "we do have a real honor to bestow tonight. In between cramming for tests, spay/neuter surgeries and Alpha Mu parties, you may have noticed an article or ten about one of the school's very own." The crowd murmured, nodded and then clapped lightly. "She made headlines in the *Washington Post*, the *New York Times* and here's one from the *Philadelphia Inquirer*." Sam clicked the controller for the next slide for the photo of a newspaper headline that read, 'Former Zoo Veterinarian Solves Mysterious Disease Outbreak: CDC Applauds Effort.'

"Please join me in a warm round of applause for the inaugural recipient of the 'Violet Marie Green, Do the Right Thing Award!' ...Doctor Green!" The crowd took to their feet and expressed their admiration with chants of VI-O-LET—VI-O-LET—VI-O-LET, shrill whistles and a catcall or two. After several moments, when it became clear that a response was expected, Violet Green stood at her seat, waved to the crowd and modestly declined Sam's invitation to speak. In her stead, Dr. Stanley Leonard Oblitzski bounded to the stage.

"I want to say just one thing, Violet Marie Green is the best friend a FRoG could have! And the best role model any vet student could emulate." Then, with his trademark hyperbole and exuberance, Stan the Path Man proceeded to embellish his own impromptu skit. He acted out the whole medical mystery, beginning with the first equine cases, "Before Violet knew it was West Nile." Transforming his body, he pantomimed gait abnormalities as he staggered across the uneven cobbles then moved on to describe, in glorious detail, the gross and microscopic postmortem lesions. He acknowledged Jack's vital contribution when he'd alerted them to the affected raptors in the Wildlife Service. And, being a consummate teacher, the previously rambunctious crowd was held in complete and rapt attention until he culminated with the "insane confrontation" at the Peaceable Kingdom. However, since Dr. Stan Oblitzski was no grandstander, he omitted the impressive roundhouse that left William Digby in a lump and concluded the presentation with, "Violet Green solved this amazing case and though she gave up her job in the process, she most certainly *Did the Right Thing*!" He raised his cup, as did those all around, "To the Mission — to Doing the Right Thing!"

The crowd clapped heartily and when the applause finally waned, Jack Doyle, led by his new companion Clancy, made his way onto center stage. Stan relinquished the mic and Jack took over, "Tonight, folks, we have another special treat. The ABC television show, 20/20, has been poking around the University of Philadelphia for the last couple of months as they develop a new series." This elicited a round of applause. "And tonight, the show's producer," Jack opened his hand to a woman in the front row, "is conducting auditions to choose the cast." This triggered a larger round. "Those interested were instructed to create a two-minute, freestyle piece entitled, 'Why I'm so special...' for performance tonight." He paused and pointed to the lights and cameras, "The 20/20 film crew has graciously agreed to record the whole of tonight's event for us. So, without further ado," he scanned the mob, "who wants to go first?"

Whether due to superior breeding and intellect, rocket-fast reflexes or a premeditated plan, a dozen hands attached to the med students were first out of the box. Similar to Jack's Witless Sampler seating chart of Room 13, two cohorts of human medical students were clustered in the wings of A1; there were nearly 20 total in attendance. Jack eyed Sam and Hoss with a grin and then pointed to the first contestant, "Mr. John A. Cadaver."

Without hesitation the guy sauntered up, brashly covered the mic with one hand and leaned into Jack's ear, "Thanks, *looooser*." then rebounded with a Hollywood smile beamed at the "producer" and launched into a soliloquy about the specialness of his being, complete with a thorough discourse on his fourth generation family tree of distinguished medical practitioners. He concluded, sheepishly and for good reason, by reading a hand-penned note from his mother stating, "My Johnny is a special boy, I knew this to be true by at least his tenth birthday..." The audience laughed uproariously as Jack ushered Mr. Cadaver offstage and then proceeded, in rapid fire succession, to showcase half a dozen more med-student victims. They performed everything from a tap rendition of *You're a Grand ole Flag*, to Abbott and Costello's *Who's on First*, to one guy in surgical scrubs doing a *Mack the Knife* solo on a squeaky clarinet. With the procession complete, Jack reconvened the "talent" as a group on stage to allow the producer, with a well-aimed cap gun, to get the lot of them to, "Dance Varmints, Dance!" As the troupe tried to synchronize their feet to the band's downbeat, the vet students could hardly control their laughter. The whole ridiculous and ultimately hilarious display came off like a cross between a prep school talent contest and a Miss America pageant — which was exactly the goal.

With a wink from Jack, the producer rose to face the crowd and, being in show business, she projected her lines with absolute clarity, "I have to admit, in all my minutes of *posing* as an ABC producer, I've never seen such raw and unbridled specialness. In fact, instead of choosing our cast, I'd like to give out another award." She signaled the band and was rewarded with a tight drumroll, "The Mount Everest Award for reaching the pinnacle of gullibility goes to ALL the human med students here tonight!" Mr. Cadaver and his buddies on stage looked to one another — stricken and crestfallen, their smiles melted as the realization set in. Sam bounded forward with a plaque just as Jack pressed the clicker to reveal a slide with one word in bold capitals, "**GOTCHA!**" Jack cupped the mic and leaning into a stupefied Mr. Cadaver, whispered, "Take a bow, my friend." The group did so with grace and egg all over their face. The ovation, which started big, grew even stronger as the scope and scale of the practical joke boomeranged around the room. Jack Doyle and the Death Row Crew had orchestrated an elaborate ruse, with multiple flyers, classroom announcements and a mock film crew for the last three months. This was a gag that would go down in history.

From there, the revelers rode the high tide watermark of a successful prank and skits were performed with aplomb. A mock advertisement for the small animal laxative, Dodecasulfate, parodying the Dr. Pepper theme song, "I'm a Pooper, She's a Pooper, He's a Pooper — Wouldn't you like to be a Pooper, too?" was followed by a faux game show, "Vet Jeopardy," which featured two well-loved vet school professors getting trounced by a first-year FRoG because the only categories were "Questions" and "Kissing Up." But the skits-night players nearly brought down the house with their rendition of Joe Jackson's rendition of a tune called, *Five Guys Named Moe*. Five singers emerged wielding medieval dissection implements including hatchets, machetes and a chainsaw. They wore scrub tops with thick block lettering "MOE" scribbled in sharpie over their left breast pockets. The audience rolled in the aisles as the first-year Death Row cast plus JJ sang and danced their way to the chorus:

> High brow, low brow, all agree
> They're the best in harmony
> I'm telling you folks you just got to see
> Five guys named Moe
> There's Big Moe... (Hoss took a bow)
> Little Moe... (Kerri blew a kiss)
> Four-eyed Moe... (JJ took a bow)
> No Moe *and*... (Sam took his turn)
> Eat Moe... (and finally, Jack)

The routine ended with the five friends on bended knee in front of Big Moe Sutton. For the second time this evening, the crowd rose in standing ovation. Big Moe, clearly moved by the display, stood, turned and addressed the congregation.

"I just wanted to thank you little moes for all your cards and well wishes. As you can see, I'll be fine." He waited out the applause and then continued, "But, I do have some news. The cops just apprehended the guys that broke into the school, and it's thanks to one of your own, Confident Moe." Then Big Moe did something he'd never done before (or since), he used a student's full name, "Anna Heywood pointed the police in the right direction." The crowd was shocked but Big Moe was just getting going. "Although the higher ups probably wouldn't want me to say this just yet, it turns out that this was an inside job. One of the first years, I think his name was Rick, sold keys and security codes to the protestors." He shook his head, "It was just a business deal." The contrast between the current pin-drop silence and the raucous laughter from just seconds before could not have been greater. Big Moe continued, "But — and here's the interesting part — once the cops started digging they discovered that this guy was an impostor. He faked his way into our school. The crowd was astonished by the revelation, murmurs swarmed, ebbed and flowed until Big Moe wobbled over to Anna and held out his hand. At his gentle urging she stood and received the third and final ovation of the evening.

Hoss and Big Moe gave Anna hugs and then bid the massive collection of students, staff and faculty to be quiet so that Anna could speak. After almost 10 full seconds of complete silence, Anna stated simply but with eloquence, "All animals deserve humane treatment. I believe in what I thought the ALM stood for — but, there has to be a better way." And then, after what seemed would be a never-ending round of affirmation, the skits regained their momentum. Anna gathered up her things and Petunia and made her way out of A1. A moment later, Jack followed with Clancy.

In the gently falling Philadelphia snow, John Fitzgerald Doyle caught up with Anna Heywood just before she exited the quad.

"Anna, wait…"

She stopped, and turned to face Jack.

Jack Doyle opened himself up, "I was wrong."

"You'll have to be more specific than that, Superman. You're wrong a lot," she replied with a smile.

Jack laughed and bowed his head, "I was wrong last night, wrong in every way."

Jack and Anna (and Petunia and Clancy) stood there in the dark as a soft gentle peace settled around them. Jack imagined he could see tears in Anna's eyes as she leaned forward and gave him a kiss on the cheek. She said, "I'll see you after the break," and then looked down at her faithful companion, "Come on Petunia, let's get back to the lab."

Jack Doyle watched as Anna Heywood, the woman who held sway over him like no other, pushed her way through the set of heavy oak doors and was gone.

◄ • ►

Though never officially acknowledged in university handbooks, Room A1 was indeed the original and enduring heart of the veterinary school. And, on a night like tonight, it even served the function. People lined up and streamed in from one side, poured into the main chamber and then were pulsed by laughter and song out into the general courtyard circulation. When this class entered A1 back in September, they were farmers and lawyers, city girls, grad students, nurses, cops and comedians. They were excited and scared. They were strangers. But on that first day, a buoyant sunlit tide ebbed into the space. It nurtured hopes, supported dreams, and now, barely four months later, the tide began to turn. A glow poured from Al's stained-glass halo. The colored shafts of light radiated outward into the night, illuminating skaters and revelers making snow angels while packs of gently padding canines looped in wide arcs.

With the requisite number of infinitely re-livable tales — the kind of stories that begin with, *I almost died laughing when...* and end in, *It was absolutely Goddamned amazing!* — seared into the collective memory bank, the evening could progress as nature intended. The Class of 1992 skits night evolved as any good party should. The beer flowed smoothly until the kegs rolled. The music, which at first throbbed a rowdy beat, slowed and softened so couples could dance the way couples should. And finally, the bonfire was lit. It was within this rhythmic glow of living light, where rising embers mingled with the pulse of twinkling stars, that we began an animal life.

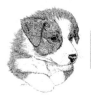

APPENDICES

Suggested Soundtrack

3 CD SET

The songs listed below represent the authors' personal (and professional) recommendations for music to accompany and enhance your reading experience. We are not offering this suggested soundtrack for sale (and it is not included with the electronic or print versions of this book). However, if you wish, you could create your own "mixed-tape" version by purchasing the individual tracks through various online sources.

DISC 1: AN ANIMAL LIFE: PART 1

Chapter 1: Dr. Green
Scene: Our opening "glimpse" of the helicopter racing over the vast Peaceable Kingdom savanna.
Song: "Wild Wild Life"
Written by: David Byrne
Performed by: Talking Heads
Album: True Stories, Sire Records, 1986
Volume: An invigorating 8

Chapter 2: Orientation
Scene: Room A1, the most hallowed hall at the University of Philadelphia's School of Veterinary Medicine. This is the real deal; the first years are gathered for the first day of their exciting new life (one they've worked towards for years).
Song: "Piano Parchment" (Opening Theme, "All Creatures Great and Small" UK series)
Written by: Johnny Pearson
Performed by: Johnny Pearson and his Orchestra
Album: All Creatures Great and Small (Original Soundtrack), Rampage Records, 1978
Volume: 5, since most of the students are nervous and half-listening

Chapter 3: The Advisors: Part I (Mike London)

Scene: Murphy's Tavern. Mike takes his first years under his wing and prepares them for the year(s) ahead.

Song: "Walk the Line"

Written by: Johnny Cash

Performed by: Johnny Cash

Album: With His Hot and Blue Guitar, Sun Records, 1956

Volume: 3, strictly background, as we don't want to compete with Mike's wise words

Chapter 4: The Advisors: Part II (Trisha Maxwell)

Scene: We open on the Kennett Square large animal facility and the western theme suggested by the opening words (and the characters) brings this to mind.

Song: Main theme from "The Good, The Bad, and The Ugly"

Written by: Ennio Morricone

Album: The Good, The Bad, and The Ugly Soundtrack, EMI America and Capitol Records, 1966

Volume: 5 and then fade

Chapter 6: That Smell

Scene: Anatomy Lab. Kerri teases the boys about their relaxed approach to the class.

Song: "(Sittin' on) The Dock of the Bay"

Written by: Steve Cropper, Otis Redding

Performed by: Otis Redding

Album: The Dock of the Bay, Volt/Atco, 1968

Volume: 4

Chapter 7: Mentoring 601

Scene: The students learn that "The Force" is in their hands.

Song: Star Wars, Main Theme

Written by: John Williams

Performed by: London Symphony Orchestra (John Williams, conductor)

Album: Star Wars Episode IV: A New Hope (soundtrack), 20th Century Records, 1977

Volume: 6, swelling

AND

Chapter 7: Mentoring 601
Scene: Trisha wonders aloud as Mike lectures on the power of True Love.
Song: "What's Love Go To Do With It?"
Written by: Terry Britten, Graham Lyle
Performed by: Tina Turner
Album: Private Dancer, Capitol Records, 1984
Volume: 7, while Mike draws. What does love have to do with it?

Chapter 8: Trust
Scene: Digby makes not-so-subtle advances while helping Violet collect semen
    from "Jam."
Song: "A Matter of Trust"
Written by: Billy Joel
Performed by: Billy Joel
Album: The Bridge, Columbia Records, 1986
Volume: 4

Chapter 9: Cramming
Scene: The first years are cramming for their first anatomy exam. Can you spell
    "P-R-E-S-S-U-R-E"?
Song: "Under Pressure"
Written by: Queen and David Bowie
Performed by: Queen and David Bowie
Album: Hot Space, EMI Records, 1982
Volume: A stressful 11!

Chapter 11: Testicle Festival
Scene: It's only been a week and a half, but it's already feeling like a lifetime of
    classes, rounds, and studying. This particular Friday Night Happy Hour at the
    Center for Large Animal Medicine couldn't have come any sooner... hey, pass
    me a beer, and don't give me any bull!
Song: "Big Ball's in Cowtown"
Written by: Hoyle Nix
Performed by: Hoyle Nix and His West Texas Cowboys
Album: Talent/Star Talent Records (No. 709), 1949
Volume: 9, toned down a bit so you can hear the calls for cow pie bingo

DISC 2: AN ANIMAL LIFE: PART II

Chapter 12: Mrs. Oliver

Scene: The first-years meet the amazing Mrs. Oliver who can "see" the students just by touch. During Clancy's eye exam, Jack is frustrated, realizing he is blind to the defects, while Anna sees them clearly.

Song: "I Still Haven't Found What I'm Looking For"

Written by: U2, Bono

Performed by: U2

Album: The Joshua Tree, Island Records, 1987

Volume: 2, Jack says he sees the cataracts, but if this song is played any louder, they'll know he's lying

Chapter 13: Dead Animal Medicine: Part I

Scene: The large animal necropsy room. Stan the Path Man does his imperson-ation of Tom Cruise in "Risky Business" while skidding across the floor.

Song: "Old Time Rock and Roll"

Written by: George Jackson, Thomas E. Jones III, Bob Seger

Performed by: Bob Seger and the Silver Bullet Band

Album: Stranger in Town, Capitol Records, 1978

Volume: 8, while Stan does a quick slide but then back down to 4

Chapter 14: Dead Animal Medicine: Part II

Scene: Trisha Maxwell rushes into the path lab with a last minute necropsy request for Stan; of course, Stan will do anything for Trisha, because she vali-dates his personal existence.

Song: "In Your Eyes"

Written by: Peter Gabriel

Performed by: Peter Gabriel and Youssou N'Dour

Album: So, Geffen Records, 1986

Volume: 1, so Trisha doesn't hear

Chapter 15: Life on the Edge

Scene: Dr. Kimball enthralls the class with her cardiac physiology lecture; Anna
　　helps Jack to find his heart (and vice versa).

Song: "I Can Feel Your Heart Beat"

Written by: Mike Appel, Jim Cretecos, Wes Farrell

Performed by: The Partridge Family

Album: The Partridge Family Album, Bell Records, 1970

Volume: 2, slowly rising to 8, then abruptly falling to 0

Chapter 16: 20/20 Vision

Scene: Sam relates the humorous details of his "cowgirl" fling to the class; Dou-
　　ble D drives him crazy!

Song: "Crazy Little Thing Called Love"

Written by: Freddie Mercury

Performed by: Queen

Album: The Game, Elektra Records, 1979

Volume: 2-6, depending upon whether or not the mic is working in Room 13

Chapter 18: Heil Vandergrift

Scene: As Dr. Vandergrift's "in-the-rough" neurophysiology lecture begins to lull
　　Jose to sleep, Death Row tees off for a game of HypnoGolf.

Song: "I'm Alright"

Written by: Kenny Loggins

Performed by: Kenny Loggins

Album: Caddyshack (soundtrack), (courtesy of Columbia Records), 1980

Volume: 1 for the golfers who bet a longer time, and 10 for those who were
　　counting on a quick drop

Chapter 20: Mr. Oliver

Scene: After taking care of Clancy, the students visit Mrs. Oliver at HUP. She and
　　Anna bond even more.

Song: "When I Fall in Love"

Written by: Victor Young and Edward Heyman

Performed by: Nat King Cole

Album: "Love is the Thing," Capitol Records, 1956

Volume: 2, background, as Mrs. Oliver quietly shares her True Love story with
　　Anna

Chapter 21: X-Ray Vision
Scene: Violet and Stan meet at the Peaceable Kingdom to try to make sense of the wave of deaths affecting numerous animal species; one common characteristic: neurologic signs prior to their demise.
Song: "Psycho Killer"
Written by: David Byrne, Chris Frantz, Tina Weymouth
Performed by: Talking Heads
Album: Talking Heads: 77, Sire Records, 1977.
Volume: 8, as they look at the maps

Chapter 22: A Note From Buck
Scene: After a circuitous and coffee-staining route from Florida to Philadelphia, Buck's thinly veiled love letter finally reaches Trisha.
Song: "Blue Ribbon Baby"
Written by: Allison Dewar and Diane Lampert
Performed by: Tommy Sands and The Raiders (original, 1958)
Album: single, "Blue Ribbon Baby," Capitol Records, 1958; compilation: The Worryin' Kind, Bear Family Records, 1992.
Volume: 2 in the background, while Trisha reads the letter

Chapter 23: Body of Knowledge
Scene: It's the Avery Banks Show, everyone!
Song: "She Blinded Me with Science"
Written by: Thomas Dolby, Jo Kerr
Performed by: Thomas Dolby
Album: Blinded by Science (EP), The Golden Age of Wireless (second edition), Capitol Records, 1982
Volume: 10, loud and brash, just like Avery herself

Chapter 24: Animal House
Scene: Avery Banks is Cleopatra, and Jack, King Tut at Alpha Mu's Halloween Party.
Song: "Walk Like an Egyptian"
Written by: Liam Sternberg
Performed by: The Bangles
Album: Different Light, Columbia Records, 1986
Volume: 10, no one can hear you anyway

AND

Chapter 24: Animal House
Scene: It's a zoo at Alpha Mu, so let's get this party started!
Song: "Burning Down the House"
Written by: David Byrne, Chris Frantz, Jerry Harrison, and Tina Weymouth
Performed by: Talking Heads
Album: Speaking in Tongues, Sire Records, 1983
Volume: 11, see above

DISC 3: AN ANIMAL LIFE: PART III

Chapter 27: Rectification
Scene: On a cold December morning, Big Moe teaches his "little moes" the fine
    art of rectal palpation, i.e., how to stick one's arm up a cow's rectum and cop
    a feel.
Song: "I Feel For You"
Written by: Prince
Performed by: Chaka Khan
Album: I Feel For You, Warner Bros. Records, 1984
Volume: varies — depending upon the student. Some can't concentrate with
    their hand up a cow when the music's too loud

Chapters 28 and 29: Can of Worms: Parts I and II
Scene: While Stan and Violet consult with Dr. O Senior about the epidemic, Anna's
    innocence and trust in the ALM is tested... or was she involved?
Song: "It's the End of the World as We Know It"
Written by: Bill Berry, Peter Buck, Mike Mills, and Michael Stipe
Performed by: REM
Album: Document, IRS Records, 1987
Volume: 1, slowly rising to 2, and then ending at 8 for each scene

Chapter 30: Mr. Right and Wrong
Scene: Murphy's Tavern. The recent happenings at the vet school invoke a som-
    ber mood.
Song: "American Pie"
Written by: Don McLean
Performed by: Don McLean
Album: American Pie, United Artists Records, 1971
Volume: 2-3, background

AND

Chapter 30: Mr. Right and Wrong
Scene: Murphy's Tavern. The mood becomes even darker as Jack openly questions Anna's loyalties.
Song: "Honesty"
Written by: Billy Joel
Performed by: Billy Joel
Album: 52nd Street, Columbia Records, 1979
Volume: 3-4, background

Chapter 32: Love is Everything
Scene: Jack races to Anna's rescue, calling out to her.
Song: "Gonna Fly Now," theme from Rocky
Written by: Bill Conti, Carol Connors, Ayn Robbins
Performed by: Bill Conti, sung by DeEtta Little
Album: Rocky-Original Motion Picture Soundtrack, United Artists, Feb 28, 1977
Volume: 8-9, expressing Jack's urgency, panic

AND

Chapter 32: Love is Everything
Scene: Jack reaches Anna to help and just as they begin to truly see each other, Avery Banks ruins the moment.
Song: "Breaking Us in Two"
Written by: Joe Jackson
Performed by: Joe Jackson
Album: Night and Day, A & M Records, 1982
Volume: A mellow 3, as Anna and Jack are once again torn apart

Ch 33: Mostly, There's Love
Scene: After a night of soft-tissue surgery with Mike at the Center for Large Animal Medicine, Trisha finds herself face to face with Buck, who has returned to see her. Suzie is ill.
Song: "Hello"
Written by: Lionel Ritchie
Performed by: Lionel Ritchie
Album: Can't Slow Down, Motown Records, 1983
Volume: 3, because Trisha and Buck have a lot to discuss

Ch 35: Violet's Choice
Scene: As Violet and Stan plan quarantine and preventative measures to pro-
    tect the animals at Peaceable Kingdom, Digby races in and Violet learns the
    ugly truth. With the help of Stan's "muscle" and a heavy heart, she leaves her
    "dream" job.
Song: "Listen To Your Heart"
Written by: Per Gessle and Mats Persson
Performed by: Roxette
Album: Look Sharp! EMI Records, 1988
Volume: starts quiet, 2, but as the realization slowly sinks in, crescendo to 10

Ch 36: Jack and Anna
Scene: Dr. Vandergrift's lab. Anna is overwhelmed by the destruction which sur-
    rounds her. Loss of animal life is compounded, in Anna's eyes, by the concur-
    rent loss of data, essentially negating their otherwise justifiable use. This major
    setback leaves her feeling even more hopeless.
Song: "Song from M*A*S*H (Suicide is Painless)"
Written by: Johnny Mandel and Mike Altman
Performed by: (uncredited)
Album: The M*A*S*H (Original Soundtrack Recording), Columbia/CBS Records,
    1970
Volume: A contemplative 3

Ch 38: The Kiss
Scene: Room A1. Anna and Jack share their first intimate kiss; for a brief moment
    they are One.
Song: "The Search is Over"
Written by: Frankie Sullivan, Jim Peterik
Performed by: Survivor
Album: Vital Signs, Scotti Brothers Records, 1985
Volume: 2, while they study and tell jokes, 10 when they kiss (yeah, it was all
    that!), but then back down to 1 after hearing the sad news

Chapter 39: Tradition
Scene: The skits night players pay tribute to their heroes.
Song: "Five Guys Named Moe" (cover by Joe Jackson)
Written by: Jerome Bresler, Larry Wynn
Performed by: Joe Jackson
Album: Jumpin' Jive, A&M Records, June 1981
Volume: 8-9, celebratory but not quite deafening

AND

Chapter 39: Tradition
Scene: The struggles of the first semester are over, trust is restored, and all is well with the world — at least for now; as the camera pulls back for an aerial shot, the bonfire illuminates the courtyard like the dawning sun of a new day.
Song: "Brand New Day"
Written by: Van Morrison
Performed by: Van Morrison
Album: Moondance, Warner Bros. Records, 1970
Volume: 2, crescendo to 8, as a quiet sense of accomplishment makes way to exuberant celebration, but then fade out to 1, as the students (eventually) head home to prepare for a brand new day and semester

Glossary of Selected Terms and Jargon

All definitions in this glossary are for edutainment purposes only (but they can and should also be used to impress your friends).

KEY

word or phrase: definition of said word or phrase; alternative definition if appropriate. *Authors' clarification, related anecdote, and/or reference to the story.*

abomasum: the last of the four compartments of the ruminant stomach. *Dr. Stan Oblitzski referred to the left displaced abomasum of Billy Stolfus, the recently deceased Angora goat.*

acidosis: a condition characterized by an abnormal increase in the acidity of the blood and extracellular fluids. *Jack developed this condition in his first, awkward encounter with Anna.*

ACVP: American College of Veterinary Pathologists; organization of board-certified veterinary pathologists, founded in 1949. *Dr. Stan Oblitzski is a board-certified pathologist and thus a member of this organization (and no one else in this organization is like Stan...).*

addax: screwhorn antelope; related to the oryx, lives in the Saharan desert; it has been listed on the IUCN Red List as endangered since 1986, but was declared critically endangered in 2000. Captive collections are important for the long-term survival of the species.

ADR: acronym for "Ain't Doin' Right." Used to indicate general, often nebulous or nonspecific signs of illness. A potential presenting complaint (PC) for animals requiring veterinary care. *Dr. Violet Green used this term to describe two flamingoes at Peaceable Kingdom suffering from a mystery illness.*

afferent: an anatomical term indicating something that bears or conducts inwards or towards a structure. The opposite of efferent. *In their studies of animal anatomy, the first-year veterinary students familiarized themselves with the various afferent and efferent pathways of structures including nerves and blood vessels.*

aliquot/blood aliquot: (in medicine) a portion of a total amount of a liquid. *In her work, Dr. Violet Green collects aliquots of blood as part of her health assessment of animals such as the immobilized giraffe and the dolphins at Peaceable Kingdom.*

ALS: Amyotrophic lateral sclerosis, also known as Lou Gehrig's disease, is a progressive neurodegenerative disease affecting nerve cells in the brain and spinal cord. *Anna Heywood was diagnosed with ALS in the year prior to starting veterinary school and faced the progressive effects of the disease during the first semester. ALS is also the focus of Dr. Even Vandergrift's research.*

AVA: American Veterinary Association *(a fictitious organization).*

Amyotrophic Lateral Sclerosis: (see **ALS** and **Lou Gehrig's Disease**)

An Animal Life: a book series, written and illustrated by a group of "little moes" and inspired by some of the greatest years of their lives. *May be an upcoming blockbuster movie or TV series.*

arbovirus: an ARthropod-BOrne virus, i.e., a virus transmitted by arthropods, such as mosquitoes; examples include EEE, WEE, yellow fever, dengue, and WNV.

ataxic: lacking coordination of voluntary muscle movements. *This was a common clinical sign in the sick and ADR animals Drs. Green and Oblitzski encountered in their work investigating the mystery illness. Ataxia can also be a result of a night at Murphy's Tavern.*

atrium: in cardiac anatomy, the atrium is the chamber that receives circulating blood from the rest of the body. *Dr. Florence Kimball referred to this structure in her discussions of cardiac physiology and heartworm infection.*

autotroph: an organism capable of self-nourishment by using inorganic materials as a source of nutrients and using photosynthesis or chemosynthesis as a source of energy.

ATP: Adenosine triphosphate carries chemical energy within cells for metabolism. It regulates many biochemical pathways. *As she struggled with the effects of ALS, Anna Heywood found her ATP stores depleted.*

atropine: An anticholinergic drug, the injectable form of which is used to treat low heart rate (bradycardia). It is frequently used as part of CPR in veterinary medicine. *One of the emergency drugs Dr. Violet Green carried with her as she prepared to examine the immobilized giraffe.*

axon: the process of a nerve cell that conducts impulses away from the body of the nerve.

ay-yuh: a response in the affirmative; Mainer slang for "yes." *"Would you like a side of lobstah with your lobstah?" "Ay-yuh."*

Banamine: flunixin; a non-steroidal anti-inflammatory drug with analgesic, and antipyretic (fever reduction) properties; used in horses, cattle and pigs.

biceps brachii: the muscle of the upper arm/foreleg on the anterior surface of the humerus, arising from the scapula. It flexes the arm. One of hundreds of muscles the first-year students must learn the function, origin, and insertion of. *Also a constant source of distraction for Kerri Feinburg during her veterinary school years.*

botulism: bacterial disease caused by *Clostridium botulinum*, which lives in soil and untreated water and can enter the body through wounds; causative agent also found in improperly canned or preserved food. Signs of illness can include respiratory difficulty, abdominal cramping, nausea, and paralysis. Blood tests are used to identify the toxin and treatment includes the administration of botulinum antitoxin.

Boxer cardiomyopathy: an inherited heart abnormality of boxer dogs characterized by the development of ventricular tachyarrhythmias (more rapid heartbeats that arise from the ventricles).

BP: blood pressure, the pressure exerted by circulating blood upon the walls of blood vessels. Measurement helps screen for hypertension (abnormally high BP) and hypotension (abnormally low BP). *Blood pressure is one of the important vital signs that Dr. Violet and her students assessed during their immobilization of the giraffe.*

Bruxism: teeth grinding. *A common clinical sign of colic in horses including those admitted to the Center for Large Animal Medicine.*

Bute: phenylbutazone; a non-steroidal anti-inflammatory drug commonly used for pain relief and fever reduction in horses.

cannon bone: in horses, the enlarged metacarpal or metatarsal of the third digit. *Dr. Daniel Linnehan performed surgery to repair a thoroughbred's shattered cannon bone and used the opportunity to teach his students the importance of post-operative recovery.*

CBC: complete blood count. *One of the lab tests that Trisha Maxwell recommended as part of the diagnostic work-up for Suzie.*

ceftiofur: cephalosporin antibiotic licensed for veterinary use; active against both Gram-positive and Gram-negative bacteria. *One of the antibiotics that Dr. Violet Green kept stocked in her Rover.*

cetacean: aquatic mammals of the Order Cetacea; includes whales, porpoises and dolphins.

chemistry panel: a blood test that measures the level of many chemicals within the body and is instrumental in assessing health, including that of organs such as the liver and kidneys. *One of the lab tests that Trisha Maxwell recommended as part of the diagnostic work-up for Suzie.*

christly: Mainer slang for "very."

chronic bog spavin: chronic synovitis of the tibiotarsal joint in horses, characterized by distention of the joint capsule.

colic: a term used broadly to describe conditions that cause a horse to exhibit signs of abdominal pain. *Horses requiring surgical treatment for colic are in good hands at the Center for Large Animal Medicine.*

cornea: the transparent convex anterior-portion of the eye, it covers the iris, pupil and anterior chamber and plays a role in refracting light onto the retina. *This is one of the anatomical structures Dr. Flo Kimball pointed out as she instructed the students about a proper ocular exam.*

corneal ulcer: an open corneal sore, with disruption of the corneal epithelium. *One of the patients presenting to the SCAVA spay/neuter and vaccination clinic appeared to have a non-healing corneal ulcer.*

corvid: birds of the family Corvidae, which include crows, ravens, jays, and nutcrackers. *Species of corvids seemed to be particularly susceptible to the mystery illness Drs. Green and Oblitzski investigated, and they were dying in large numbers.*

CRI: continuous rate infusion; a specific quantity of drug is added to a specific volume of fluid and administered at a specific rate; administration via CRI permits one to maintain steady-state concentrations of a drug. *Mike London's treatment orders for a patient with Boxer cardiomyopathy included CRIs of Lasix and dopamine.*

CRT: capillary refill time; the rate (in seconds) at which blood refills empty capillaries; it can be used to help assess the quality of peripheral perfusion, with a prolonged CRT indicating decreased perfusion. *Measurement of CRT featured in the assessment of several patients, including a giraffe, a dog, and William Digby.*

Dead Man Talking: see **HypnoGolf**.

Demodex canis: one of approximately 65 species of parasitic mites that live in or near the hair follicles of mammals, *Demodex canis* lives on dogs and causes demodectic mange, also known as demodicosis.

depressor labii: a facial muscle that depresses the lower lip and moves it laterally. *As Anna reacted to Jack's fumbling attempts to make amends for his unintentionally insulting behavior, this muscle proved critical to her facial expression. Nothing says "I'm pissed" better than a depressed* depressor labii.

DJD: degenerative joint disease, also known as osteoarthritis. *One of the many reasons a horse might end up with a new life "serving "students at the Center for Large Animal Medicine's teaching barns.*

DMT: Dead Man Talking; see **HypnoGolf**.

dopamine: a drug used in the treatment of severe hypotension, acute heart failure, and certain types of kidney failure.

drongo: Aussie slang for "idiot"; U.S. equivalents also include "dumbass," "buffoon," and "moron."

dura mater: the tough, fibrous, outermost layer of tissue covering the brain and spinal cord.

Dx: abbreviation for "diagnosis" (i.e., the cause of a disease or lesion).

DDx: abbreviation for "differential diagnoses" (i.e., different possible causes for a disease and/or lesion).

Eastern Equine Encephalitis: an important viral disease transmitted by the bite of infected mosquitoes that can infect a wide range of animals including mammals, birds, reptiles and amphibians; horses particularly susceptible to infection, with mortality rates of 70-90%; though rare in humans, EEE is one of the most severe mosquito-transmitted diseases in the United States with approximately 33% mortality and significant brain damage in most survivors. *Dr. Violet Green discussed this as one of the differentials for horses with neurological signs.*

EEE: see **Eastern Equine Encephalitis**.

EKG: an electrocardiogram, also known as an ECG; measures the heart's electrical activity and helps identify cardiac abnormalities, including arrhythmias. *An EKG serves as a common feature in the monitoring of patients at VHUP, the Peaceable Kingdom, the Center for Large Animal Medicine, and HUP.*

efferent: bears or conducts outwards or away from a structure; the opposite of afferent.

emerging infectious diseases: diseases caused by an organism (e.g., a bacterium, fungus, parasite, or virus) that have increased in incidence in the past 20 years and threaten to increase further in the future; includes diseases caused by newly identified microorganisms, newly identified strains of a known organism, or a known infection that spreads to a new geographic area or population. *The mystery illness that Drs. Green and Oblitzski investigated ultimately fell under this heading. Surprisingly, the CDC does not yet consider Rick Larson an emerging infectious disease.*

encephalitis: acute inflammation of the brain; causes include, but are not limited to, viral, bacterial, parasitic, or fungal infection. *Doctors treating Mrs. Oliver at HUP had ruled out all known causes of encephalitis.*

endotracheal tube: a catheter placed into the trachea to facilitate oxygen and carbon dioxide exchange and/or for more controlled administration of gas anesthesia.

entropion: a turning in of the edges of the eyelid (usually the lower eyelid) so that the eyelashes rub against the eye surface. *Anna squinted at Jack so severely, she induced a voluntary entropion.*

epinephrine: also known as adrenalin, a naturally occurring hormone involved in many bodily functions; as a drug, epinephrine is used in the treatment of conditions such as asthma, anaphylaxis, and cardiac arrest.

epizootic: disease affecting a large number of animals at approximately the same time within a particular region or geographic area; an epidemic.

EPM: Equine Protozoal Myeloencephalitis; a central nervous system disease caused by the one-celled parasite *Sarcocystis neurona*; considered a common neurological disease of horses in the Americas; horses are considered an aberrant (abnormal) host of this parasite; opossums are definitive, reservoir hosts, but other mammals, including raccoons, armadillos, skunks and cats are intermediate hosts; parasite can infect any portion of the central nervous system, so almost any neurological sign is possible. *A differential for horses displaying neurological signs, including Buck's beloved Suzie.*

equine stay apparatus: the system of tendons, ligaments, and deep fascial tissue that holds a horse's legs straight and "locked in place" with minimal exertion. *Big Moe risked life and limb testing the first-years' knowledge of the stay apparatus.*

ES: Emergency Service; The ES's at VHUP and HUP provide for those requiring urgent medical care.

Esbilac: milk replacer formulated for puppies but used in other species as well. *Dr. Green lovingly reared the twin snow leopards on a steady diet of Esbilac.*

Euglena: one-celled, flagellated organism of the genus *Euglena*, characterized by the ability to feed both by autotrophy, like plants, and heterotrophy, like animals.

femur: thigh bone, one of the primary long bones of the leg/hind limb, situated between the pelvis and the knee. *The first years were responsible for knowing all the muscles, tendons, ligaments, nerves, and blood vessels associated with this and every other bone in future patients.*

fetlock: common name for the metacarpophalangeal joint (in the foreleg) and the metatarsophalangeal joint (in the hind leg) of horses and other large animals; formed by the joint between the cannon bone and the longer pastern bone. *William Digby noted a hyperextension of the giraffe's fetlocks as one of the first signs that the M99 is taking effect.*

fimbriated: having a fringe or border of hair-like or finger-like projections. *Anna palpated the fimbriated lining of Clover's rumen as she assisted Jack in the large animal palpation lab.*

fish-sicle: slang term for frozen fish used, after thawing, to feed marine mammals.

flatlander: Mainer term for someone not from Maine; *aka an "outta-state-ah."*

flavivirus: genus of viruses belonging to the family Flaviviridae; includes yellow fever, dengue, and WNV; most are transmitted by the bite of an infected mosquito or tick (arthropods) and thus are also classified as arboviruses. *One of the types of viruses that doctors considered in their work-up of Mrs. Oliver's illness.*

flehmen: a behavioral response found in many male mammals when they detect particular smells, characterized by a curling of the upper lip and a raising of the head; behavior thought to facilitate exposure of the vomeronasal organ to pheromones. *One of the signs noted in horses presenting to the Center for Large Animal Medicine with colic. Prior to veterinary school, Rick Larson was briefly jailed for exposing his vomeronasal organ in public.*

flexor carpi radialis: muscle of the forelimb that acts to flex the carpus (*wrist*).

fluoroscopy: an imaging technique used to obtain real-time moving images of the internal structures of a patient through the use of a fluoroscope. *One of many diagnostic tools available at the Peaceable Kingdom's state-of-the-art animal clinic.*

footrot: a necrotic infection originating from a lesion in the interdigital skin that leads to a cellulitis in the digital region. *One of the large animal ailments being treated back in the heyday of the old vet school quad and one that is still a problem today.*

formalin: a solution of formaldehyde gas dissolved in water; a 10% neutral buffered formalin solution is commonly used for fixing and preserving biologic specimens for pathologic and histologic examination. *Reportedly, Joan Rivers applies a formalin-based "rejuvenating" cream every second Wednesday.*

frog: in the horse, a portion of the underside of the hoof which plays a role in shock absorption; if spelled "FRoG," a lovingly derogatory acronym for "Front Row Geek"; any tailless, stout-bodied amphibian of the order Anura. *Trisha palpated Suzie's frog as part of her lameness exam.*

fuzzies: slang for young mice that have fur but are not yet very mobile.

gastrocnemius: muscle of the calf of the leg, the action of which extends the foot and bends the knee. *Sam (aka "Yankee Moe") Stone demonstrated that cutting the gastrocnemius has no impact on the stay apparatus. Unless, of course, you "yankee some moe" on it.*

gelding: a castrated (formerly male) horse/equine. *A descriptor applying to some of the horses presenting to the Center for Large Animal Medicine.*

gemsbok: an antelope of the *Oryx* genus that is native to arid regions of Southern Africa and which has long, rapier-shaped horns and striking black and white facial markings.

GI anastomosis: gastrointestinal reconnection; a gastrointestinal anastomosis is performed after the removal of a diseased or damaged section of the intestine and involves the surgical and functional reconnection of the remaining sections. *One of the procedures included in the junior-year student surgeries.*

glycogen: a polysaccharide, $(C_6H_{10}O_5)_n$ that is the main form of carbohydrate storage in animals and is found primarily in the liver and muscle tissue; glycogen is readily converted to glucose as needed by the body to satisfy its energy needs.

hacky sack: a popular way for veterinary students to pass time between classes (at least in the late 1980's), this game involved players standing in a circle and kicking a small "foot bag" or "hacky-sack" between them without letting it touch the ground. *It sated the students' desire to brag about playing a sport while also minimizing the risk of serious injury, death or breaking a sweat.*

HBC: acronym for "Hit By Car," a potential presenting complaint for animals that, pleonastically enough, were hit by a car and require veterinary care. *A common presenting complaint for patients admitted through VHUP's ES.*

HCT: hematocrit, a diagnostic measure which represents the percentage volume of blood made up of red blood cells (RBCs). *Suzie's HCT of 60% on presentation to the Center for Large Animal Medicine indicated that she is very likely dehydrated.*

heartworm: a parasitic infection with the roundworm *Dirofilaria immitis*, spread by the bite of mosquitoes; definitive host is the dog, but many other species can be infected; adult stage of the heartworm typically resides in the pulmonary arteries, though occasionally the worm migrates to the right side of the heart; symptoms of infection can include coughing, exercise intolerance, weight loss, and congestive heart failure. *Dr. Florence Kimball made it her mission to educate her students and the public about the evils of heartworm infection.*

hemangiosarcoma: a highly malignant cancer arising from the lining of blood vessels; particularly common in dogs, where it is most often found in the spleen, liver, and right heart.

heparin: an anti-coagulant (i.e., prevents blood from clotting). *Heparin is especially helpful for students who are just learning how to draw blood from any number of species and from any number of blood vessels (heparin helps keep the blood from clogging their needle and making them look silly).*

hepatoencephalopathy: also known as hepatic (liver) encephalopathy; a condition in which decreased liver function leads to the accumulation of toxic substances normally metabolized and detoxified by the liver; clinical signs are often neurological and can include disorientation, seizures, and coma. *Dr. Violet Green included this as one of the differentials for horses with neurological signs.*

heterotroph: an organism that, unlike autotrophs, cannot synthesize its own food and is dependent on complex organic substances for nutrition.

hip dysplasia: abnormal formation of the coxofemoral joint (i.e., the hip joint), common in large and giant breed dogs (e.g., Great Danes, Labrador Retrievers, Golden Retrievers, and German Shepherds) that can eventually cause crippling lameness and painful arthritis of the joints.

homunculus brain: a sensory map representing each part of the body in proportion to its number of sensory neural connections rather than its actual size. *Anna's blushing description of the disproportionate representation of sensory nerve endings in the lips, tongue, and cheek triggered Jack to action.*

hoof tester: a tool shaped like a pair of large pincers that is used to squeeze the hoof to locate the pain or tenderness; one of the blades is placed on apparently normal hoof and the other on the part to be tested; if there is a flinch response when the handles are squeezed, this is taken as an indication of pain at one of the pressure sites. *Dr. Linnehan made use of the hoof tester during his lameness exam.*

hook and pinworm ova: the eggs of two types of roundworms (hookworm and pinworm).

HUP: acronym for Hospital of the University of Philadelphia *(a fictitious place in this book).*

hydatid cyst: the larval cyst stage of the tapeworms *Echinococcus granulosus* and *E. multilocularis;* a zoonotic disease, the tapeworms' definitive host include dogs, and intermediate hosts include sheep and cattle; humans can become accidental hosts and develop large cysts within their liver, lungs, and in other organs. *The liverwurst and mini-marshmallow mock-ups purportedly served at the Alpha Mu Halloween Party were decidedly less infectious than the real thing.*

hyperemic response: an increase in the quantity of blood flow to a body part (hyperemia) in response to some stimulus. *Dr. Oblitzski left his mark (quite literally a reverse "P") on William Digby's face. John, Paul, Ringo, and George played two shows as "The Reverse Hyperemic P's" before they decided the name was too wordy.*

hypertensive decompensation: deterioration in a patient's condition due to a poorly controlled elevation in blood pressure.

HypnoGolf: aka "Dead Man Talking"; HypnoGolf is a challenging variant of golf played by veterinary students, most often during "in-the-rough" lectures; in HypnoGolf, players predict when a specific student will fall dead asleep, and whoever is closest to the "hole" without going over wins; betting is mandatory. *Jose was a legend, critical to the Class of 1992's HypnoGolf club regulars because he was guaranteed to fall asleep during almost any class.*

Hx: abbreviation for "patient history."

IgG: one of the main classes of antibodies produced by B-cells (a type of immune cell); measurement of immunoglobulin G can be a diagnostic tool for certain conditions, including multiple sclerosis.

IgM: one of the main classes of antibody produced by B-cells (a type of immune cell), this class is produced relatively rapidly and appears early on in an infection.

immunoassays: a biochemical test that measures the presence or concentration of a substance in a complex solution (often in blood serum or urine) using the substance's reactivity to specific antibodies.

iris: the structure of the eye controlling the size of the pupil (and therefor the amount of light admitted) and responsible for giving the eye its color.

isoflurane: a type of inhalation/gas anesthetic.

IZA: International Zoo and Aquarium Association *(a fictitious organization).*

laparotomies: surgeries involving incisions through the abdominal wall to allow access to the abdominal cavity. *One of the procedures included in the junior-year student surgeries.*

Lasix: furosemide; a diuretic drug used in the treatment of congestive heart failure. *It is part of the treatment protocol Dr. Kimball and Mike London used to treat a patient with Boxer cardiomyopathy with heart failure.*

lead shank: (aka, lead chain) a line with a chain attached that used in a variety of ways to safely control horses. *A required piece of equipment for all fourth-year students at the Center for Large Animal Medicine.*

left displaced abomasum: also known as an LDA; a condition in which a gas-filled abomasum moves into an abnormal position left of the ventral midline. *Dr. Oblitzski's necropsy of Billy Stolfus confirmed the suspicion of LDA.*

lens: the structure of the eye that, together with the cornea, helps refract (bend) light to be focused on the retina; has an ellipsoid, biconvex shape and is made up of three parts: the capsule, epithelium, and fibers.

lenticular cataracts: an opacity within the body of the lens not affecting the lens capsule. *Dr. Kimball noted some clouding in the center of Clancy's right lens.*

Lou Gehrig's Disease: (see **ALS**).

lysosome: a membrane-bound organelle in the cytoplasm of most cells containing various hydrolytic enzymes that function in intracellular digestion; lysosomal lysis represents one of the manifestations of cellular aging.

M99: etorphine; also known as Immobilon; a semi-synthetic opioid often used to immobilize large mammals. It is 1,000 to 3,000 times more potent than morphine as an analgesic; a small amount can cause serious harm to a human if accidentally injected or deposited on exposed skin or mucous membranes. *Dr. Green used M99 to immobilize a giraffe for examination and blood sampling.*

M50-50: diprenorphine; also known as diprenorfin, Revivon; an opioid antagonist, M50-50 is used to reverse the effects of powerful opioids such as M99.

mast cell tumor: a cancer consisting of mast cells — immune cells involved with allergic and hypersensitivity reactions.

mastitis: inflammation of the mammary tissues. *The most common disease of dairy cattle in the U.S. and one of the large animal ailments being treated back in the heyday of the old vet school quad.*

MC4: the fourth metacarpal bone, lateral to the third metacarpal (cannon) bone; also known as a splint bone. *As Trisha performed her lameness exam on Suzie, she noted pain on palpation of MC4.*

medial canthus: the medial angle or corner of the eye where the upper and lower eyelids meet.

meningitis: inflammation of the meninges, the membranes that surround the spinal cord and brain.

meningoencephalitis: inflammation of the brain and meninges. *Meningoencephalitis is a common clinical finding in WNV disease cases.*

mental foramen: an opening on the lateral part of the body of the mandible (lower jaw bone) through which the mental nerve and blood vessels pass. *The point of impact of Dr. Oblitzski's well-placed inaugural punch. "Dr. Oblitzski's Inaugural Punch" sounds like something Murphy's Tavern should be serving in bottles.*

mitochondria: membrane-enclosed organelles found in the cytoplasm of eukaryotic cells, they are responsible for generating most of the cell's energy via production of adenosine triphosphate (ATP). *One of the many victims in formalin's path of destruction.*

Mount Augustus: considered the world's largest monolith (or rock), it rises approximately 866m above the surrounding plain in Western Australia. *At the Peaceable Kingdom, it wears a khaki shirt and cargo shorts.*

mouse-sicle: a frozen mouse used after thawing to feed a predator (such as a bird or snake). *Hoss thawed some mouse-sicles to feed Hootie the formerly great horned owl, who was acting decidedly "off" due to illness.*

myelin: a biological insulating material that surrounds an axon (the primary impulse-bearing nerve structure) and helps speed up the transmission of nerve impulses.

myomere (skeletal muscle): segments of skeletal muscle separated from neighboring segments by fibrous connective tissue.

naloxone: a drug (opiate antagonist) used to counter the effects of opioid drugs, for example morphine, or as a reversal for accidental M99 (etorphine) injection in humans.

navicular bone: distal sesamoid; articulates with the distal phalanx (PIII) and middle phalanx (PII), and lies completely within the hoof; critical for weight bearing. *During the lameness exam, Trisha tried her best to push deeply into Suzie's frog to assess if there was any tenderness in or around the navicular bone.*

necropsy: an autopsy for animals; careful examination/dissection of a dead animal to determine cause of death or changes resulting from disease. *For Dr. Oblitzski, necropsy is the ultimate physical exam in pathology, aka "dead animal medicine."*

necrotic: dead/dying; *(as in "you are necrotic to me").*

necrotizing myocarditis: inflammation of the heart that results in death of tissue.

neuroglia: important support cells for nerves and neurons.

NIC-U: Neonatal Intensive Care Unit (ICU for newborns). *When Dr. Stan visited Dr. Violet at Peaceable Kingdom, she showed him the video monitor of baby addax in the NIC-U.*

nippers: a farrier's (equine hoof care specialist's) tool used to trim a horse's hoof wall.

orbicularis oculi: the muscles in the face which function to close the eyelids. *After Anna — with Petunia's help — navigated through the revolving door, her orbicularis oculi drew her eyelids together as she prepared to verbally disembowel Jack.*

ophthalmoscope: an important handheld piece of medical equipment used to examine the eye. *Jack had problems working the ophthalmoscope during Clancy's eye exam.*

orthopod: term for an orthopedic surgeon; a surgeon who works primarily on the musculoskeletal system. *Trisha told Buck that a "real" orthopod (perhaps Dr. Linnehan?) should also examine Suzie.*

palpebral reflex: an automatic response causing the eyelids to close when the medial canthus is touched; this evaluates the integrity of the facial (cranial nerve VII) and trigeminal (cranial nerve V) nerves. *Dr. Green checked the snow leopard "Peeka's" palpebral reflex to assess her depth of anesthesia, i.e., was she sufficiently knocked out for the artificial insemination?*

patellar ligament: the continuation of the central portion of the tendon of the quadriceps femoris (the "quad") muscle distal to the patella, extending from the patella to the tuberosity of the tibia; part of the equine stay apparatus.

PCV: packed cell volume; a commonly measured blood parameter used to determine the relative amount of red blood cells present in a blood sample.

PBR: Pabst Blue Ribbon, a wallet-friendly beer; among the rodeo crowd, Professional Bull Riders.

PE: physical examination; a critically important component of a full diagnostic work up; cf necropsy. *Learning how to perform a comprehensive physical examination is one of the professional "Holy Grails" for veterinary students; a head-to-tail (or head-to-butt, if no tail is present) assessment and use of all the senses (except for maybe taste) and multiple forms of "scopes."*

perineal urethrostomy: a surgical procedure commonly used in male cats that involves widening the urinary tract (urethra) and removing the penis to make obstruction (as by urinary stones) less likely. *During the annual SCAVA spay/neuter and vaccination clinic, Spartacus the cat was a potential candidate for perineal urethrostomy to prevent further obstruction.*

peripheral nerve: a nerve that is outside of, and not considered part of, the brain or spinal cord (the central nervous system).

peroneal nerve: a nerve located in the hind leg, it innervates muscles that flex the hock and extend the digit.

peroneus tertius: the muscle which originates on the fibula, inserts on the 5th metatarsal, is innervated by the deep peroneal nerve, and moves the foot. The peroneus tertius is not technically part of the passive stay apparatus in horses, but is involved in flexing the hock joint when the stifle joint flexes during movement.

pigeon: a common and fairly abundant "urban wildlife" bird that has also been domesticated; known by some as a "rat with wings," infected pigeons can also spread zoonotic diseases including the fungal disease cryptococcosis. *And they can, of course, make lovely pets.*

pinkies: slang for baby mice that do not yet have hair.

pissah: a New England term that can be used to describe something really awesome *("that Philly cheesesteak with broccoli rabe was wicked pissah!")* or very crappy *("I just got rumen juice in my hair, what a pissah!").*

pred: abbreviation for prednisone, an oral, synthetic anti-inflammatory corticosteroid drug. *Hootie the owl received pred to help with any inflammation that could be the cause of his clinical signs.*

primum non nocere: (Latin) "First, do no harm," one of the most critical, and often challenging principles of veterinary and human medicine. *During the "vet-school-survival" session with their first years, Mike reminded them of the importance of this principle.*

proglottid: a segment of a tapeworm that contains a sexually mature reproductive system and which can be disturbing to see in the feces of animals *(and/or people, Jose...). A little known fact: sexually immature tapeworms are known as "rookieglottids."*

propofol: a short-acting, milky-white, intravenously administered hypnotic agent used for induction and maintenance of general anesthesia.

Przewalski's horse: a species of once-extinct, wild horse, native to Mongolia/central Asia, which has been reintroduced into these areas. *Dr. Green questioned the wisdom of her employer's purchase of 39 of these horses for the Peaceable Kingdom.*

pupillary light reflex: an automatic response that controls the diameter of the pupil, in response to, and in order to regulate, the intensity of light that falls on the retina of the eye; greater intensity light causes the pupil to become smaller (allowing less light in), whereas lower intensity light causes the pupil to become larger (allowing more light in). *During a thorough eye exam, this will help rule in, or out, various sensory and motor diseases of the eye.*

purple top tube: a glass container (tube) with a purple rubber top which contains EDTA, a substance that prevents clotting; purple top tubes are used commonly for complete blood cell counts and blood smear diagnostics. *Not to be confused with "purple tube top," an essential wardrobe item for Prince's back-up singers.*

rabies: a zoonotic, viral disease that attacks the central nervous system of mammals and causes brain inflammation; typically spread by a bite from an infected animal; for people, rabies is almost invariably fatal if post-exposure treatment is not provided prior to the onset of severe symptoms. *Rabies can be a rule out for any unusual neurologic disease signs, although in many cases it is less likely, as Trisha explained to the first years during necropsy of the Clydesdale Bud.*

RBCs: acronym for red blood cells.

red top tube: a glass container (tube) with a red rubber top, this container has no additives; used for serum samples intended to measure blood chemistries and serology (antibodies), among other diagnostics.

retina: the delicate multilayered light-sensitive membrane lining the inner posterior chamber of the eyeball, containing the rods and cones, structures necessary for visual perception and connected by the optic nerve to the brain.

Salter-Harris type IV bone fracture: a break that involves the growth plate of the bone as well as the bone on each side of that growth plate; any fracture through a growth plate can be a challenge to fix, because the bone will continue to change in size. *During weekly grand rounds, the student's presentation of Dr. Green's reduction of a Salter-Harris type IV fracture in a black rhino was particularly fascinating because of the accompanying video.*

sartorius: a narrow ribbon-shaped muscle and the longest muscle in the body, extending from the pelvis to the calf of the leg, it acts to flex the thigh and rotate it laterally (toward the outside) and to flex the leg and rotate it toward the middle. *The sartorius is only one of the thigh muscles that Jack visualized during Avery Banks' "presentation."*

SCAVA: Student Chapter of the American Veterinary Association; the student affiliation of the American Veterinary Association *(both are fictitious organizations).*

sclera: the tough, white outer coat of the eyeball, covering approximately the posterior five-sixths of its surface, connected anteriorly to the cornea and posteriorly to the external sheath of the optic nerve.

scolex: the anterior, or "head" end of a tapeworm which contains suckers and/ or hooks used for attachment. *Trisha previously dressed as a tapeworm, complete with scolex and throw-pillow proglottids, for the Alpha Mu Halloween party during her second year of veterinary school.*

semimembranosus: one of the hamstring/thigh muscles; the semimembranosus helps extend the hip joint and bend the knee.

semitendinosus: one of the hamstring/thigh muscles; the semitendinosus helps to extend (straighten) the hip joint and flex (bend) the knee joint; helps medially rotate the knee. *During the "Testicle Festival," Jack, Hoss, and Sam are mesmerized by Miss Colorado's semimembranosus and semitendinosus, visible courtesy of her tight denim jeans.*

serosanguinous: containing blood and serous fluid. *Some serosanguinous fluid was spit up by the Stryker saw during Dr. Oblitzski's necropsy of Trisha's Clydesdale case.*

shit: a synonym for fecal matter; aka feces, poop, doo doo, crap, poo poo; also a popular term used to indicate surprise, both good and bad. *Can be mistaken for vanilla icing when one is somewhat inebriated and sees bird feces with uric acid on the tiara of a hot veterinarian (seriously, we're not shitting you).*

sinoatrial node: the sinoatrial node (also commonly spelled sinuatrial node, abbreviated SA node or SAN, also called the sinus node) is the impulse-generating (pacemaker) tissue located in the right atrium of the heart, and thus the generator of normal sinus rhythm; a group of cells positioned on the wall of the right atrium, near the entrance of the superior vena cava; these cells are modified cardiac myocytes which possess some contractile filaments, but do not contract. *Dr. Flo Kimball, as per usual, made learning about the importance of the SA node's role in coordinating heart chamber contractions fun!*

splint bones: term referring to metacarpal or metatarsal II and IV, which are remnants of two of the five toes of prehistoric horses, and which run down either side of the cannon bone (metacarpal or metatarsal III).

***Star Wars*: ground-breaking sci-fi movie franchise, created by Obi-Wan-George-Lucas**; the first installment, *Episode IV (A New Hope)* was **THE SCI-FI FILM of the 70s**; the genius and wisdom of this first movie is under appreciated by many current Gen-X'ers, Gen Y'ers (Milleniums), and Gen Z'ers; subtly steeped in ancient veterinary lore and life lessons; "The Force" guides and binds all veterinary students and veterinarians to "the Mission" of our profession as they are the "Jedi Knights" of the animal world; introduced ancient, yet frighteningly modern galactic veterinary equipment, including the Lightsaber; *Episodes V (The Empire Strikes Back) and Episode VI (Return of the Jedi)* have fairly obvious parallels with veterinary school. *A veterinary colleague and mentor of ours who will remain nameless (unless we are asked in private) watched this movie 28 times when it first came out.*

sternocephalicus: a long, narrow muscle that extends from the manubrium sterni (upper part of the sternum) to the mandible, forming the ventral border of the jugular groove; it splits at the middle of the neck, becoming narrower and thinner as the segments move up the neck; the branches pass under the parotid gland and end at a flat tendon at the mandible. *Dr. Kimball used this landmark during class to show the first years how to find their pulses.*

stringhalt: a sudden flexion of one or both hind legs in the horse, most easily seen while the horse is walking or trotting, backing up, or suddenly frightened, and feet are held high. *Some of the "retired" horses used for teaching purposes have stringhalt.*

Stryker saw: an oscillating (vibrating) electric saw which cuts and removes casts, and does not cut skin; a variant, the oscillating electric bone saw cuts bone but not skin. *A great gag gift for the novice veterinary student, as Dr. Oblitzski demonstrated during large animal necropsy!*

superficial digital flexor: muscle that originates on the humerus and the caudal side of the radius, travels distally to become the superficial digital flexor tendon; flexes the carpus and lower joints. *Kerri reminded her male colleagues that this is one of the components of the equine passive stay apparatus.*

tetanus: a medical condition characterized by a prolonged contraction of skeletal muscle fibers, commonly caused by infection with the bacterium *Clostridium tetani.*

theriogenology: branch of veterinary medicine dealing with reproduction (*i.e., sex and "sexy time" for animals*). *During their theriogenology rotation, Mike learned to appreciate and become friends with one of his class's "FRoGs."*

thoracic excursion: expansion of the chest/thorax as by respiration.

tinback: a metal folder used to hold patient records and to write on. *Use of the tinback makes vet students feel more "official."*

TMS: Trimethoprim-sulfamethoxazole; a broad spectrum potentiated sulfonamide antibiotic; aka TMP-SMZ, TMP-Sulfa, SXT.

TPR: temperature, pulse, and respiration; important biological data essential for a thorough physical exam. *Even human doctors assess these.*

True Love: difficult to define, easy to spot. *For more information and contextual examples, see Chapters*: *4, 6, 7, 11, 15, 20, 22, 24, 27, 32, 33, 34, 35, 36, 37, 38, and 39.*

twitch: a device, consisting of a stick-like handle with a loop of chain or rope on the end, or a metal ring with a rope loop which is wrapped around the upper lip of the horse and tightened; is a humane method of restraint and believed to work through release of endorphins that act to calm the horse. *Although twitches are considered a humane method of restraint, they are often not necessary, especially by those with "horse-sense" and/or skilled clinicians like Drill Sergeant Dan. When Nothing Ventured's owner immediately placed a twitch on his ailing horse for a simple lameness exam, Dan was disgusted.*

Tx: abbreviation for "treatment."

ulnarus lateralis: a muscle of the forelimb which originates on the lateral side of the humerus, inserts into the accessory carpal bone and on the proximal side of the lateral splint bone; it flexes the carpus, extends the elbow.

ungulates: a term generally used to describe hoofstock, including horse, zebra, donkey, giraffe, cattle, antelope, sheep, goat, and pig species.

vector: an organism that transmits an infection from one host to another; e.g., mosquitoes are vectors for heartworm disease and many other important diseases.

ventricle: a chamber of the heart receiving blood from the atrium; the right ventricle receives oxygen-depleted blood from the right atrium, and pumps it to the lungs while the left ventricle receives oxygenated blood from the left atrium and pumps it throughout the body.

veterinarian: a professional who has obtained a doctorate in veterinary medicine (in the US, DVM or VMD; equivalent degrees in other countries) and has the legal authority to practice veterinary medicine with all non-human animals; cf "human physician," or "MD" or "DO" aka "single species" and often "single species, single organ" doctors.

veterinary caduceus: the term used to describe the symbol of the veterinary profession, although technically not the Greek god Hermes' "caduceus"; comprised of the staff of Aesclepius (ancient Greek physician)--symbolized by a snake encircling a wooden staff — overlain by a capital "V" (for Veterinary).

veterinary medical ethics: a system of moral principles that apply values and judgments to the practice of veterinary medicine; veterinary medical ethics combines veterinary professional ethics and the subject of animal ethics; a critical reflection on the provision of veterinary services in support of the profession's responsibilities to both non-human and human animals. *Veterinarians and veterinary students know this better as "how to 'Do the Right Thing.'"*

veterinary nurse: the veterinary patient's best friend; the veterinary student's best friend and mentor, OR his/her worst nightmare. *It's all in the student's attitude! Just ask Rick Larson.*

VHUP: acronym for the Veterinary Hospital of the University of Philadelphia *(a fictitious place in this book).*

vinblastine: a drug used to treat specific types of cancer including Hodgkin's lymphoma and breast (mammary) cancer.

Wawa: a-24/7-convenient-as-hell-being-right-down-the-street-from-the-vet-school store stocked with coffee, Coke, Jolt, snacks, and other stay-awake essentials; frequented by "woke-up-too-late-to-make-my-own- breakfast-but-starving" first and second years and obscenely late night/early morning Emergency Service shifts; the word means "Canada Goose" in Ojibwe (a major Native American tribe).

WEE: see **Western Equine Encephalitis**; *half of a pig call (as in SU-WEE).*

Western Equine Encephalitis: a zoonotic, mosquito- and tick-borne viral disease that can affect numerous animals (including horses) and people; infected horses will appear quiet and depressed, and later show more neurologic signs. *WEE, EPM, and EEE were among the differentials for Buck's horse Suzie's neurologic signs.*

West Nile Virus (see this book's "Afterword" section).

wicked: in New England slang, a term meaning "very" or, sometimes, "cool." *"That witch with the urinary tract infection sure is a "wicked pissah."*

WNV: West Nile Virus (see this book's "Afterword" section).

x-ray dosimeter badge: a monitoring device worn by faculty, staff, and students operating near a radiography (x-ray) unit and used to measure cumulative radiation exposure.

YAG laser/Nd: YAG laser: Neodymium-doped yttrium aluminum garnet; $Nd{:}Y_3Al_5O_{12}$; a type of laser with a ridiculously complicated "official" name, used commonly for soft tissue surgeries.

zoonotic: a disease that can spread from animals to humans or humans to animals and cause disease in both; two of the most famous zoonotic diseases are rabies and avian influenza. *Dr. Green expressed concern to her boss (Davaris) over the possibility that they were in the middle of a zoonotic outbreak.*

Afterword

West Nile virus (WNV) is a mosquito-borne zoonotic arboviral disease. First discovered in Uganda in 1937, WNV has spread globally and is now considered an endemic pathogen in Africa, Asia, Australia, the Middle East, Europe, and the US.

The emergence of WNV in the US manifested with unexplained human deaths due to encephalitis in the New York City region in the late summer of 1999. Concurrently, New York area zoos were noting unexplained deaths in bird species including Chilean flamingoes, an owl, a bald eagle and local wild crows. Dr. Tracey McNamara, a veterinarian and at the time the head of the Department of Pathology at the Bronx Zoo, was the first to suspect a link between the human and animal deaths — this was a critical step in the identification of WNV and in formulating prevention measures. Her role exemplified the need to foster better communication between the veterinary and public health communities. WNV spread across the US in approximately 4 years. By 2011 there were 31,414 reported human cases of West Nile Virus, including 1,426 deaths, in the US (as per the CDC). The impact on avian populations has also been severe. It is estimated that hundreds of thousands of birds have been killed in the US alone and studies suggest that crow populations have fallen by at least 30% nationwide.

Horses appear to be particularly susceptible to the virus and they represent almost 97% of all reported non-human, mammalian cases of WNV disease. In 1999 there were 25 equine cases limited to the area around New York City, but by 2002 there were more than 15,000 equine cases from 41 states. The incubation period for West Nile virus in horses appears to be 3 to 15 days. In the US it is estimated that 10-39% of infected horses develop clinical signs, which include fever, ataxia, depression, stupor, weakness of limbs, partial paralysis, recumbency (inability to rise), convulsions, blindness, colic, and intermittent lameness, or death. The mortality rate for horses exhibiting clinical signs of WNV infection is approximately 33%. An equine vaccine was given limited approval in 2001 and was used in regions with WNV activity. The vaccine received full licensure in 2003 and is now the primary method of reducing the risk of infection in horses.

Mosquitoes are the major transmission vectors for WNV, with birds acting as the major vertebrate reservoir hosts. Other identified routes of viral transmission for humans include blood transfusion, organ transplantation, breastfeeding, and transplacental transmission. Most WNV disease is associated with the mosquito season, peaking in the late summer and early fall. Approximately 80% of persons infected with WNV will remain asymptomatic. Mild symptoms of infection, which can include fever, nausea, muscle aches, and skin rash, are noted in 20% of infected persons. Less than 1% of humans infected will develop severe illness, including meningitis or encephalitis. People most at risk include the elderly and those with suppressed immune systems. No specific treatment for WNV exists and no human vaccine is currently available. Disease prevention efforts are focused primarily on vector control, including community-based mosquito control programs and encouragement of personal protection measures to reduce the incidence of mosquito bites.

As of this writing, WNV presents an ever-growing threat. By Sept 2012, the Center for Disease Control had the highest number of annual cases seen by the month of September since 2003.

Acknowledgments

First and foremost, the authors want to thank our immediate families for decades of loving support and encouragement during our pursuit of *An Animal Life*. Specifically: Priscilla Krum and Mary Margaret Sloan, Bob and Millie Krum; Drs. Procopio and Gregoria Yanong, sisters Rosemarie Y. Mangan and Roselynn Y. Espina and their wonderful families; JT and Edeltraut Moore, Christina Moore, and Janine Czarnecki; and, John and Geraldine Hogan. We love you dearly.

We are immeasurably grateful for the amazing experiences we shared as veterinary students at the University of Pennsylvania, School of Veterinary Medicine between 1988-1992. Penn's faculty and staff are truly second to none. To our upperclassmen advisors — your survival tips worked! To those who followed us — we are proud to see your continued dedication to the "Mission" of friendship, love, unbridled Friday Night Happy Hours and, of course, Doing the Right Thing. And to all veterinarians, past, present, and future, thank you for your tireless commitment to improving the health and welfare of animals, people, and our planet.

Russell Ball, Marc Pickard, Greg Lewbart, and Brent and Becky Whitaker were early readers (and supporters) of this work. We sincerely thank you. Then, a focus group of intrepid readers made up of: Marc Pickard, Craig Watson, Joanne Spurlino, LeeBeth Cranmer, Mark Mills, Laura Bennett, Sue Kirincich, and Susan Hill gave us wise and wonderful feedback. Again, we are more than grateful for your time, effort and kindness.

Finally, HK needs to single out Mary Margaret Sloan for her unfailing support and encouragement of this project — it could not have happened without you.

Biographies

Dr. Howard Krum MS, VMD, MA

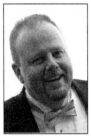

Some would say Howard's youth was particularly ill-spent (e.g., his parents). But, raised on a family farm in Northeastern Pennsylvania, he was most happy in the streams, rivers, lakes and ponds within striking distance on his Sears Free Spirit bike. In fact, that bike, which shimmied wildly at speeds over 2 mph and always pulled to the left, routinely caused Howard to detour from the perfectly good one-room school house he was supposed to attend. Despite his "best efforts" at two-wheeled navigation, he usually ended up where he could study/catch two or three bluegill, a yellow perch and some calico bass.

In the early 1970's, if you were a kid who liked animals and wanted to pursue *An Animal Life*, adults reflexively pronounced, "You should be a veterinarian!" Then, in the same breath they'd say, "But nobody gets into to vet school…" establishing a dream and dashing hopes in one fell swoop. Regardless, the idea of becoming a veterinarian sounded almost perfect: vets studied science, helped animals and even got to work outside sometimes. But, in Howard's case there was a catch — even though dogs, cats, cows and horses were interesting to him, he wanted to work with fish. So it wasn't until 1987, when he was studying fish circadian rhythms in graduate school at Southern Illinois University, that things started to come together; that was when he learned about the emerging field of *aquatic animal medicine*. Before he'd even finished his thesis, he applied to the University of Pennsylvania's School of Veterinary Medicine. This decision yielded the four best consecutive years of his professional life thus far.

Along with canine anatomy, ruminant physiology, comparative biochemistry and small animal orthopedic surgery, in veterinary school Howard got to study aquatic animals at both the Marine Biological Laboratory in Woods Hole and the National Aquarium in Baltimore (NAIB). After graduating from Penn in 1992, a benefactor helped him create a veterinary internship working with Dr. Brent Whitaker at NAIB. His good fortune continued because after this internship he was hired as the first full-time veterinarian by the New England Aquarium (NEAq) to develop their veterinary services department. At NEAq he and his awesome crew worked with nearly every species under the sun — humpback whales, harbor seals, jellyfish, sea turtles, bluefin tuna, lobster, lumpfish and herring — and created award-winning public exhibits. It was an amazing and formative experience. Subsequently, Howard signed on to help launch both the Georgia Aquarium and the Georgia Sea Turtle Center. He has been featured on the PBS TV series *Scientific American Frontiers* with Alan Alda. His work with stranded sea turtles, large whales and dolphins has been recognized on the *NBC Nightly News,* various local TV news stations and in numerous newspaper outlets including the Boston Globe. And his contributions to help create the world's largest aquarium were chronicled in the award-winning documentary, "Window To Wow/The Opening of the Georgia Aquarium" (produced by WXIA-TV Atlanta).

With a long-standing goal to combine his love for animals, science and creative communication, Howard enrolled in the Writing Seminars at Johns Hopkins University where he studied science writing, creative nonfiction and fiction writing. He graduated in 2002 with a MA and ultimately led the science communications and outreach program for the Massachusetts Ocean Partnership. He has published numerous scientific articles and penned the chapter, "When Whale Sharks Fly" in *The Rhino With Glue-on Shoes and Other Surprising True Stories of Zoo Vets and Their Patients* (Bantam/Dell Publishing Company, Random House Book Group). In fact, Howard loves writing so much, he's been known to compose emails and to-do lists on a daily basis. At present, he lives in Vermont with his wonderfully fabulous wife, Mary Margaret, their sweet dog Mola and a really-good kitten, Lucky George.

Dr. Roy P. E. Yanong VMD

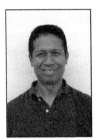

A first-generation-Filipino-American-Chicagoan, Roy Yanong's MD parents bought him his first doctor's kit at age five, "subtly" luring him and his two sisters toward human medicine. But a genetic predisposition to all things aquatic; a steady diet of James Herriot, Jacques Cousteau, and Marlin Perkins (with the oft "endangered" Jim Fowler); wet, winged, and tail-wagging pets; and frequent trips to aquaria, zoos, and wild animal parks in Chicago and Florida veered Roy toward *An Animal Life*.

Disguised as a pre-med student at Yale University, Roy majored in Molecular Biophysics and Biochemistry. But in his second year, he made the fateful phone call, "Pa, I want to become a veterinarian." Silence. Pause. "Okay. If that will make you happy…" Yes, it did, and that summer, the fun began with gainful employment at both the Lincoln Park Zoo and a local vet clinic.

After college, Roy needed a break from the classroom and soon found himself ankle deep in the low-tide, sulfurous mud flats of Boston Harbor. There he studied leukemia in soft-shell clams (yes, clams have blood) while working as a research technician for Tufts University. But there's only so much blood you can get from a clam... so two years later he hung up his muddy waders and entered the University of Pennsylvania's School of Veterinary Medicine where he concentrated in aquatic animal medicine. His most memorable experiences (in addition to meeting great mentors and friends) include the Aquavet ® summer programs in Woods Hole; externships at the National Aquarium in Baltimore, SeaWorld Orlando, and the Bronx Zoo; a summer working with aquatic animal veterinarians in the Philippines; and, of course, skits and Friday Night Happy Hours. He proudly received his VMD in May 1992.

After graduation, he was hired by 5-D Tropical, Inc., a large ornamental fish farm in Plant City, Florida, where he was plunged into the aquarium fish industry. He worked as staff veterinarian there for four and a half years. In 1996, he joined the University of Florida/IFAS Tropical Aquaculture Laboratory in Ruskin where he works today, providing extension, research, and educational programs in fish health management, including on-site veterinary assistance and disease diagnostic support for aquaculturists throughout the state. He also works closely with the Florida Fish and Wildlife Conservation Commission and Florida's Department of Agriculture and Consumer Services. Roy is currently and officially an associate professor and extension veterinarian in the Fisheries and Aquatic Sciences program of the School of Forest Resources and Conservation, headquartered on UF's main campus in Gainesville, and faculty in the UF College of Veterinary Medicine's Aquatic Animal Health Program.

Roy works with colleagues to promote the advancement of aquatic animal medicine through courses, internships, externships, outreach and scientific publications, continuing education sessions, and other venues, including his entertaining Aquariumania podcast (available online at http://www.petliferadio.com/aquariumania.html).

Over the years, Roy has participated in a number of local, state, and national fish health-related committees. He is currently the Chair of the Aquatics Working Group for the American Veterinary Medical Association's Panel on Euthanasia; a former member and Chair of the AVMA's Aquatic Veterinary Medicine Committee; and a past member of the AVMA's Animal Agriculture Liaison Committee.

In addition, he is President-Elect for the newly formed American Association of Fish Veterinarians, a member of a number of other aquaculture and fish health organizations, and on the Fluid Design Foundation's science team.

Roy lectures nationally and internationally, for industry, scientific meetings, and aquarium societies. Work has taken him to Canada, the Dominican Republic, Honduras, Singapore, Malaysia, and, most recently, Indonesia. He has published his research findings in refereed journals; authored book chapters, fish medicine reviews, and outreach articles; and written for industry, hobbyist, and aquarium trade magazines.

Dr. Yanong's adjunct pursuits include singing, high-intensity doodling, comedy writing, eating, and travel (not necessarily in that order of priority). Although he freely admits mediocrity in most of these endeavors, he keeps trying. To "sharpen the saw," he enjoys fishing, canoeing, kayaking, scuba diving, sprint triathlons, and, of course, quality time with family and friends.

Dr. Scott Moore VMD

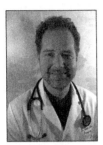

Despite childhood experiences that included being stalked by an alligator and bitten by a moray eel, Scott developed an affinity for animals at an early age.

Though it took him five years to graduate from Swarthmore College with a degree in biology, it was only because he took a year off to work for the School for Field Studies in Kenya (and not because he was "slow," as his co-authors might claim). After carefully honing his stunningly accurate impression of the tree hyrax's nocturnal vocalization, he returned to the US to attend the University of Pennsylvania's School of Veterinary Medicine. With the intention of pursuing a career in zoo and wildlife medicine, he completed externships at the Bronx Zoo, the National Zoo, and the Durrell Wildlife Conservation Trust on the isle of Jersey.

After graduating from veterinary school with honors in 1992, Scott completed an internship in small animal medicine and surgery at Friendship Animal Hospital outside of Washington, D.C., where the challenge and intensity of emergency medicine got its hooks in him and never let go. He has been a small animal, emergency veterinarian at the Hope Center for Advanced Veterinary Medicine since March 1995.

In 2011, he was honored to have been chosen by his colleagues as one of "Virginia's Top Veterinarians" in the Emergency and Critical Care category. Though he'd dreamt of making it into Teen Beat, he settled for a mention in *Virginia Living* magazine. He's had a few television appearances over the years and loves it when people tell him he looks like Tom Hanks or sounds like Jeff Bridges (though, admittedly, these admirers are usually vision and/or hearing impaired). And despite having a French bulldog, he is married to a wonderful woman. They live in Northern Virginia where Dr. Moore still occasionally dreams of days vaccinating Chinese river otters. While he has not had as scintillating a post-graduate career as Drs. Krum and Yanong, he dresses better. And though he is not nearly as pretty as Dr. Hogan, he is significantly less likely to be kicked by a horse.

Dr. Patricia Hogan VMD, Diplomate ACVS

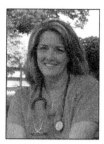

Patty Hogan was one of those countless numbers of girls born every year, afflicted from birth, with that incurable disease called "horse-crazy." From the time she could remember, Patty was obsessed with horses – loving them, drawing them, even trying to be them – she could whinny with the best of them and often allowed her six brothers and sisters the opportunity to lasso and ride her around their backyard in suburban New Jersey.

Patty began working with racehorses at the age of 10, learning to care for and drive standardbreds at a small fair track near her home. She parlayed her love of the horse into a lifelong career caring for horses as a veterinary surgeon, seeking to repair their most serious injuries. After graduating from veterinary school in 1992, Patty pursued specialized training in equine surgery, completing a rigorous internship and three-year residency before setting up shop back in New Jersey. For the past 17 years, Patty has focused on addressing the medical and surgical needs of the standardbred and thoroughbred racehorse in the northeastern portion of the United States. Her past surgical successes reads like a "who's-who" list of racing's athletes – ranging from the famous (like Kentucky Derby winners Smarty Jones and Mine That Bird), to the not-so-famous but oh-so-beloved (like Brussel Sprout and George The Animal).

In 2005, Patty was honored by the American Veterinary Medical Association as the recipient of the "President's Award" for her treatment of Smarty Jones as an example of extraordinary commitment to animal health and welfare, bringing credit and honor to her and her colleagues. As a recognized authority on equine orthopedics, Patty was named to the faculty of the Association for the Study of Internal Fixation of Fractures' Equine Principles of Fracture Management Course, held annually at The Ohio State University. This course offers veterinarians the most current information on the art and science of equine fracture repair.

Patty also played a role in the "On Call" program of the American Association of Equine Practitioners. This program provides veterinary expertise for live media coverage of major equine sporting events. She was most often "On Call" for Harness racing at the Meadowlands Racetrack and has served as a member of the broadcast team for CBS Sports, ESPN, and the Fox Network.

Patty spends her days at her own little surgical boutique, Hogan Equine, on a beautiful farm across the street from her house. She lives in animal heaven on 38-acres with her husband Eddie, a legend in his own right in the world of harness racing, and their two fabulous dogs, many feline friends, and numerous standardbred horses.

An Animal Life — No Contest

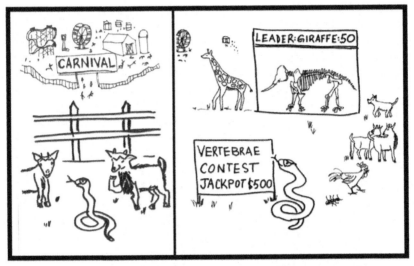

"Cyrus is so low...."   The kids said Cyrus was a loser, he'd show them...

CPSIA information can be obtained at www.ICGtesting.com
Printed in the USA
BVOW06s0056250216

437888BV00012B/246/P